UICC International Union Against Cancer

Manual of Adult and Paediatric Medical Oncology

Edited by
S. Monfardini (Chairman)
K. Brunner D. Crowther S. Eckhardt
D. Olive S. Tanneberger A. Veronesi
J. M. A. Whitehouse R. Wittes

With 25 Figures and 184 Tables

Springer-Verlag Berlin Heidelberg New York
London Paris Tokyo

UICC

3, rue du Conseil-Général
CH-1205 Geneva
Switzerland

Telephone: (022) 20 18 11
Telex: 429724 uicc, ch
Telegraph: Cancerunion, Geneva

Previously published by the UICC
as Manual of Cancer Chemotherapy

ISBN-13: 978-3-540-15347-4 e-ISBN-13: 978-3-642-82489-0
DOI: 10.1007/978-3-642-82489-0

Library of Congress Cataloging in Publication Data
Manual of adult and paediatric medical oncology. At head of title: UICC, International Union Against Cancer. "Previously published by the UICC as Manual of cancer chemotherapy." Includes bibliographies and index. 1. Cancer-Chemotherapy-Handbooks, manuals, etc. 2. Tumors in children-Chemotherapy-Handbooks, manuals, etc. 3. Antineoplastic agents-Handbooks, manuals, etc. I. Monfardini, S. (Silvio) II. International Union against Cancer. III. Manual of cancer chemotherapy. [DNLM: 1. Antineoplastic Agents-therapeutic use-handbooks. 2. Neoplasms-drug therapy-handbooks. 3. Neoplasms-prevention & control-handbooks. QZ 39 M294] RC271.C5M25 1987 616.99'4061
86-29766

2121/3145-543210

Editors

Monfardini, S., Dr., (Chairman)
Centro Riferimento Oncologico
Via Pedemontana, 33081 Aviano (Pordenone)
Italy

Brunner, K., Prof.
Onkologie-Abteilung, Inselspital
Freiburgstraße, 3010 Bern
Switzerland

Crowther, D., Prof.
Manchester University and Christie Hospital
and Holt Radium Institute
Winslow Road, Manchester M20 9BX
U.K.

Eckhardt, S., Prof.
National Institute of Oncology
XII. Ráth Gyorgy-u 7–9, Budapest 1525
Hungary

Olive, D., Prof.
Service de Médécine Infantille II, Hopital d'Enfants
Allée du Morovan, 54120 Vandoeuvre-Les-Nancy
France

Tanneberger, S., Prof.
Akademie der Wissenschaften der DDR
Robert-Roessle-Institut
Lindenberger Weg 80, 1115 Berlin-Buch
G.D.R.

Veronesi, A., Dr.
Centro Riferimento Oncologico
Via Pedemontana, 33081 Aviano (Pordenone)
Italy

Whitehouse, J. M. A., Prof.
CRC Medical Oncology Unit, Centre Block CF 99
Southampton General Hospital
Southampton S09 4XY
U. K.

Wittes, R., Dr.
Division of Cancer Treatment, Dept. of Health, Education and Welfare, National Institute of Health
Bethesda, MD 20205
USA

This publication was made possible by a grant from the National Cancer Institute (NIH).

Foreword

It is a very special honour for me to be able to present this handbook of medical oncology, which under diverse headings and origins covers such a vast spectrum of experience. I believe the reader will be struck in particular by the impressive volume of information available, especially with regard to childhood tumours, which represent, today, an immense "laboratory of hope". It is in this very field that we oncologists have been able to obtain the most consoling results in recent years.

I feel sure that all those who read these chapters will find that their oncological competence is enriched and also in a certain sense that their wish to contribute to progress in cancer research and treatment has been renewed.

In conclusion, my most heartfelt congratulations go to the authors for the excellent job they have done, as well as my admiration for having been able to concentrate so much precious and innovative information into so little space.

Umberto Veronesi

Preface

Since 1976, the UICC has been holding chemotherapy courses in all parts of the world, excluding North America and Australia. The Manual of Cancer Chemotherapy, originally devised as a didactic tool to be used by course participants, expanded itself in the successive editions to a comprehensive, although schematic, textbook of medical oncology. Recently, it was suggested by the course Faculties and attendees that preclinical data, epidemiology and non-medical management might receive more attention in the courses, which accordingly, are now becoming more interdisciplinary. This was reflected also in the production of this edition of the Manual, with an effort to cover more widely the various aspects of Oncology, beginning from the title, converted into "Manual of Adult and Paediatric Medical Oncology". The change in character of the book, together with the necessity of appropriate updating, have implied an extensive restructuring of most chapters, which have been entirely rewritten. It has been tried, however, to comply with the original "telegraphic" style of the Manual as delineated in the Introduction. The table and graph form proved in fact quite appropriate for this purpose and was very well accepted by the readers. Every effort has been made in order to prevent misprints and errors; however, as far as drug dosage and schedule are concerned, readers are invited to check manufacturers' instructions before administration.

The authors hope that the present edition of the Manual will prove of help in the development of the fight against cancer, particularly in developing countries, by providing an updated and relatively unexpensive source of reliable information.

January 1987 Silvio Monfardini

Table of Contents

Appendices

Introduction

Following the progress in the management of patients with malignant diseases over the past thirty years, a new type of physician has emerged in the field of clinical oncology - the cancer chemotherapist or, to give him a more comprehensive definition, the medical oncologist - whose principal activity is the treatment of neoplastic disease by means of chemotherapy, endocrine therapy and immunotherapy.

As a result of the broad-based interaction that has developed between the various disciplines involved in the care of the cancer patient, the medical oncologist has become an essential component in the team that makes the initial management decision and has responsibility for co-ordinating the selection of appropriate therapy in the event of relapse following primary treatment or where the disease is already disseminated on first presentation.

Moreover, there has recently also been a growing trend towards the use of chemotherapy in earlier stages of neoplastic disease than was previously the case. Since all cancer patients are entitled to receive optimal management regardless of economic, social or geographic considerations, it is necessary to develop new health care delivery structures and new facilities for the training of young physicians in the field of medical oncology on completion of their internal medicine training programme.

The First Part of this Manual contains basic data on the various antitumour drugs available as well as explaining the principles of endocrine therapy and immunotherapy, but also deals with such fundamental problems as the initial evaluation of the patient, the evaluation of the response to treatment and the management of complications occuring in patients with advanced neoplastic disease.

The Second Part deals with the therapeutic strategy for adult tumours of individual sites, with particular emphasis on the clinical practice of chemotherapy. The Third Part deals with paediatric tumours whilst the Fourth Part covers tumours of specific importance in Africa and Asia.

The data have intentionally been presented almost exclusively in table and graph form and no attempt has been made to be comprehensive in coverage; on the contrary, only the absolute essentials have been given. The objective of this "telegraphic" approach is:

(a) to provide access to the most important concepts in the least time-consuming manner;
(b) to facilitate the rapid transfer of recommended chemotherapeutic regimens and the necessary precautions related to them into clinical practice;
(c) to stimulate readers to acquire deeper and more extensive knowledge of this discipline by further reading of the recommended publications listed in Appendix 3.

The need for such education programmes is all the more urgent in those countries where, although the practice of the more traditional forms of cancer treatment such as surgery and radiotherapy is of a high standard, knowledge of and practical experience in the clinical use of antitumour drugs are still at an early stage. Yet even in countries which have a relatively long history in this field, the chemotherapeutic treatment of cancer is largely limited to a small number of specialized centres; in such cases it is also vital that the development of new treatment modalities in specialized centres should be backed up by the integration of chemotherapy into the cancer management resources available to the population as a whole.

Previous editions of this Manual have been utilized for UICC Postgraduate Courses on Clinical Cancer Chemotherapy held throughout the world and translations have been published in Portuguese, Spanish, Turkish, Serbo-Croat and Italian.

Part I

General Aspects

1 The Development of Cancer Chemotherapy

1.1 Historical Development of Cancer Chemotherapy

1.1.1 Period 1946–1960

Introduction of single-drug chemotherapy mainly on an empirical basis.

First encouraging results from the treatment of leukaemias and malignant lymphomas. Generally poor results in the treatment of advanced solid tumours.

Establishment of critical criteria for the clinical development of new drugs: criteria of response; toxicity; performance status; optimum tolerated dose.

1.1.2 Period 1960–1970

Development of knowledge of cell kinetics and application of kinetic concepts to the design of chemotherapy schedules. These have not so far been shown to be of more benefit than empirical schedules outside of experimental systems.

Broadening of the experimental basis for clinical chemotherapy.

Introduction of pharmacokinetic concepts into clinical chemotherapy.

First developments in the field of combination chemotherapy.

Introduction of the concept of the controlled randomized clinical trial into clinical chemotherapy assessment.

Improvement of treatment results in the acute leukaemias, particularly acute lymphoblastic leukaemia of childhood. Significant progress obtained in the treatment of Hodgkin's disease and certain non-Hodgkin lymphomas.

Demonstration of sensitivity of some solid tumours to anticancer drugs.

1.1.3 Period 1970 to Date

Development of the concept of the combined modality approach: improved co-operation between the surgeon, radiotherapist and medical oncologist.

Early indication of a definitive role for adjuvant chemotherapy in management of certain subgroups of patients with cancer of the breast; exploration of possible role in other tumours.

Recognition, in long-term survivors, of the late toxicities of anticancer drugs particularly when combined with radiotherapy.

Experimental immunotherapy - renewed interest development in 1960s with the availability of syngeneic animal populations.

Development of the concepts of immunotherapy in man, despite failure to demonstrate tumour-specific antigens. Widespread application - failure to demonstrate clear beneficial effect.

Sect. 1.1.4 below shows, on a time scale, the introduction of the cytostatic drugs in wide clinical use in recent years. For a list of common abbreviations of the most widely used cytotoxic agents, see Appendix A.

1.1.4 Growth in the Number of Cytostatic Drugs in Clinical Use in Recent Years

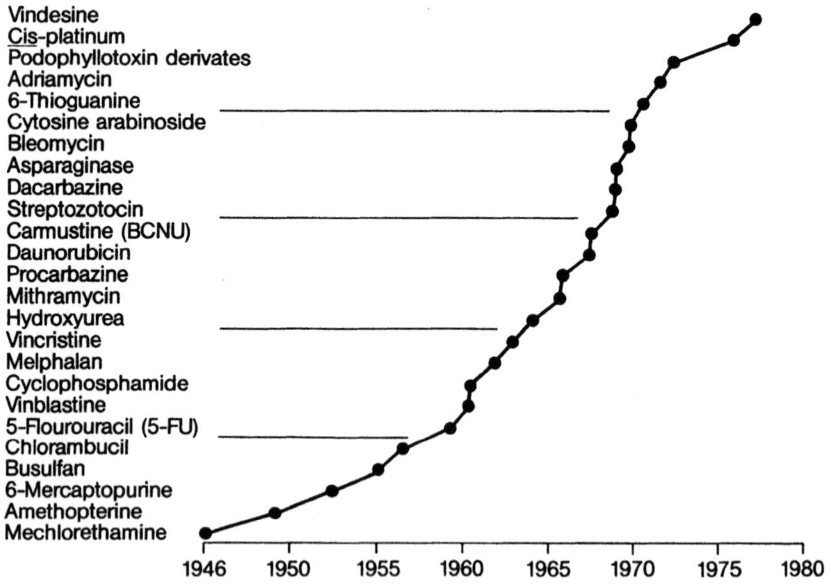

1.1.5 New Drugs Widely Used Since 1972 (Some Not Yet Commercially Available)

Dibromomannitol	Lomustine (CCNU)	Streptozotocin
5-Azacytidine	Methyl-CCNU	Razoxane (ICRF 159)
Hexamethylmelamine	Rubidazone	Teniposide (VM-26)

1.2 Procedure for the Development, Testing and Use of Chemotherapeutic Drugs

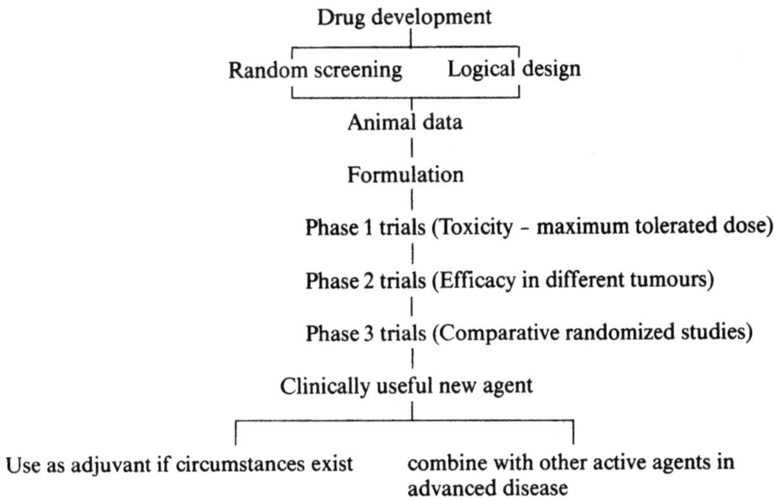

1.3 Clinical Evaluation of New Drugs

1.3.1 Selection of New Potentially Active Drugs from Preclinical Data

The decision to evaluate a new compound in man depends on a number of factors, in particular therapeutic activity in animals bearing cancer.

Other considerations include tolerable toxicities in normal rodents and other animals, the feasibility of producing the compound in large quantities, cost, pharmaceutical formulation, stability and activity via oral route of administration.

Screening Models. Most of the new compounds submitted to experimental screening procedure are tested for therapeutic activity by means of transplanted mice. The table below shows the experimental tumours most commonly used in the USA and Europe. The increase in survival time or the reduction of tumour weight with regard to a non-treated control group are the parameters on which is based the selection of new drugs for human use. The predictive value of these models for activity in specific human tumours is generally low.

The experimental tumours most commonly used in the USA and Europe and the parameters on which are based the selection of new drugs for human use

Tumour	Parameters
Leukaemia P388	Survival
Leukaemia L1210	Survival
Melanoma B16	Survival
Lewis lung carcinoma	Survival
Colon carcinoma 38	Survival
Mammary carcinoma CD8F1	Tumour weight
Mammary M × 1 (xenografts)	Tumour weight
Lung L × 1 (xenografts)	Tumour weight
Colon C × 1 (xenografts)	Tumour weight

Preclinical Toxicity. There is evidence that the mouse can be used as a predictor of quantitative drug toxicity in man. The following guidelines are useful in this context:

a) Two schedules should be employed: single dose and daily times 5.
b) LD_{10}, LD_{50} and LD_{90} should be computed with these two schedules.
c) The minimum observation period must be 28 days.

In addition, dogs may be treated with one-tenth of the LD_{10} for mice, single dose and daily times 5, and observed for 60 days. Clinical examination, blood and chemistry parameters and histopathology are performed at specific times.

1.4 Procedure for Clinical Evaluation

1.4.1 Components of a Trial Protocol

Introduction and scientific background for the study
Study objectives (with references)
Patient selection

Study design (including schematic diagram)
Treatment programme
Procedures in event of response, no response, or toxicity
Required clinical and laboratory data
Criteria for evaluating the effect of treatment
Statistical considerations
Informed consent procedure
Record forms to be kept
Study co-ordinator

1.5 Procedure for Phase I Clinical Trials

As with any therapeutic intervention, experimental drugs are given to patients with therapeutic intent. The chief scientific end-point of the phase I study is to determine maximum tolerated dose (MTD) for the schedule and route chosen, and to determine if human toxicity is predictible, reversible and treatable. The evaluation of antitumour activity is not the role of a phase I study, but actively pursued if occurring. The starting dose in man is taken as one-tenth of the LD_{10} in mice.

Patients entered must have cancer known to be unresponsive to therapy of proven value, or a tumour which has become resistant to available treatment.

These patients must not have major hepatic, renal or bone marrow dysfunction and have a survival expectancy of at least 2 months. It is recommended to enter three patients in sequence at each dose level. It is customary to start with large dose escalations, and to decrease increments at the first sign of toxicity. Doses should not be increased in individual patients, since it would then be impossible to know whether a toxicity was due to a cumulative dose or administered dose.

Data related to drug toxicity are often summarized on a numerical scale from 0 to 4. An attempt to standardize the reporting of drug toxicity data is presented in Sect. 3.15.

1.6 Phase II Clinical Trials

Phase II studies are intended to determine the percentage of patients who will respond to treatment with the drug, and in whom there will be significant tumour shrinkage. Two options are open to the investigator.

1. Drug-Orientated Study. This requires a large number of patients with a variety of malignancies to be treated with a particular drug. Drugs that were identified by this 'classical' approach include 5-FU, cyclophosphamide, methotrexate and Adriamycin.

2. Disease-Orientated Study. In this situation, the prognostic variables which may influence response interpretation are anticipated in the study design. These studies may be structured either in a randomized controlled fashion or a non-randomized sequential manner.

Where two groups of patients are to be compared, then the patients entering each group must be categorized using characteristics known to be of prognostic importance, so that equal numbers of patients with important prognostic factors are included in each arm. This is the process of 'stratification'. Several designs may be used for testing new agents in phase II studies. After stratification, patients may be randomized between two alternative drugs, one of which may be an agent of known activity. Alternatively, two new drugs may be tested. In either case, a point may be reached (such as in the case of disease progression), when a cross-over trial of treatment should be initiated, i.e. the drug in the arm is substituted for the other. Alternatively a new drug may be substituted for both.

Antitumour activity in phase II trials is usually measured by estimating objective tumour regression. Several categories of measurability in solid tumours can be considered as shown in the following table (see also Sect. 3.9).

Measurability in solid tumours

Category of parameter	Example
1. Measurable clinically	
a) Bidimensional	Cutaneous lesions, round lung metastasis
b) Unidimensional	Hepatomegaly
2. Non-measurable clinically	
a) Evaluable	Abdominal masses that can be palpated but not measured clinically
b) Non-evaluable	Lesions not clinically detectable

The criteria for objective response are based on measurements recorded in metric notation using a ruler or a caliper. For bidimensionally measurable lesions, the area is approximated by multiplying the longest diameter by the perpendicular diameter. When multiple lesions are present, a sum of the product is then used. The definition of objective response, given under Sect. 3.10, takes into account the inaccuracy of the measurements. Decrease of less than 50% in total tumour size should not be used to indicate response.

The incorporation of a time factor is essential in studying responses. Short responses are of little significance and are more subject to measurement errors. In general, it is required that a response lasts for a minimum of 4 weeks. In expressing the results, it is essential to define numerator and denominator. Deletion of patients from the denominator for a variety of reasons such as: lost to follow-up, early death, toxic death, inadequate data, failure to complete therapy, refusal by the patient to go on, etc., must be specified. It is recommended to use at least the three following denominators to report results:

a) Registered and eligible. (N.B. The number of patients registered and entered in the study but subsequently found to be ineligible and the reasons for their ineligibility must be reported.)
b) Registered, eligible and treated. This includes all patients who were registered, were eligible and were given therapy regardless of how little or how much therapy was given.
c) Registered, eligible and adequately treated.

When other denominators are used, they should be clearly defined.

1.7 Procedure for Phase III Clinical Trials

The purpose of these studies is to define the role of a new drug or regimen in therapeutic practice. These trials are randomized, comparative studies between the new regimens and the standard therapy. An essential feature of the design is stratification by prognostic factors; these can be grouped into six major categories:

1. Demographic (age, sex ...)
2. Prior therapy
3. Clinical stage
4. Histology
5. Performance status
6. Institution

Any imbalance in this distribution between the treated groups of patients may bias the final comparison between regimens.

Results in phase III trials are often reported in terms of duration of an event; these can be survival time, disease-free interval, time to progression, etc. Disease-free interval is the time from curative treatment to recurrence.

To define this time precisely, it is essential to specify the frequency of examination and the duration of follow-up. Time to recurrence or to death should be measured from the first day of therapy.

The analysis of disease-free interval curves or of survival data entails the use of sophisticated mathematical techniques which should be handled by a professional statistician.

Large sample sizes are generally needed to compare anticancer treatments. Multicentre trials are often performed in order to access enough patients in a relatively short period of time. With large sample sizes, it may become necessary to organize a centralized "data centre" to monitor and analyse the data.

Further Reading

1. Armitage P, Bardelli D, Galton DAG, Gehan EA, Higgins GA, Magnus K, Miller AB, Pocock ST, Saracci R (eds) (1978) Methods and impact of controlled therapeutic trials in cancer. Part 1. UICC technical report series, Vol 36, UICC, Geneva
2. Cascinelli N, Davis HL Jr, Flamant R, Kenis Y, Lalanne CM, Muggia F, Rozencweig M, Staquet M, Veronesi U (eds) (1981) Methods and impact of controlled therapeutic trials in cancer. Part 2. UICC technical reports series, Vol 59, UICC, Geneva
3. Flamant R, Fohanno C (eds) (1978) Controlled therapeutic trials in cancer. UICC Information Office and list of registered trials. UICC technical report series, Vol 32, UICC, Geneva
4. Flamant R, Fohanno C (eds) (1982) Evaluation of methods of treatment and diagnostic procedures in cancer. UICC technical report series, Vol 70, UICC, Geneva
5. Mihich E, Laurence DJR, Laurence DM, Eckhardt S (eds) (1974) UICC Workshop on new animal models for chemotherapy of human solid tumours. UICC technical report series, Vol 15, UICC, Geneva
6. Muggia FM, Staquet MJ, Rosencweig M, McGuire W (1980) Methodology in Phase II clinical trials in cancer. In: Carter SK, Sakurai Y (eds) Recent results in cancer research, Springer Berlin Heidelberg New York
7. Staquet M (1972) The design of clinical trials in cancer therapy. Presses scientifiques Européennes, Brussels
8. Staquet M (1978) Randomized trials in cancer: A critical review by sites. Raven Press, New York
9. UICC Committee on International Collaborative Activities (1981) The international cancer patient data exchange system. Two-year progress report. UICC technical report series, Vol 58, UICC, Geneva
10. UICC Committee on International Collaborative Activities (1982) The international cancer patient data exchange system - system manual. UICC technical report series, Vol 68, UICC, Geneva
11. World Health Organization (1979) Reporting results of cancer treatment. WHO Offset Publication No 48, Geneva

N.B. For additional reading, see Appendix C.

2 Basic Concepts in Cancer Chemotherapy

2.1 General

Chemotherapy is planned on the basis of observed differences between normal and tumour cells in response to antitumour agents used both singly and in combination. Part of the difference between normal and neoplastic cells can be explained by consideration of proliferative characteristics; however, it must be emphasized that cell kinetics cannot explain all the consequences of tumour cell exposure to a drug, since these are also dependent upon pharmacokinetics, biochemistry and tumour biology.

The proliferation of tumour cells is not entirely autonomous, neither is it constant; it varies with the size of the tumour and is related to its blood supply. Animal studies show that the characteristics of tumour cell proliferation have an important influence on the response to chemotherapy. Skipper has reviewed some of the principles concerned and the following generalizations can be made.

2.2 Cell Division

The entire process of cell division (the cell cycle) begins following mitosis and is conventionally divided into four phases. A knowledge of the phases of the cell cycle is important in the use of specific chemotherapeutic agents.

The Cell Cycle (See Sect. 2.6). M is mitosis; G1 is the first gap (G, gap); S is the DNA synthetic phase; and G2 is the second gap. Cells can either cycle continuously or go into a G0 phase in which the cell is "dormant". Following a suitable stimulus the cell then begins to divide (recruitment).

2.3 Tumour Growth

During tumour growth, the time taken for the mass to double in volume is known as the *doubling time*. This is extremely variable and may be as short as a few days in the leukaemias to 100–200 days in some solid tumours.

The doubling time of a tumour increases with the tumour mass up to a critical point, while the thymidine-labelling index decreases. The growth of most experimental tumours can be described as Gompertzian (after the statistician who first described the mathematics) rather than linear.

The response to chemotherapy is reflected by the change in the thymidine-labelling index (the number of cells synthesizing DNA).

The shorter the doubling time at the onset of treatment, the better the initial response to chemotherapy is likely to be.

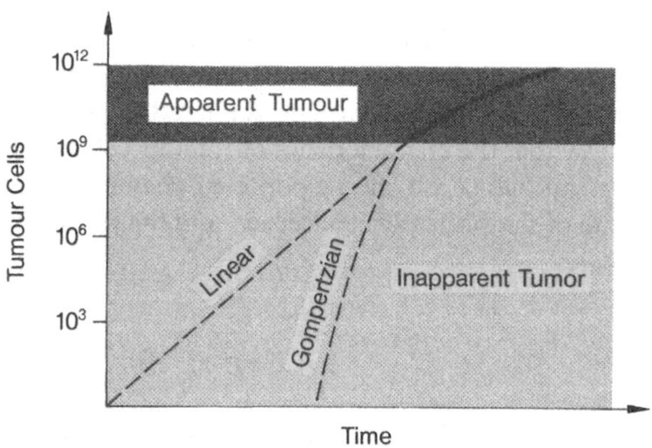

Animal tumours do not grow in a linear manner. As they become larger, the growth rate slows. Though few data are available for human tumours, there are suggestions that the above generalizations may apply to human cancer, and proliferation studies may come to be helpful in the choice of chemotherapy and in predicting duration of remission and survival.

A human tumour is inhomogenous in space and time. It is possible to divide the cancer cells within each tumour into several compartments. These compartments include the *growth fraction*. It is this fraction of cells that is actively dividing. Small tumours tend to have a high growth fraction, while larger tumours have a small growth fraction. The second growth compartment of the tumour is known as the *clonogenic fraction* or the stem cell compartment. This compartment is composed of tumour cells which, though not in division at the time, are capable of dividing if given an appropriate stimulus (G0 cells). These cells cannot be killed by drugs which act predominantly on dividing cells. But if the growth fraction is reduced by effective treatment, the cells in the clonogenic compartment are recruited into the growth fraction. The last fraction of cells is the *non-clonogenic compartment* composed of end cells. These cells are actually dead or, though viable, unable to divide.

Non-proliferating compartment		Proliferating compartment
Non-clonogenic fraction	←	Growth
Clonogenic fraction	⇄	Fraction

2.4 The Tumour-Drug Response

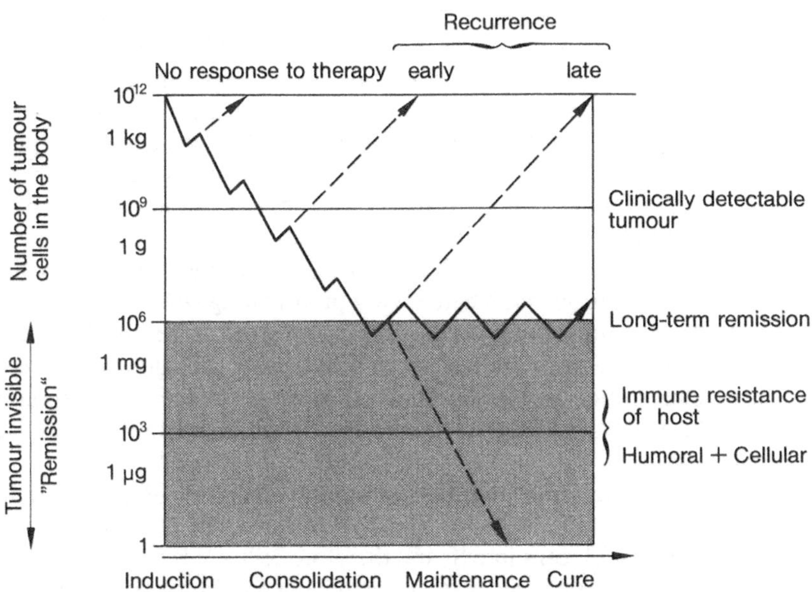

2.5 Cycle Specificity/Phase Specificity of Cytotoxic Drugs

Cytotoxic drugs cause three patterns of response when the surviving fractions of normal and tumour clonogenic cells are plotted against the dose of anticancer drugs.

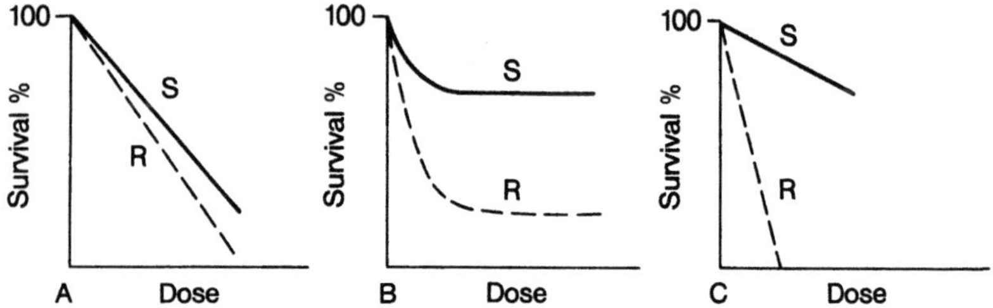

S, Slowly poliferating cells (i.e. haemopoietic normal);
R, Rapidly poliferating cells (i.e. tumour)

1. *Cell cycle-non-specific* drugs **(A)** kill cells whether or not they are in cycle.
2. *Cell cycle-(phase-)specific* drugs **(B)** show a higher killing rate in rapidly than in slowly proliferating cells, but there is a proportion of cells which are not killed even with massive increases of dose. Phase-specific agents exert an increasingly toxic effect with prolonged exposure of the cells to an effective concentration while in the sensitive phase. This results from an accumulation of cells in that phase (provided the drug does not prevent entry). Given over a short period, even at high dose level, these agents are not very toxic. Cells not in the sensitive phase at the time of the brief exposure will be minimally affected.
3. *Cell cycle-(non-phase-)specific* drugs **(C)** kill increasing numbers of cells with increasing dose, but where slowly proliferating cells are less sensitive to drug treatment than the rapidly growing cells. The toxicity of cycle-specific drugs for both malignant and normal cells depends on the drug concentration and the duration of exposure. To achieve maximum effect it is therefore logical to administer the drugs intermittently at the highest dose.

Some drugs interfere with progression from one phase of the cell cycle to another. Cytosine arabinoside and hydroxyurea, for example, inhibit the progression of G_1 cells into S_1 and therefore cells not is S are protected. This protective effect can be overcome by giving the drug intermittently at intervals that permit the non-S-phase cells to enter S during the drug-free period.

This classification of antitumour agents has limitations in determining therapeutic strategies in the management of human cancers, but it has been of considerable value in defining the kinetic basis of drug toxicity.

2.6 Phase Specificity of Some of the Cytotoxic Drugs

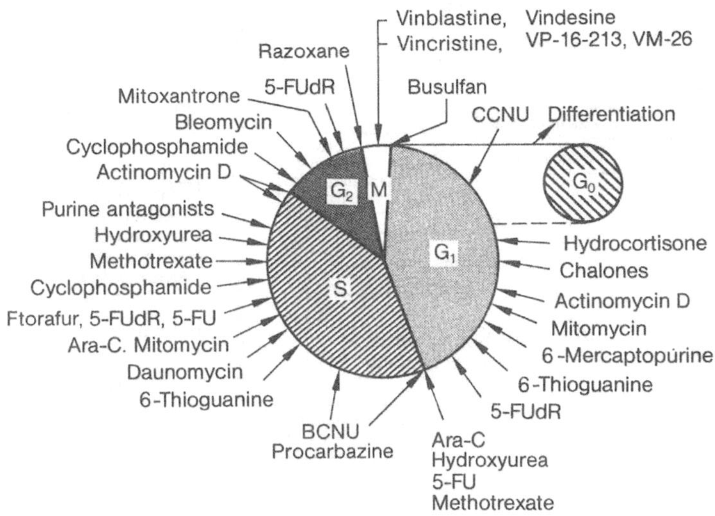

5-FUdR, 5-fluoro-2'-deoxyuridine; VP-16-213, etoposide; VM-26, teniposide; 5-FU, 5-fluoruoracil; BCNU, carmustine; CCNU, lomustine; ara-C, cytosine arabinoside

2.7 Classification of Antitumour Agents According to Their Effect on the Cell Cycle

Predominantly non-phase-specific	*Predominantly phase-specific*
Alkylating agents	*Vinca* alkaloids
Nitrosoureas	Hydroxyurea
Anthracyclines	Cytosine arabinoside
Dacarbazine (DTIC)	Methotrexate
Mitomycin C	6-Mercaptopruine
Actinomycin D	6-Thioguanine
Dibromodulcitol	Procarbazine
Cis-platin	Podophyllotoxins - VM-26
Carboplatin	- VP-16-213

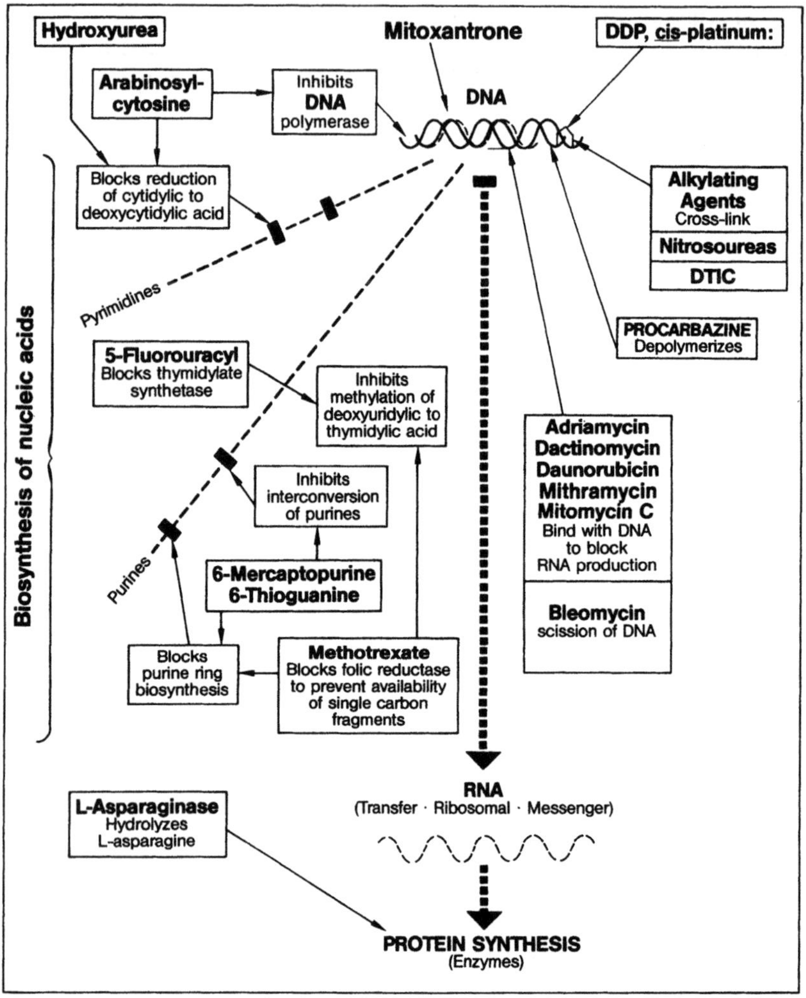
Hydroxyurea
Mitoxantrone
DDP, cis-platinum:
Arabinosyl-cytosine
Inhibits DNA polymerase
DNA
Blocks reduction of cytidylic to deoxycytidylic acid
Alkylating Agents Cross-link
Nitrosoureas
DTIC
Pyrimidines
Biosynthesis of nucleic acids
PROCARBAZINE Depolymerizes
5-Fluorouracyl Blocks thymidylate synthetase
Inhibits methylation of deoxyuridylic to thymidylic acid
Adriamycin
Dactinomycin
Daunorubicin
Mithramycin
Mitomycin C
Bind with DNA to block RNA production
Inhibits interconversion of purines
Purines
6-Mercaptopurine
6-Thioguanine
Bleomycin scission of DNA
Blocks purine ring biosynthesis
Methotrexate Blocks folic reductase to prevent availability of single carbon fragments
RNA
(Transfer · Ribosomal · Messenger)
L-Asparaginase Hydrolyzes L-asparagine
PROTEIN SYNTHESIS
(Enzymes)

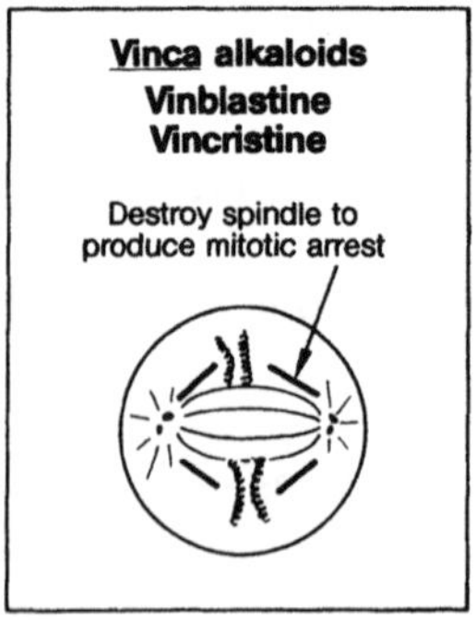
Vinca alkaloids
Vinblastine
Vincristine
Destroy spindle to produce mitotic arrest

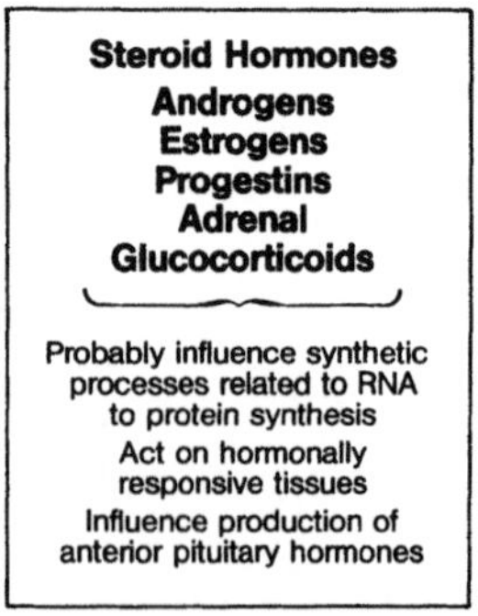
Steroid Hormones
Androgens
Estrogens
Progestins
Adrenal
Glucocorticoids
Probably influence synthetic processes related to RNA to protein synthesis
Act on hormonally responsive tissues
Influence production of anterior pituitary hormones

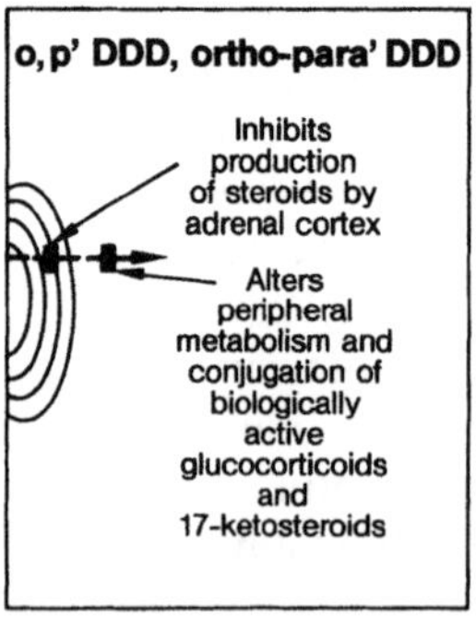
o,p' DDD, ortho-para' DDD
Inhibits production of steroids by adrenal cortex
Alters peripheral metabolism and conjugation of biologically active glucocorticoids and 17-ketosteroids

2.8 Mechanisms of Action of Anticancer Drugs at the Cellular Level (Modified from Krakoff)

2.9 Drug Metabolism

Most anticancer agents are metabolized in the body, usually to products which are inactive having lower lipid solubility. These are then excreted. In some instances, active metabolites are produced (e.g. cyclophosphamide).

2.9.1 Drug Absorption, Distribution and Excretion

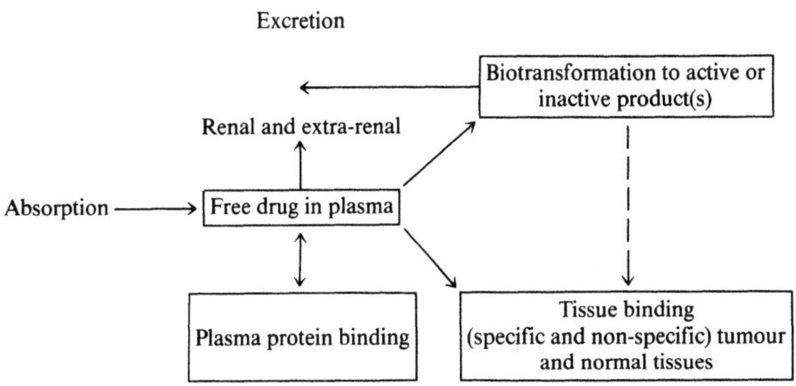

Anabolic activation is particularly important in the case of antimetabolites. The role of anabolic and catabolic activation and deactivation is of great importance since it may form the basis of selective activity in different cell types (normal and malignant).

Usually, drug metabolism occurs in two phases:

1. Biotransformation – involving hydroxylation, oxidation, reduction or hydrolysis
2. Conjugation – e.g. with sulphate, acetyl or a glucuronyl group

Drug metabolism occurs chiefly in the liver but may also take place in the plasma, gastrointestinal tract, kidneys and lungs. For this reason, hepatic function is an important consideration in the choice of dose of some antitumour agents. The anthracyclines (e.g. Adriamycin and daunorubicin) are excreted mainly in the bile and these drugs produce enhanced toxicity in patients with hepatic failure or biliary obstruction.

2.10 Drug Excretion

Most antitumour agents are excreted in the bile and urine. Drugs not bound to albumin are filtered by the glomerulus. The proximal tubule possesses two pump systems which transport drugs from plasma to urine, one for the acidic and the other for the basic drugs. Acidic drugs compete with one another for the secretory mechanism and probenecid can be used to reduce the elimination of acidic drugs (e.g. penicillins and, possibly, anticancer agents such as methotrexate). Passive reabsorption of lipid-soluble drugs and the non-ionized fraction of drugs which are weak electrolytes takes place in the renal tubule. Elimination of weak acids by the kidney is increased by alkalinizing the urine. The reverse is true for weak bases. Active tubular resorption of ions and various solutes can also take place in the proximal tubule.

Excretion in tears, sweat, saliva and in the breath is relatively unimportant but may be the cause of unusual toxicity such as the conjunctivitis seen following the use of high-dose methotrexate. Several host-dependent factors have important influences on drug absorption, distribution, metabolism and excretion. Illness which affects renal and hepatic function, bone marrow reserve or gastrointestinal function may well have a marked influence on the efficacy and toxicity of a drug. Methotrexate, for example, is largely excreted in the urine and its toxicity may be markedly enhanced in patients with renal failure. Biliary excretion is the major route of elimination of anthracycline antibiotics (Adriamycin, daunorubicin) and, in patients with biliary tract obstruction, major modifications of drug dosage are necessary to prevent excessive toxicity.

2.10.1 Mechanism of Renal Excretion

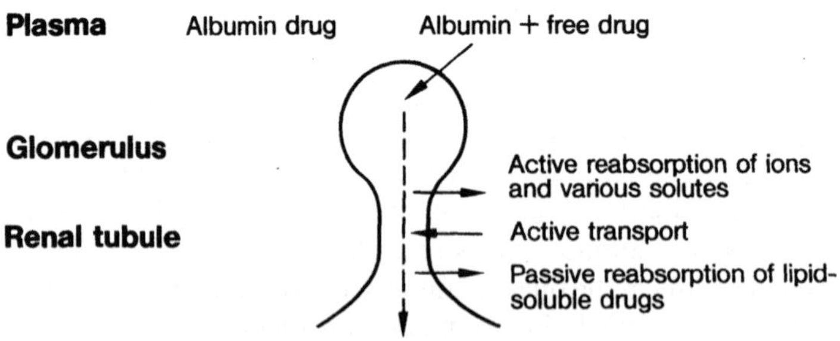

2.11 Drug Resistance

1. Intrinsic (Primary) Resistance. Factors responsible are pharmacological, biochemical or kinetic features of the particular tumour.

2. Acquired (Secondary) Resistance. Factors responsible are:
Selective killing (leaving resistant cells)
Adaptive change by tumour cells (to some extent mutation)

a) Insufficient drug uptake by cancer cell caused by inhibited active or passive membrane transport
(Methotrexate, daunorubicin, doxorubicin, melphalan?, dactinomycin)
b) Increased drug inactivation
(6-Mercaptopurin, ara-C, alkylating agents)
c) Insufficient drug activation
(Ara-C, 5-FU)
d) Non-specific interaction with non-essential targets
(Melphalan)
e) Increased production or decreased requirement of the target enzyme or metabolite
(*L*-Asparaginase)
f) Change in the conformation of an enzyme rendering it insensitive to the drug
(Ara-C)
g) Increased utilization of an alternative biochemical pathway – 'salvage'
(Anti metabolites)
h) Rapid repair of a drug-induced lesion
(Alkylating agents, mitomycin C)
i) Increased drug release from tumour cells
(Anthracyclines?)
k) Change in proliferative characteristics of the tumour population
(All drugs)

Most data on anticancer drug resistance come from animal studies. In man the factors responsible for human drug resistance have been poorly investigated. Nevertheless, also for man it is accepted that the acquired tumour resistance to cytostatic drugs is a frequent cause of treatment failure.

2.12 Theoretical Basis for the Effects of Combination Chemotherapy

1. Drugs with differing toxicities to various tissues and different mechanisms of action may, when used in combinations:

a) Increase tumour cell kill without a corresponding increase in host toxicity:

⟶ *improved preferential killing*

b) Allow for more rapid host recovery and better selectivity:

⟶ *more rapid preferential killing*

c) Kill various segments of neoplastic cells in different phases of the cycle:

⟶ *more complete remission, delay of resistant cell populations*

2. Additive toxicity to host tissues without synergistic tumour cell kill results in decreased effectiveness of combinations, or even preferential killing of normal host cells.

2.13 Problems of Schedules in Combination Chemotherapy

1. *Choice of drugs used in combinations:*
   a) Empirical basis:
      - Drugs most effective in a tumour type, when used alone
      - No cross-resistance, different mechanism of action
      - Toxicity spectrum of drugs differing from each other: no additive toxicity

   b) Information from animal models: gives little direct information
2. *Route of administration:* High i.v. dose vs daily oral dose, etc.
3. *Schedules of administration:*
   - Pharmacological and cytokinetic considerations
   - Intermittent vs continuous
   - Simultaneous vs sequential
   - Influence of immunosuppression
   - Host recovery
4. *Tumor cell burden:* Induction - maintenance
5. *Resistance:* Previous treatments, killing of various phase-related sections of the neoplastic cell population, in order to prevent resistance
6. *Miscellaneous factors:*
   - Biological differences of neoplastic cells
   - Age and sex of the host
7. *Practical considerations:*
   - Feasibility of experimental designs
   - Ambulatory patients
   - Distance of treatment centre

2.14 Theoretical Advantages of Chemotherapy for Patients with Small Cell Mass (Minimal Residual Disease)

1. Experimental animals with tumours are more easily cured by chemotherapy when the tumour mass is small.
2. Small tumour foci are associated with better drug access to the tumour cells.
3. Low tumour mass is associated with reduced cell cycle times and greater susceptibility to most chemotherapeutic agents.
4. Host has minimal immunosuppression.
5. Better tolerance of drug effects on normal cells (toxicity).
6. Reduced likelihood of competitive inhibitors for the chemotherapeutic agent.
7. Potentially reduced number of drug-resistant mutants.

Further Reading

1. Kuemmerle HP, Berkarda B, Karrer K, Mathe G (eds) (1984) Antineoplastic chemotherapy. (Clinical Chemotherapy; Vol III) Thieme-Stratton Inc, New York, 587 S
2. Knobf MKT, Fischer DS, Welch-McCaffrey D (1984) Cancer Chemotherapy-Treatment and care. 2nd ed. GK Hall Med Publ, Boston, 343 S
3. Greenspan EM (1982) Clinical interpretation and practice of cancer chemotherapy. Raven Press, New York, 666 S
4. Brunner KW, Nagel GA (Hrsg) (1985) Internistische Krebstherapie. 3. völlig überarb Aufl. Springer, Berlin Heidelberg New York, 576 S
5. Tanneberger St (ed) (1986) Experimentelle und klinische Chemotherapie. Akademie-Verlag, Berlin, Gustav Fischer Verlag, Stuttgart New York 1980
6. Calman KC, Smyth JF, Tattersall M (1980) Basic Principles of Cancer Chemotherapy. Macmillan Press, London Basinstoke
7. Carter StK, Bakowski MT, Hellmann K (1981) Chemotherapy of Cancer. J Wiley & Sons, New York London Sydney Toronto

3 Evaluation of the Cancer Patient and the Response to Treatment

3.1 Essential Investigations

3.1.1 Clinical History

1. Onset of first symptoms of primary and/or metastatic disease.
2. Description of first symptoms, development of symptoms: pain, fatigue, performance status, paraneoplastic syndromes, etc.
3. Weight change during the last 3 months.

3.1.2 Clinical Examination

1. Size and extent of primary or metastatic disease: measurement of all measurable tumour manifestations in two perpendicular diameters for follow-up documentation during therapy.
2. Clinical check-up for all organ systems for possible metastatic involvement or functional disturbances: all clinically palpable lymph nodes, liver, spleen. Physical examination of lung and heart, abdominal palpation, rectal and gynaecological examination, skeletal system.

3.1.3 Routine Laboratory Investigations

1. Sedimentation rate, haemoglobin, WBC with differential count, platelets.
2. Bone marrow aspiration and/or biopsy is indicated in all leukaemias, in malignant lymphoma, multiple myeloma and other haematological neoplastic disorders. In solid tumours, it is indicated if peripheral haematological values show abnormalities, such as unexplained anaemia, immature white or red cells, which often are a first sign of diffuse bone marrow infiltration, or low platelet counts.
3. Laboratory investigations to assess organ functions: blood urea nitrogen (BUN), creatinine, alkaline phosphatase, serum glutamic-oxalacetic transaminase (SGOT), serum glutamic-pyruvic transaminase (SGPT), gamma-glutamyl transpeptidase (gamma-GT).

Further laboratory investigations are indicated according to clinical symptoms and signs of suspected abnormalities (see also under Sect. 3.7).

3.1.4 Radiodiagnostic Procedures

1. Routinely: chest x-ray; bone scan in all diseases with a high incidence of bone metastases (breast cancer, lung cancer, hypernephroma, thyroid cancer, prostatic cancer) and in all cases where bone pain suggests skeletal involvement.
2. Other radiodiagnostic procedures should be performed according to symptoms, clinical findings or abnormal laboratory investigations.
3. Abdominal lymphography is indicated in all malignant lymphomas, in gynaecological cancer, testicular cancer or whenever involvement of lower retroperitoneal lymph nodes is suspected.
4. Skeletal survey may be performed instead of bone scan in asymptomatic patients with neoplastic disease which has a high incidence of osseous metastases, as mentioned above.
5. Liver scan: when metastatic liver disease is suspected. Liver scans have a high percentage of false-positive and false-negative findings. Sonogram of the liver may be superior.
6. Thyroid scintigram: in suspected or manifest thyroid cancer.
7. Sonogram: useful to evaluate size and extent of abdominal disease.
8. Computed tomography (CT): this radiological technique is rapidly becoming a quite accurate method of detecting metastases in a wide variety of locations [mainly lungs, liver and central nervous system (CNS)].

During any systemic therapy or follow-up after curative treatment all the above-mentioned routine examinations should be performed at regular intervals, even if normal. All pathological findings are monitored also at regular intervals, with routine and special investigations where necessary.

All normal and pathological findings should be documented on special flow and tumour measurement sheets (see Sect. 3.16).

3.2 General Prognostic Factors in Neoplastic Disease

Factors which determine the natural course of the disease, cure rate in localized disease, or survival and, possibly, response to therapy in metastatic disease may be either tumour-related or host-related.

3.2.1 Tumour-Related Factors

1. Histology, histological subtype and histological grading (degree of anaplasia)
2. Tumour mass, tumour cell burden at the time of diagnosis
3. Proliferative characteristics (growth fraction) of the tumour cell, tumour doubling time
4. Stage of the disease at diagnosis: size of primary tumour, relation of primary tumour to neighbouring organ structures, involvement of regional lymph nodes

3.2.2 Host-Related Factors

1. Age and sex
2. Weight loss, general disease symptoms (unfavourable)
3. Duration of disease symptoms before diagnosis
4. Time interval between primary diagnosis or first treatment and occurrence of metastases (short interval unfavourable)
5. Anaemia
6. Fever, infection at start of treatment
7. Bone marrow reserve at start of chemotherapy
8. Other organ failure: kidney, liver, etc.
9. Nutritional status at start of therapy

3.3 The TNM Classification and Its Purpose

The UICC believes that it is desirable to reach agreement on the recording of accurate information of the extent of the disease for each site because the precise clinical description and classification of malignant neoplasms may serve a number of related objectives. These objectives have been stated to be:

1. To aid the clinician in the planning of treatment
2. To give some indication of prognosis
3. To assist in evaluation of treatment results
4. To facilitate the exchange of information between treatments
5. To contribute to the continuing investigation of human cancer

To meet these objectives there is a need for a system of classification whose basic principles are applicable to all sites, regardless of treatment, and which may be supplemented later by information which becomes available from histopathology or surgery.

The TNM system is based on the assessment of:

1. The extent of the primary tumour T
2. The condition of the regional lymph nodes N
3. The absence or presence of distant metastases M

The addition of numbers to these three components (e.g. T1, ... etc., N0, N1, ... etc., M0, M1, ... etc.) indicates the extent of the malignant disease.

Other supplementary symbols are also used for specific purposes.

3.4 General Rules of the TNM System

The general rules applicable to all sites are as follows:

1. In all cases, confirmation of malignancy by histological examination is obligatory. Any cases not so proved must be recorded separately.
2. All cases are identified by T, N and M categories which must be determined and recorded prior to definitive treatment. They are to remain unchanged, though they may be qualified by additional histopathological or surgical information.
3. In the clinical assessment of a patient, numerous investigations may be done. It is important to distinguish obligatory investigations from those which add refinement to the diagnosis of the extent of malignant disease. For each site classified, minimum criteria for TNM classification are listed. The regional lymph nodes and in some cases the juxta-regional lymph nodes for each site are defined.
4. After assigning T, N and M categories (with degrees of extension), these may then be grouped into a number of clinical stages.

3.5 TNM Brochure of Checklists

Written or dictated clinical notes more often than not omit details subsequently required for case analysis in both prospective and retrospective studies and for the communication of treatment experiences to others without ambiguity. This difficulty can be overcome by incorporating the required information in a checklist.

The TNM checklists published by the UICC facilitate the routine acquisition of information on the anatomical extent of disease in an uniform fashion. They document an organized description of the essential features of the primary tumour (T), the regional and (where indicated) juxta-regional lymph nodes (N), and distant metastases (M).

The checklist is largely self-classifying and self-staging: where all of the boxes applicable to a given patient have been checked by the examiner, the TNM profile for the patient will simply be the highest corresponding TNM category and stage group. The completed checklist should become part of the patient's medical record.

3.6 Example of a TNM Checklist - Ovary

3.7 Biochemical Markers for Malignant Disease

Findings from numerous investigators suggest that many genes, acquired at early stages of evolution, may appear during ontogeny, are repressed after birth and can be reactivated and expressed in neoplasia.

These gene products, although not entirely specific for the cancer concerned, can be used as a diagnostic tool and may provide a measure for the amount of tumour present and changes following treatment.

1. Foetal Substances:
   Carcinoembryonic antigen (highest in gastrointestinal cancer)
   Alpha-foetoprotein (hepatoma, teratoma)
2. Enzymes:
   Histaminase (medullary carcinoma, thyroid)
   Acid phosphatase (cancer of the prostate)
   Amylase (cancer of the pancreas)
   Alkaline phosphatase isoenzymes (e.g. Regan isoenzyme)
3. Hormones:
   Choriogonadotrophic hormone (gestational choriocarcinoma, germ cell tumours)
   Adrenocorticotrophin, Antidiuretic hormones } cancer of the bronchus (frequently oat cell), pancreatic cancer
   Parathormone (parathyroid tumours, cancer of the bronchus, pancreas)
   Erythropoietin (cerebellar haemangioblastoma, hepatoma, testicular tumours, hypernephroma)
   Insulin (insulinoma)
   Thyroid-stimulating hormone (TSH) (choriocarcinoma)
   Gonadotrophins, follicle-stimulating hormone (FSH), luteinizing hormone (LH) (hepatoma, teratoma)
   5-Hydroxy indoleacetic acid (carcinoid)
   Noradrenaline metabolites (phaeochromocytoma, neuroblastoma)
   Calcitonin (medullary cancer, thyroid)

OVARY

ICD-O T-183.0

Centre .... Case No. .... Ident. No. ....

Patient .... Reg. Year ....

Date of Birth .... Age .... Sex .... Ann. Month ....

PRE-TREATMENT CLINICAL CLASSIFICATION (TNM)

→Please check one or more items in each section. Note minimum requirements for classification on reverse side.

Site and Extent of Tumour

Site: ....

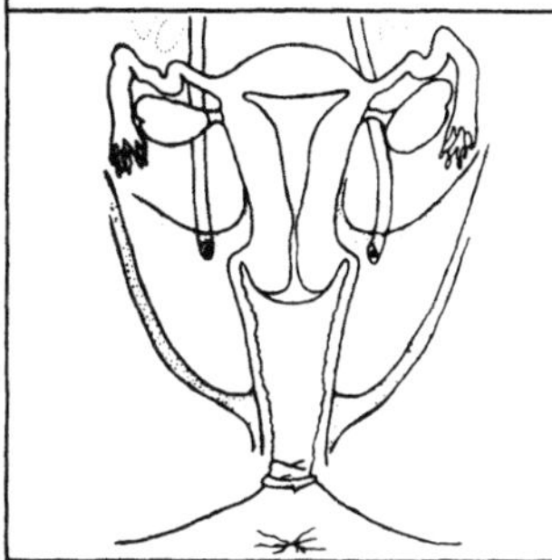

Regional lymph nodes:

Histologically: negative ☐ positive ☐

Histological diagnosis ....

Degree of differentiation:

High ☐ Med. ☐ Low ☐ Not assessed ☐

PRIMARY TUMOUR

Ovary	Ascites	Capsule	Tumour on Surface	Pelvic or other Extension	Category	Stage
No evidence or primary tumour ☐					T0	—
One ☐	None ☐	Intact ☐	None ☐	None ☐	T1a1	Iai
		Ruptured ☐	Present ☐		T1a2	Iaii
Both ☐	None ☐	Intact ☐	None ☐	None ☐	T1b1	Ibi
		Ruptured ☐	Present ☐		T1b2	Ibii
One or Both ☐	Present* ☐	*Containing malignant cells or with positive peritoneal washings		None ☐	T1c	Ic
	None ☐			Uterus ☐ Tubes ☐	T2a	IIa
	None ☐			Other pelvic tissues ☐ Visceral peritoneum ☐	T2b	IIb
	Present* ☐			Uterus/Tubes/ Pelvic Tissues ☐	T2c	IIc
		In true pelvis →		Small bowel/Omentum ☐	T3	III
		Beyond true pelvis →		Intraperitoneal extension ☐		
Primary tumour not assessed ☐					TX	—

REGIONAL LYMPH NODES

	Category	Stage
No evidence of involvement ☐	N0	I
Evidence of involvement ☐	N1	III
Regional lymph nodes not assessed ☐	NX	—

DISTANT METASTASES

	Category	Stage
No evidence of distant metastases ☐	M0	I
Evidence of distant metastases (specify) ☐	M1	IV
Distant metastases not assessed ☐	MX	—

Category: T N M Stage G

Information obtained: Before admission ☐ At Centre ☐ Examiner Date:

POST-SURGICAL HISTOPATHOLOGICAL CLASSIFICATION (p.TNM)

→Please check one or more items in each section. Note minimum requirements for classification on reverse side.

Site and Extent of Tumour

Site: ....

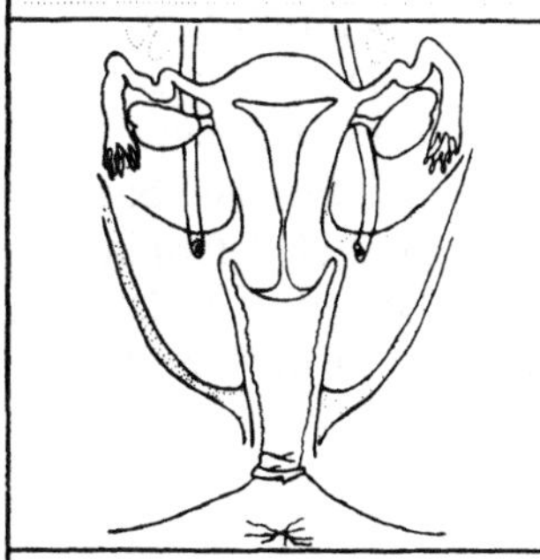

Regional lymph nodes:

Histologically: negative ☐ positive ☐

Histological diagnosis ....

Degree of differentiation:

High ☐ Med. ☐ Low ☐ Not assessed ☐

PRIMARY TUMOUR

Ovary	Ascites	Capsule	Tumour on Surface	Extension Pelvic or other	Category	Stage
No evidence or primary tumour ☐					pT0	—
One ☐	None ☐	Intact ☐	None ☐	None ☐	pT1a1	Iai
		Ruptured ☐	Present ☐		pT1a2	Iaii
Both ☐	None ☐	Intact ☐	None ☐	None ☐	pT1b1	Ibi
		Ruptured ☐	Present ☐		pT1b2	Ibii
One or Both ☐	Present* ☐	*Containing malignant cells or with positive peritoneal washings		None ☐	pT1c	Ic
	None ☐			Uterus ☐ Tubes ☐	pT2a	IIa
	None ☐			Other pelvic tissues ☐ Visceral peritoneum ☐	pT2b	IIb
	Present* ☐			Uterus/Tubes/ Pelvic Tissues ☐	pT2c	IIc
		In true pelvis →		Small bowel/Omentum ☐	pT3	III
		Beyond true pelvis →		Intraperitoneal extension ☐		
Primary tumour not assessed ☐					pTX	—

REGIONAL LYMPH NODES

	Category	Stage
No evidence of invasion ☐	pN0	I
Evidence of invasion ☐	pN1	III
Regional lymph nodes not assessed ☐	pNX	—

DISTANT METASTASES

	Category	Stage
No evidence of distant metastases ☐	pM0	I
Evidence of distant metastases (specify) ☐	pM1	IV
Distant metastases not assessed ☐	pMX	—

Category: pT pN pM Stage G

Information obtained: Before admission ☐ At Centre ☐ Clinician Date:

AHS

4. Immunoglobulins:
   IgM — Macroglobulinaemia
   IgA, G, D, E; Light chains – lambda and kappa — multiple myeloma
5. Other:
   Melanin and precursors (melanoma)

3.8 Evaluation of Response to Treatment

This may be considered at three levels:
1. Evaluation of objective response
2. Evaluation of subjective or not-strictly-objective disease parameters
3. Evaluation of toxicity

3.9 Evaluation of Objective Response

The guidelines proposed by the Treatment Committee of the Breast Cancer Task Force in the USA and the guidelines proposed for breast cancer as the outcome of a UICC project have served in large measure as the basis for the criteria of response recommended here. In the past, some groups and investigators have reported decreases of less than 50% in tumour size as responses, but it is often not possible to determine this with precision. It is recommended that only complete or partial responses as defined below should be used. This will reduce the variability between the results reported by different investigators. While it is recognized that in some treatment trials, shorter durations of response may be useful, in general 4 weeks should be used as the minimum duration of reported response. Objective response can be determined clinically, radiologically, biochemically or by surgicopathological staging. The method of determining response should therefore always be specified. The use of a 25% increase in one or more measurable lesions or the appearance of a new lesion is recommended for defining progression of disease.

3.9.1 Measurable Disease

All measurements should be recorded in metric notation, using a ruler, or calipers.
1. *Bidimensionally measurable:* surface area approximation – multiply the longest diameter by the greatest perpendicular diameter; multiple le-

sions for a single organ site - sum the products of the diameters of all measured lesions.

2. *Unidimensionally measurable:* liver involvement due to tumour involvement - sum of the three distances of the inferior liver edge from the xiphoid notch and the right and left costal margins in the respective midclavicular lines; other lesions where only one dimension is measurable - record that single dimension.

3.9.2 Unmeasurable Disease

There are many forms of unmeasurable disease, and only a few are mentioned as examples: lymphangitic pulmonary metastases; skin involvement in breast cancer (documented by photograph when possible); and abdominal masses that can be palpated but not measured.

3.10 Definition of Objective Response

3.10.1 Measurable Disease

1. Complete Response (CR). The disappearance of all known disease, determined by two observations not less than 4 weeks apart.

2. Partial Response (PR). Decrease of 50% or more in total tumour size of the lesions which have been measured to determine the effect of therapy by two observations not less than 4 weeks apart. In addition, there can be no appearance of new lesions or progression of any lesion.

3. No Change (NC). A 50% decrease in total tumour size cannot be established nor has a 25% increase in the size of one or more measurable lesions been demonstrated.

4. Progressive Disease (PD). A 25% or more increase in the size of one or more measurable lesions, or the appearance of new lesions.

3.10.2 Unmeasurable Disease

1. CR. Complete disappearance of all known disease for at least 4 weeks.

2. PR. Estimated decrease in tumour size of 50% or more for at least 4 weeks.

3. NC. No significant change for at least 4 weeks. This includes stable disease, estimated decrease of less than 50%, and lesions with estimated increase of less than 25%.

4. PD. Appearance of any new lesion not previously identified or estimated increase of 25% or more in existing lesions.

3.10.3 Bone Metastases

A separate set of response criteria is necessary for bone metastases.

1. CR. Complete disappearance of lesions on x-ray or scan.

2. PR. Partial decrease in size of lytic lesions, recalcification of lytic lesions, or decreased density of blastic lesions.

3. NC. Because of the slow response of bone lesions the designation "no change" should not be applied until at least 8 weeks have passed from start of therapy.

4. PD. Increase in size of existing lesions or appearance of new lesions.
N. B. Occurrence of bone compression or fracture and its healing should not be used as the sole indicator for evaluation of therapy.

3.11 Determination of Overall Response in Solid Tumours

If both measurable and unmeasurable disease is present in a given patient, the result of each should be recorded separately. Note that an overall assessment of response involves all parameters. In patients with measurable disease, the poorest response designation shall prevail. NC in unmeasurable lesions will not detract from a PR in measurable lesions but will reduce a CR in measurable lesions to PR overall. If in the totals of responses by organ site there are equal or greater numbers of CR plus PR than of NC designations, then the overall response will be partial. If PD exists in any lesions or when a new lesion appears, then the overall results will be PD.

3.12 Duration of Response

The period of *complete response* lasts from the date the CR was first recorded to the date thereafter on which PD is first noted. In those patients who only achieve a *partial response,* only the period of overall response should be recorded. The period of *overall response* lasts from the first day of treatment to the date of first observation of PD.

3.13 Miscellaneous Evaluation

A. Performance status – two main examples of classification:

Swiss Cooperative Group		*Karnofsky*	
0	Able to carry on normal activity	100	Normal; nor complaints, no evidence of disease
		90	Able to carry on normal activity, minor signs of symptoms of disease
1	Patient able to live at home with tolerable tumour manifestation	80	Normal activity with effort; some signs or symptoms of disease
		70	Cares for self, unable to carry on normal activity or to do active work
2	Patient with disabling tumour manifestations, but less than 50% of time in bed	60	Requires occasional assistance but is able to care for most of his needs
		50	Requires considerable assistance and frequent medical care
3	Patient severely disabled and more than 50% of time in bed, but able to stand up	40	Disabled; requires special care and assistance
		30	Severely disabled; hospitalization is indicated, although death not imminent

A. Performance status – two main examples of classification:

Swiss Cooperative Group	*Karnofsky*
4 Patient very sick and bedridden	20 Very sick; hospitalization necessary, active supportive treatment is necessary
	10 Moribund, fatal processes progressing rapidly
5 Dead	5 Dead

B. Pain, specific organ symptoms, appetite, etc.:
Scale: 0, no symptoms
1, mild
2, moderate
3, severe
4, extremely severe, life-threatening

C. Weight changes

D. Change of initially pathological laboratory parameters:
Kidney function
Liver function
Other organ functions
Specific laboratory parameters of the disease
Sedimentation rate

3.14 Evaluation of Toxicity

The management of malignancies frequently requires the use of treatment modalities which are associated with significant toxic effects. The acceptability of specific therapy can be assessed by comparing its benefits with its potential cost in terms of toxicity. For this reason, the documentation of toxicity is a crucial part of reporting treatment results. For purposes of classification, toxic effects are best divided into acute plus subacute, and chronic or late, rather than in terms of specific treatment modalities.

3.14.1 Acute and Subacute Toxic Effects

Grading of acute and subacute toxic effects has several important advantages:

1. It permits comparison of toxicity between treatment programmes.
2. It permits computerized storage and analysis of such toxicity data.

3. It allows uniform treatment modification within a therapeutic programme.

The attachment of clinical significance (e.g. mild, moderate, severe, life-threatening) to a grade should be avoided. A five-grade system (grades 0–4) is recommended for general use. No attempt has been made to be all-inclusive and investigators will undoubtedly need to add some toxic manifestations (see Sect. 1.6).

3.14.2 Chronic and Late Toxic Effects

Chronic and late toxic effects are becoming more common as more effective treatments result in longer survivals. The severity of these manifestations is less easily quantified than that of acute effects. It is suggested that the following format should be used in reporting these toxic effects:

1. Organ site or system affected
2. Timing in relation to presumed causative therapy
3. Nature of toxicity or disability (including second malignancy)
4. Magnitude of symptoms
5. Impact on performance status (see Sect. 3.13)
6. Therapy required
7. Response to therapy

It is recommended that patients should be evaluated annually for chronic and late toxicity.

3.14.3 Death Due to Treatment

Several forms of cancer treatment can result in or contribute to death. Such deaths must be reported separately.

3.15 Toxicity Criteria for the Patient Flow Sheet Used by Eastern Cooperative Oncology Group

		0	1	2	3	4
Hemat	WBC X 10^3	≥4.5	3.0–<4.5	2.0–<3.0	1.0–<2.0	<1.0
	Neut X 10^3	≥1.9	1.5–<1.9	1.0–<1.5	0.5–<1.0	<0.5
	Plt X 10^3	≥130	90–<130	50–<90	25–<50	<25
	Hgb gm%	≥11	9.5–10.9	<9.5		
	Hct %	≥32	28–31.9	<28		
	Clinical			Sx of anemia	Req transfusions	
	Hemorrhage	None	Minimal	Mod–Not debilitating	Debilitating	Life threatening
	Infection	None	No active Rx	Requires active Rx	Debilitating	Life threatening
GU	BUN mg%	≤20	21–40	41–60	>60	Symptomatic uremia
	Creatinine	≤1.2	1.3–2.0	2.1–4.0	>4.0	
	Proteinuria	Neg	1+	2+–3+	4+	
	Hematuria	Neg	Micro-Cult ⊖	Gross-Cult ⊖	Gross+Clots	c̄ obst uropathy
Hepatic	SGOT	<1.5Xnl	1.5–2 X normal	2.1–5 X normal	>5 X normal	
	Alk Phos	<1.5Xnl	1.5–2 X normal	2.1-5 X normal	>5 X normal	
	Bilirubin	<1.5Xnl	1.5–2 X normal	2.1–5 X normal	>5 X normal	
	Clinical				Precoma	Hepatic coma
Other GI	N & V	None	Nausea	N & V controllable	Vomiting intractable	
	Stomatitis	None	Soreness	Ulcers–can eat	Ulcers–cannot eat	
	Diarrhea	None	No dehydration	Dehydration	Grossly bloody	
Pulm	PFT	Nl	25–50% decrease in Dco or VC	>50% decrease in Dco or VC		
	Clinical		Mild Sx	Moderate Sx	Severe Sx-Intermittent O_2	Assisted vent or continuous O_2
Cardiac		Nl	ST–T changes	Atrial arrhythmias	Mild CHF	Severe or refract CHF
		Nl	Sinus tachy >110 at rest	Unifocal PVC's	Multifocal PVC's	Ventric tachy
					Pericarditis	Tamponade
Neuro	PN	None	Decr DTR's	Absent DTR's	Disabling sens loss	Resp dysfunction 2° to weakness
			Mild paresthesias	Severe paresthesias	Severe PN pain	
			Mild constipation	Severe constipation	Obstipation	Obstipation req surg
				Mild weakness	Severe weakness	Paralysis–confining pt to bed/wheelchair
					Bladder dysfunct	
	CNS	None	Mild anxiety	Severe anxiety	Confused or manic	Seizures
			Mild depression	Mod depression	Severe depression	Suicidal
			Mild headache	Mod headache	Severe headache	Coma
			Lethargy	Somnolence	Cord dysfunction	
				Tremor	Confined to bed due to CNS dysfunct	
				Mild hyperactivity		
Skin		Nl	Transient erythema	Vesiculation	Ulceration	
			Pigmentation, atrophy	Subepidermal fibrosis	Necrosis	
			Alopecia–mild	Alopecia–severe		
Allergy		None	Transient rash	Urticaria	Serum sickness	Anaphylaxis
			Drug fever ≤38°C (≤100.4°F)	Drug fever >38°C (>100.4°F)	Bronchospasm–req parenteral meds	
				Mild bronchospasm		
Fever		≤37.5°C	≤38°C (≤100.4°F)	>38°C (>100.4°F)	Severe c̄ chills (>40°C)	Fever c̄ hypotension
Local Tox		None	Pain	Pain + Phlebitis	Ulceration	

1. The toxicity grade should reflect the most severe degree occurring during the evaluated period, not an average.
2. When two criteria are available for similar toxicities, e.g. leukopenia, neutropenia, the one resulting in the more severe toxicity grade should be used.
3. Toxicity grade = 5 if that toxicity caused the death of the patient.
4. Refer to detailed toxicity guidelines or to study chairman for toxicity not covered on this table.

Sx, symptoms; Rx, therapy; N & V, nausea and vomiting; PFT, pulmonary function test; DCO, diffusing capacity for CO; VC, vital capacity; Nl, normal; PVC, premature ventricular contractions (extrasystoles); CHF, congestive heart failure; PN, peripheral neuropathy; DTR, deep tendon reflexes

3.16 Patient Measurement Form Used by Eastern Cooperative Oncology Group

Date of Observation							
Day of Study							
Observer's Initials							
GIVE COORDINATES FOR ALL MEASUREMENTS (Include Liver and Spleen) — Lesions Measured							
Liver (cm)							
Spleen (cm)							

Did new lesions appear during treatment? YES............ NO............

Give coordinates for new lesions: ....

INDICATE ON DIAGRAM ALL MEASURABLE AND PALPABLE LESIONS AT START OF THERAPY
(Include Liver and Spleen)

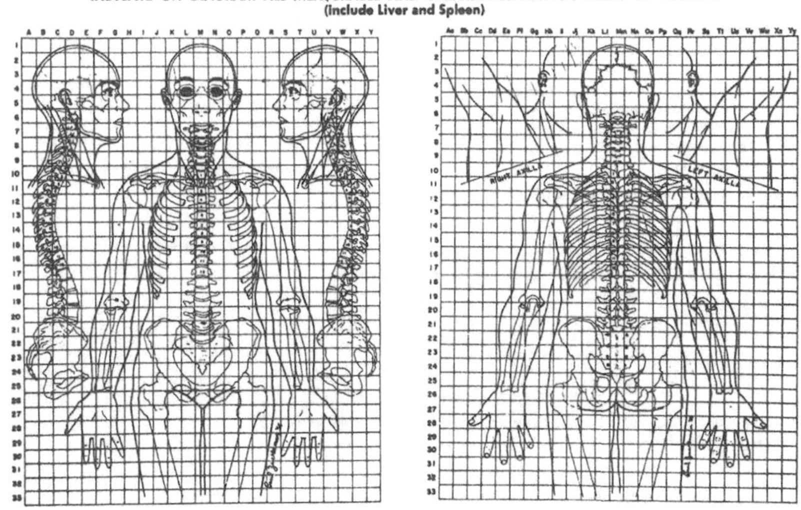

Patient Name .... Institution ....

Protocol # EST .... Page .... of .... pages

ECOG FORM C
3/69

3.17 Patient Summary and Evaluation Report Used by Eastern Cooperative Oncology Group

1. STUDY TREATMENT

Treatment	NSC #	Quantity	Unit	Base	Schedule	Route	Total Amount Drug Given

2. ABNORMALITIES OCCURRING DURING TREATMENT

	Degree** 0-5	Due To	
		Disease	Treatment
Pain			
G.I.			
Nausea			
Vomiting			
Diarrhea			
Infection			
Bleeding			
Skin & Muc. Memb.			
Neurologic			
Respiratory			
GU			
Blood			
Liver			
Other (specify)			

3. TREATMENT MODIFICATION

	Number of days at dose modification
None	
Decreased	
Increased	
Interrupted	
Stopped	
Reason for modification:	

4. ORGAN INVOLVEMENT AT END OF TREATMENT

Bone		Soft Tissue	
Skin		Lymph Nodes: regional	
Liver		distant	
CNS		OTHER (specify)	
Lungs			

5. OBJECTIVE RESPONSE TO TREATMENT

	Onset Date	Duration No. of days	Relapse Date
Comp. Response			
Part. Response			
No Change			
Progression			

6. Did additional metastasis develop during treatment
YES .... NO ....
If, YES, specify ....

7. Date treatment started ....
Date treatment ended ....
Date off study or phase ....

8. Did Patient benefit from treatment? Indicate:
Marked improvement ....
Moderate improvement ....
No improvement ....
Worsening ....

9. SURVIVAL: Alive .... Dead .... Unknown ....
Date last known to be alive ....
Date of death ....
Autopsy YES .... NO .... UNKNOWN ....

10. Did patient have other complicating disease?
YES .... NO ....
Explain: ....

11. Future plans for treatment of patient.
....

12. INVESTIGATOR'S SUMMARY (use reverse side for additional space)

13. PROTOCOL: Followed .... Minor deviation .... Case invalidated YES .... NO ....
Reason for invalidation ....

....
SIGNATURE (senior investigator) (Date)

....
Institution

Patient Name ....
Protocol # EST ....
Page ...... of .... pages

**KEY

0—None or Normal
1—Mild
2—Moderate
3—Severe
4—Life-Threatening
5—Lethal

ECOG FORM D
3/69

3.18 Patient Flow Sheet Used by Eastern Cooperative Oncology Group

B2 Page____ of____

Patient's Name______________________ Hosp. or Soc. Sec. No.______________________

Institution______________________ Protocol Number______________________

							REMARKS (R_1, R_2, R_3, etc.)
PROTOCOL TREATMENT	1. Date 197____(mo./day)						
	2. Initials						
	RECORD ACTUAL DOSE; IF MODIFIED OR NOT GIVEN, EXPLAIN						
	3. Rx 1 (dose/day)						
	4. Rx 2 (dose/day)						
	5. Rx 3 (dose/day)						
	6. Rx 4 (dose/day)						
	7. Rx 5 (dose/day)						
OTHER THERAPY	SPECIFY AMOUNT; GIVE DETAILS						
	8. Antibiotics/Analgesics						
	9. Radiation (rads/day)						
	10. Transfusions (units)						
	11.						
PATIENT STATUS	12. PERFORMANCE STATUS*						
	13. Weight (kg)						
	14. Temperature						
ABNORMALITIES (Grade 0-5**)	CIRCLE REACTIONS DUE TO PROTOCOL THERAPY						
	15. Anemia						
	16. Hemorrhage						
	17. Infection						
	18. GU						
	19. Hepatic						
	20. Nausea & Vomiting						
	21. Other GI						
	22. Pulmonary						
	23. Cardiac						
	24. Neurologic–PN						
	25. Neurologic–CNS						
	26. Skin						
	27. Allergy						
	28. Fever						
	29. Pain						
	30. Other (specify)						
LABORATORY VALUES	REFER TO PROTOCOL FOR TEST SCHEDULES						
	31. HGB (gm %)]						
	32. HCT (%)						
	33 WBC (x 1000)						
	34. Neutrophyls (%)						
	35. Lymphs (%)						
	36. Platelets (x 1000)						
	37. Retic (%)						
	38. BUN (mg %)						
	39. Serum Creatinine (mg %)						
	40. Alk. Ptase (units)						
	41. Bilirubin (mg %)						
	42. SGOT (units)						
	43. SGPT (units)						
	44. LDH (units)						
	45. Uric Acid (mg %)						
	46. Total Protein (gm %)						
	47. Albumin (gm %)						
	48. Abnormal Protein (gm %)						
	49. Calcium (mg %)						
	50. Phosphorus (mg %)						
	51.						
SKIN TESTS†	52. PPD Int (mm)						
	53. Mumps (mm)						
	54. Varidase (dose & mm)						
	55. Dermatophytin 0 (1:100) (mm)						
	56. Other:						

† Measure at 48 hours induration as the mean of two diameters measured at right angles in mm.

* PERFORMANCE STATUS KEY	** ABNORMALITY KEY
0–Normal activity	0–None or Normal
1–Symptoms but ambulatory	1–Mild
2–In bed < 50% of time	2–Moderate
3–In bed > 50% of time	3–Severe
4–100% bedridden	4–Life-Threatening
	5–Lethal

3.19 Common Causes of Mistakes in the Clinical Evaluation of Response

1. Not accurate recording of initial picture
2. Lack of periodic review and recording of measurable lesions
3. Lack or inaccurate utilization of patient measurement forms

Further Reading

1. TNM classification of malignant tumours (1980) A brochure of checklists, UICC Technical Report Series, Vol 51. First Edition, Geneva
2. Staquet MJ (ed) (1975) Cancer Therapy: Prognostic Factors and Criteria of Response. Raven Press, New York
3. Flammant R, Fohanno C (1978) Controlled Therapeutic Trials in Cancer. UICC Information Office and List of registered Trials. UICC Technical Report Series, Vol 32. UICC, Geneva
4. Armitage P et al. (1978) Methods and Impact of Controlled Therapeutic Trials in Cancer. Part 1. UICC Technical Report Series, Vol 36. UICC, Geneva

4 Complications of the Disease and Their Treatment

4.1 Complications in Advanced Neoplastic Disease

These may be classified as follows:

Complications as direct manifestations of invasive tumour growth
Complications as indirect manifestations of the neoplastic disease
Complications unrelated to the neoplastic disease
Complications due to treatment of the disease

4.2 Complications as Direct Manifestations of Invasive Tumour Growth

4.2.1 Compression or Obstruction of Vital Organs

1. Superior vena cava syndrome:
   Central lung cancer
   Mediastinal lymphoma
2. Spinal cord compression:
   Bone metastases (breast cancer)
   Malignant lymphoma
   Multiple myeloma
3. Increased intracranial pressure:
   Brain tumours
   Brain metastases
   Neoplastic meningitis
4. Intestinal obstruction (ileus):
   Abdominal cancers
5. Obstructive jaundice:
   Abdominal cancers, mainly pancreas and colon
6. Urinary tract obstruction:
   Urogenital cancers
   Intestinal cancers

7. Inferior vena cava syndrome and compression of other blood vessels:
   Urogenital cancer
8. Compression of the bronchial tree:
   Post-stenotic pneumonia

4.2.2 Manifestations of Invasive Tumour

1. Pain syndromes:
   Invasion of nerves and nervous plexus
   Bone pain from bone metastases
   Pancoast's syndrome of the lung
   Capsular pain from massive hepatic infiltration
2. Loss of endocrine functions by destruction of endocrine organs:
   Diabetes insipidus from metastases of the hypophysis
   Addison's syndrome from adrenal metastases and hepatic failure
3. Bone fracture

4.2.3 Erosions and Perforations

1. Blood vessels:
   Bleeding
   Haematuria
2. Tracheo-bronchial fistula
3. Recto-vaginal or recto-vesical fistula
4. Bowel perforation

4.3 Complications as Indirect Manifestations of the Neoplastic Disease

4.3.1 General Manifestations

1. Pain
2. Fever
3. Weight loss
4. Fatigue
5. Loss of appetite and weight
6. Tumour cachexia

4.3.2 Haematological Complications

1. Anaemia: Haemolytic, aplastic, iron deficiency (bleeding)
2. Leukaemoid reaction: Bone marrow infiltration by tumour cells
3. Leukopenia, thrombocytopenia, pancytopenia
4. Erythrocythaemia: Renal cell carcinoma
5. Thrombocytosis
6. Coagulation defects: Fibrinolytic syndrome (disseminated intravascular coagulation)

4.3.3 Immunological Complications

1. Non-specific immune deficiency (humoral or cellular): Infections, septicaemia
2. Defects of granulocyte mobilization and phagocytosis
3. Hypo- or hypergammaglobulinaemia, paraproteinaemia
4. Hyperviscosity syndrome: Multiple myeloma
5. Amyloidosis: Multiple myeloma
6. Specific immune deficiencies in malignant lymphomas and chronic lymphocytic leukemia

4.3.4 Metabolic Complications

1. *Hypercalcaemia* in metastatic bone disease or, rarely, caused by secretion of a parathormone-like substance (high serum phosphate levels):
   Symptoms and signs:
   Polyuria, polydipsia, dehydration
   Muscular atony: Constipation, anorexia, nausea, vomiting
   CNS symptoms: Somnolence, disorientation, coma
   Deterioration of kidney function, anuria
2. *Hyperuricaemia* with uric acid nephropathy: Due to increased cell metabolism and cell turnover, aggravated by massive therapeutic cell lysis, mainly in haematological neoplasia

4.3.5 Endocrine Paraneoplastic Syndromes (Ectopic Secretion of Hormones by Tumours)

1. Cushing's syndrome: Adrenocorticotrophin(ACTH)-like substance
2. Salt loss syndrome (Schwartz-Bartter): Ectopic anti diuretic hormone – hyponatraemia, water intoxication, coma. Mainly in oat cell carcinoma
3. Hypoglycaemia by insulin-like substances: Retroperitoneal sarcomas, ovarian cancers

4. Ectopic parathyroid hormone: Hypercalcaemia
5. Ectopic thyroid-stimulating hormone (TSH): Hyperthyroidism
6. Ectopic erythropoietin: Erythrocythaemia (renal cell cancer)
7. Ectopic gonadotrophins:
   Choriocarcinoma
   Testicular cancers
   Ovarian teratoma
   Mediastinal teratoma
   Rarely, hepatoma
   May produce gynaecomastia. Important for monitoring therapeutic response

4.3.6 Neuro-Muscular Paraneoplastic Syndromes

1. Neuromuscular disorders
2. Carcinomatous myopathy: Polymyositis, dermatomyositis
3. Myasthenic syndrome: Malignant thymoma
4. Carcinomatous peripheral neuropathy
5. Carcinomatous myopathy
6. Subacute cerebellar degeneration
7. Encephalopathy associated with carcinomas
8. Progressive multifocal leukoencephalopathy

4.3.7 Dermatological Paraneoplastic Disorders

1. Erythema gyaratum serpens
2. Acrodermatosis (psoriasis-like)
3. Acanthosis nigricans: Abdominal adenocarcinoma, mainly stomach
4. Dermatomyositis
5. Thrombophlebitis migrans

4.3.8 Osseous Paraneoplastic Syndromes

1. Osteoarthropathy
2. Polyarthritis
3. Myelofibrosis
4. Myelosclerosis

4.4 Treatment of Direct and Indirect Manifestations

4.4.1 Principles

The first responsibility of the physician faced with direct or indirect manifestations of invasive tumour growth is a careful evaluation of what the prognosis will be after the complication has been dealt with. The aggressiveness of management of the complication should be directly proportional to the probability of cure or long-range remission of the cancer. Thereby it must be taken into account that in addition to the potentially curable cancer patient who may be successfully managed in case of complications, there are numerous patients for whom the quality of life can be substantially improved even though they are not curable (compression of spinal cord, pathological fractures).

Often (mainly direct manifestations of invasive tumour growth) complications of cancer can be reversed only when the cancer itself is controlled. In other cases, management of the complications may delay or interfere with definitive therapy of cancer. In any case, attention must be given to the initiation at the earliest possible time of definitive anti tumour therapy.

4.4.2 Management of Hypercalcaemia

1. Long-term control only by reduction of the tumour burden.
2. Rehydration (because of hypercalcaemia associated with hypervolaemia).
3. Avoid furosemide before rehydration is completed.
4. Give 3–4 l saline/day (forced saline diuresis with > 10 l/day + furosemide not recommended).
5. Corticosteroids only if a direct antineoplastic effect can be expected.
6. Calcitonin excellent (4–8 IU/kg/two-four times daily).
7. There is no longer much justification for:
   Low-calcium diet
   Mithramycin
   Indomethacin
   Chelating agents
   i.v. Phosphates.
8. Diphosphonates are new and promising agents: disodium etidronate (EHDP), disodium clodronate (Cl_2MDP).

4.4.3 Prevention of Hyperuricaemia

1. Increased fluid intake
2. Alkalinization of urine (sodium bicarbonate)
3. Allopurinol (Zyloric – inhibitor of xanthinoxidase): prophylactic dose 300 mg daily

4.5 Complications Unrelated to the Neoplastic Disease

Cancer patients may have other unrelated intercurrent diseases. There is a tendency to ascribe every symptom and sign in a cancer patient to his neoplastic disease and to overlook other unrelated diseases. Proper diagnosis of another unrelated disease can only be made by careful evaluation of all symptoms and signs and by unbiased differential diagnosis.

4.6 Complications Due to the Treatment of the Disease

1. Complications of surgery:
   Lymphoedema, etc., usually well-recognized
2. Complications of radiotherapy:
   a) Cardiopathy
   b) Acute and late constrictive pericarditis
   c) Acute and chronic pulmonary radiation syndrome
   d) Radiation myelitis
   e) Radiation neuropathy
   f) Radiation nephropathy
   g) Radiation strictures of the gut after abdominal radiation
   h) Malabsorption
3. Specific toxicities of cytostatic drugs

4.7 General Conclusions on the Management of Complications in Advanced Neoplastic Disease

It is crucial for the general management of the cancer patient that specific complications due to treatment procedures are recognized as such and are clearly differentiated from direct or indirect complications of the disease process itself or a possible unrelated intercurrent disease.

This implies:

1. Broad medical knowledge
2. Knowledge of the natural course of all neoplastic diseases
3. Specific knowledge and experience of all forms of treatment and their complications, especially the side effects and toxicities of the various cytostatic drugs

4.8 Supportive Care

Supportive care is essential in all forms of malignant disease, but patients with acute leukaemia (particularly acute myelogenous leukaemia), and certain other forms of malignant disease in which there is severe impairment of bone marrow reserve, require more intensive and specialized support. The following sections are concerned with these aspects.

4.9 Supportive Care Measures in Acute Leukaemia

4.9.1 Essential

1. Good general medical care
2. Treatment of fluid and electrolyte imbalance
3. Prophylactic non-absorbable antibiotics p.o.; early intensive treatment of infection
4. Treatment of haemorrhage and anaemia – whole-blood or packed-cell transfusion, platelet transfusions
5. Allopurinol to prevent hyperuricaemia
6. Treatment of local and other general complications of disease
7. Granulocyte transfusion in infected neutropenic patients if after 48 h of intensive antibiotic treatment there is no adequate response

4.9.2 Controversial

1. Prophylactic granulocyte transfusion: helpful in infected neutropenic patients, controversial as a prophylactic measure
2. Isolation units: helpful in reducing incidence of infection. Role compared with "clean nursing" not fully assessed.
3. Prophylactic platelet transfusions in patients with platelet counts. $\leq 15\,000/\mu l$: advisable when period of thrombocytopenia likely to be short

4.10 Investigation of Fever in a Granulocytopenic Patient

The following measures should be taken within 1 h of a fever (38 °C or more) being noticed:

1. History and examination (special emphasis - skin, mouth, axillae and perineum).
2. Laboratory culture: Swab - Throat
   - Nose
   - Vagina
   - Any apparently infected site

   Mid-stream specimen of urine
   Blood culture
   Sputum, when possible
   Stool culture - only if indicated
   CSF examination - only if indicated
3. Chest x-ray as soon as feasible.
4. If no apparent site of infection is discovered, antibiotic therapy should be started using a regime such as that described under Sect. 4.11.
5. CSF examination for spores (i.e. *Cryptococcus*) should be carried out where unexplained deterioration of mental function or low-grade fever in an immunosuppressed patient persist.

N.B. Negative cultures do not rule out serious systemic bacterial or fungal infection. Discuss with the laboratory the advisability of both aerobic and anaerobic cultures and examination for fungi or yeasts.

4.11 Management of Pyrexia in a Granulocytopenic Patient (Once Investigations Are Complete)

Neutrophil count $< 0.5 \times 10^9/l$

1. With i.v. access and no allergy to penicillin:
   Gentamicin 120 mg i.v. stat followed by 120 mg i.v. 8-hourly.
   Refer to nomogram for patients who weigh less than 70 kg or more than 80 kg or who have concomitant renal failure.
   Carbenicillin 5 g i.v. 6-hourly (infuse separately in 100 ml water over 15-min period). (Often tobramycin + ticarcillin recommended).
2. With i.v. access and allergy to penicillin:
   Gentamicin as above, + cefuroxime 1.5 g three times daily
   Reduce by 50% if evidence of renal failure
   Other alternatives:

- Azlocillin + Amikacin
- Cefotaxime + Amikacin
- Ticarcillin + Amikacin
- Erythromycin 600 mg (60 ml of a 1% solution at 10 mg/l) given 6-hourly. If *no response* after 48–72 h of parenteral antimicrobials, take a throat swab in Stuart's medium and another set of blood cultures containing β-lactamase (obtainable from bacteriology laboratory).

4.12 Herpes Virus Infection (Simplex or Zoster)

The use of i.v. therapy is indicated only where evidence of dissemination exists. Cytomegalovirus does not respond.
Take vesicle fluid or lesion swab into virus transport medium before commencing therapy.

Adenine arabinoside

Herpes-specific immunoglobulin – available from blood transfusion

4.13 Fungal Infection

Take fungal blood cultures before commencing therapy.
A combination of amphotericin and 5-fluorocytosine is used and should be maintained for a least 6 weeks.

5-Fluorocytosine:

a) Oral – 200 mg/kg/day in four divided doses
b) i.v. As for oral but as a 20- to 40-min infusion
c) Reduce dose in renal failure

Amphotericin:

A starting dose of 0.25 mg/kg/day by slow infusion over 6 h, increasing to a standard dose between 0.5 and 1.0 mg/kg/day depending on toxicity

4.14 Management of the Sore Mouth

Each patient should be the responsibility of a specific nurse. Teeth should be cleaned either with an electric toothbrush or cotton wool tipped swabs after each meal, followed by a diluted Oraldene mouthwash. Bland soft foods are advisable. Benzocaine or lignocaine lozenges 4-hourly or before meals, or lignocaine gel applied before meals may reduce local pain. An AAA benzocaine spray may be used, but in some cases effective analgesics (including opiates) may be required.

Hydrogen peroxide 1 in 4 is effective in removing slough from a dirty mouth, but should not be continued longer than necessary. In severe cases, 2-hourly mouth toilet with sodium bicarbonate and Oraldene is given with white vaseline or glycerine and lemon for cracked lips.

4.14.1 Specific Mouth Problems

Simple Aphthous Ulcers. Dissolve a hydrocortisone tablet locally every 4 h.

Methotrexate. Ulcers may appear if insufficient folinic acid rescue has been given.

Adequate dose of folinic acid in tablet form or i.v. will usually prevent this; however in the established case, folinic acid mouthwash 1 in 200 will help.

Adriamycin- or Bleomycin-Induced Mucositis. Stop the drug.

Moniliasis. Mild infection – Amphotericin lozenges (Fungilin) dissolved slowly in the mouth every 4 h. If no response after 3 days, change to nystatin.

Severe cases – Povidone-iodine (Betadine) 2-hourly followed after 15 min by nystatin suspension, 2 ml, swilled around the mouth and swallowed.

Ketoconazole (R 41400) or gentian violet are alternatives.

4.15 Prophylaxis for Infection in Patients with Acute Myeloblastic Leukaemia

Synthesis of data from major studies (updated) in terms of prophylaxis for infection in patients with acute myeloblastic leukaemia (AML). Randomized studies [all compared with untreated controls]

Conclusion. Isolation and sterilization do not appear to offer substantial clinical benefit.

	Type of prophylaxis	No. of cases	No. of remissions	No. of deaths due to infection	No. of cases of infection
National Cancer	A	38	=	=	=
Institute	I+A	32	=	↓	↓
(Bethesda, USA)					
Memorial	A	28	↑	=	=
Sloan-Kettering					
(New York, USA)					
Baltimore CRC	A	19	↑	↓	↓
(Baltimore, USA)	I+A	24	↑	↓	↓
Roswell Park	I	22	=	=	↓
(Buffalo, USA)	A	28	=	↓	=
	I+A	27	=	↓	↓
Jules Bordet	A	14		=	↓
(Brussels, Belgium)	I+A	16		=	↓
Leukaemia Research	A	46	=	↓	↓
Fund (London, UK)					

A, gut prophylactic antibiotics; I, isolation unit; =, no change; ↑, statistically significant increase; ↓, statistically significant decrease

Further Reading

1. Yarbro JW, Bomstein RS (1980) Oncologic Emergencies. Grune & Stratton, New York
2. Stadmik L (1980) Nutrition Information for Cancer Patients. Delaware Cancer Network, Wilmington
3. Klastersky J (ed) (1982) Infections in Cancer Patients. (Monograph Series of the EORTC; Vol 10) Raven Press, New York, 220 S
4. Klastersky J, Staquet MJ (1981) Medical Complications in Cancer Patients. (Monograph Series of the EORTC; Vol 7) Raven Press, New York, 317 S
5. Seifter EJ, Bell WR (1984) Coagulation Disorders in the Cancer Patient. Futura Publ Comp, Mount Kisco New York, 212 S

5 Present Achievements of Cancer Chemotherapy and Drugs Currently Used for Different Diseases

5.1 Present Achievements in Anticancer Chemotherapy for Generalized Malignant Disease

1. Examples of disease where chemotherapy may produce potential cure:
   Acute lymphoblastic leukaemia (in childhood)
   Burkitt's lymphoma
   Hodgkin's disease
   Retinoblastoma
   Wilms' tumour
   Diffuse large-cell non-Hodgkin lymphomas
   Malignant trophoblastic choriocarcinoma
   Embryonal rhabdomyosarcoma
   Ewing's sarcoma
   Testicular tumours
2. Examples of disease where chemotherapy may produce increase in survival:
   Acute leukaemia (adults)
   Breast carcinoma
   Chronic leukaemias - chronic myelocytic leukaemia (CML), chronic lymphocytic leukaemia (CLL)
   Multiple myeloma
   Non-Hodgkin lymphomas (low-grade histology)
   Ovarian cancer
   Small-cell lung cancer
   Neuroblastoma
   Endometrial carcinoma
   Prostatic carcinoma
3. Examples of disease where chemotherapy may produce objective response, which is of appreciable value:
   Osteosarcoma
   Thyroid carcinoma
   Head and neck tumours
   Gastric carcinoma

Soft-tissue sarcomas
Melanoma
Malignant gliomas
Bladder carcinoma

4. Examples of disease where chemotherapy may produce a poor response which is short-lived:
   Non-small-cell bronchial carcinoma
   Oesophageal carcinoma
   Intestinal carcinoma (colon, rectum)
   Hepatocellular carcinoma
   Cervix carcinoma
   Hypernephroma

5.2 Present Achievements with Adjuvant Chemotherapy

1. Examples of disease in which adjuvant chemotherapy is of documented value for prolonged survival:
   Wilms' tumour
   Ewing's sarcoma
   Rhabdomyosarcoma in childhood
2. Examples of disease in which adjuvant chemotherapy is showing promising results:
   Breast cancer
   Certain lymphomas
   Brain tumours (in childhood)
   Bronchogenic carcinoma (small-cell)
   Osteogenic sarcoma
   Testicular carcinoma

5.3 Principal Cytotoxic Drugs and Hormones Effective in Various Solid Tumours and Haematological Malignancies

Type of Tumour	Cytotoxic Drug, or Hormone
Breast cancer	Adriamycin, cyclophosphamide, methotrexate, 5-fluorouracil, mitomycin C, vincristine, dibromodulcitol Progestins, anti-oestrogens, oestrogens, androgens, corticosteroids
Ovarian cancer	Melphalan, cyclophosphamide, Adriamycin, 5-fluorouracil, methotrexate, *cis*-platinum, hexamethylmelamine
Cancer of the endometrium	Progestins Cyclophosphamide, 5-fluorouracil, Adriamycin
Cancer of the cervix	Cyclophosphamide, vincristine, 5-fluorouracil, Adriamycin, bleomycin
Cancer of the vulva	Bleomycin
Gestational choriocarcinoma	Methotrexate, 6-mercaptopurine, actinomycin D, cyclophosphamide, Adriamycin, vinblastine, vincristine
Testicular carcinomas	Actinomycin D, vinblastine, bleomycin, cyclophosphamide, iphosphamide, Adriamycin, vincristine, *cis*-platinum, etoposide (VP-16-213)
Seminoma	Cyclophosphamida, Adriamycin, vinblastine, bleomycin, *cis*-platinum
Penis cancer	Bleomycin
Prostate cancer	Oestrogens, progestins, Estracyt, cyclophosphamide, 5-fluorouracil. Adriamycin, *cis*-platinum
Bladder cancer	Adriamycin, teniposide (VM-26), 5-fluorouracil, *cis*-platinum, cyclophosphamide
Brain tumours	Nitrosoureas, procarbazine, vincristine, methotrexate, VM-26
Thyroid cancer	Thyroid hormones Adriamycin, cyclophosphamide, 5-fluorouracil
Head and neck cancer	Methotrexate, bleomycin, *cis*-platinum, dibromodulcitol
Lung cancer (non-small-cell)	Cyclophosphamide, Adriamycin, *cis*-platinum, 5-fluorouracil, mitomycin C, methotrexate, procarbazine, vindesine
Lung cancer (small-cell)	Cyclophosphamide, Adriamycin, *cis*-platinum, vincristine, nitrosoureas, hexamethylmelamine, procarbazine, VP-16-213
Oesophageal cancer	Bleomycin, methotrexate, *cis*-platinum
Gastric cancer	5-Fluorouracil, mitomycin C, Adriamycin, carmustine (BCNU), vincristine
Colorectal cancer	5-Fluorouracil, nitrosoureas
Pancreatic carcinoma	5-Fluorouracil, streptozotocin, nitrosoureas, mitomycin C, Adriamycin
Primary hepatic carcinoma	5-Fluorouracil, Adriamycin, mitomycin C

Type of Tumour	Cytotoxic Drug, or Hormone
Adrenal cortex carcinoma	Ortho-para DDD (o,p-DDD), aminoglutethimide
Malignant insulinoma	Streptozotocin, 5-fluorouracil
Carcinoid tumours	5-Fluorouracil, cyclophosphamide, streptozotocin
Squamous cell skin cancer	Bleomycin, topical 5-fluorouracil
Malignant melanoma	Dacarbazine, nitrosoureas, vindesine, vinblastine, procarbazine, actinomycin D
Neuroblastoma	Cyclophosphamide, Adriamycin, vincristine, dacarbazine, nitrosoureas
Retinoblastoma	Cyclophosphamide, vincristine
Wilms' tumour	Actinomycin D, vincristine, Adriamycin
Ewing's sarcoma	Cyclophosphamide, Adriamycin, actinomycin D, vincristine
Osteogenic sarcoma	Adriamycin, high-dose methotrexate with "leucovorin rescue", carminomycin
Soft-tissue sarcomas	Adriamycin, dacarbazine, cyclophosphamide, vincristine, actinomycin D, methotrexate
Hodgkin's disease	Nitrogen mustard, vinblastine, procarbazine, Adriamycin, vincristine, bleomycin, prednisone, dacarbazine, nitrosoureas, VP-16-213, prednimustine
Non-Hodgkin lymphomas	Cyclophosphamide, vincristine, Adriamycin, bleomycin, prednisone, methotrexate, cytosine arabinoside, nitrosoureas, procarbazine, vinblastine, VP-16-213
Burkitt's tumour	Cyclophosphamide, methotrexate, vincristine, cytosine arabinoside
Acute lymphoblastic leukaemia (ALL)	Prednisone, vincristine, daunomycin, Adriamycin, methotrexate, 6-mercaptopurine, L-asparaginase, cytosine arabinoside, cyclophosphamide
Actue myeloblastic leukaemia (AML)	Cytosine arabinoside, daunomycin, Adriamycin, 6-thioguanine, methotrexate, 6-mercatopurine, cyclophosphamide, amsacrine (m-AMSA)
CML	Busulfan, phenylalanine mustard, dibromomannitol
CLL	Chlorambucil, cyclophosphamide, prednisone
Multiple myeloma	Phenylalanine mustard, cyclophosphamide, prednisone, procarbazine, nitrosoureas, Adriamycin, vincristine
Polycythaemia rubra vera	busulfan, hydroxyurea, dibromomannitol

Further Reading

De Vita, V.T., Hellman, S., Rosenberg, S.A., (1982) Cancer. Principles and Practice of Oncology. J.B. Lippincott Co., Philadelphia-Toronto

Frei, E., Holland, J. (1973) (eds.). Cancer Medicine. Lea & Fabiger, Philadelphia

Haskell, C.M. (1980) (Ed.). Cancer Treatment. Saunders, Philadelphia

6 The Chemotherapeutic Drugs and Their Characteristics[1]

N. B. Generic names are used throughout this chapter.

6.1 Alkylating Agents

6.1.1	Generic name:	Busulphan (Myleran)
	Dosage:	Continuous 0.5–10 mg daily, according to FBC Intermittently 50–250 mg as a single dose
	Precautions:	May cause prolonged myelosuppression
	Administration:	Oral 0.5-mg, 2-mg tablets
	Toxicity:	Myelosuppression (nadir 2–4 weeks, recovery 4–8 weeks) Infertility and amenorrhoea Pigmentation Gynaecomastia Cataracts Nausea and vomiting Pulmonary fibrosis
	Monitoring tests:	Regular full blood count
	Metabolism and excretion:	Excreted in the urine as methanesulfonic acid
	Storage:	Room temperature
6.1.2	Generic name:	Chlorambucil (Leukeran)
	Dosage:	5–15 mg daily continuous treatment Or occasionally 20·100 mg/day intermittently
	Administration:	Oral 2-mg, 5-mg tablets
	Toxicity:	Myelosuppression Nausea and vomiting Indigestion

[1] A nomogram for calculating body surface area is given in Appendix B.

		Hepatic Pulmonary
	Metabolism and excretion:	Unknown, probable extensive metabolism and renal excretion of metabolites
	Storage:	Room temperature
6.1.3	Generic name:	Cyclophosphamide (Endoxan, Cytoxan)
	Dosage:	50-200 mg orally daily (when used in combinations) Or 300-600 mg/m^2 i. v. every 3 weeks
	Administration:	i. v. bolus + N. (normal) saline flush Oral - 50-mg tablets
	Precautions:	Patients should increase fluid intake (> 3 l/day) to avoid cystitis
	Toxicity:	Myelosuppression (nadir 1-2 weeks, recovery by 3-5 weeks) Alopecia Sterility Nausea and vomiting (especially with high doses i. v.) Haemorrhagic cystitis (consider mesnum, see sect. 6.1.5) Mucositis Amenorrhoea Cardiomyopathy (only with high-dose therapy Syndrome of inappropriate antidiuretic hormone secretion (SIADH) pulmonary fibrosis
	Monitoring tests:	Full blood count
	Metabolism and excretion:	Renal excretion. Activated in liver
	Storage:	Tablets - room temperature Powder - 100-mg, 200-mg, 500-mg, 1000-mg vials room temperature Solution - refrigerated, 24 h
	Interactions:	Allopurinol, anaesthetic agents, barbiturates, chloramphenicol, chloroquine, corticosteroids, dapsone, hypoglycaemic drugs, neuromuscular blockers

6.1.4	Generic name:	Dibromodulcitol (mitolactol, DBD)
	Trade Name:	None
	Presentation:	50- and 100-mg tablets
	Mode of administration:	Oral
	Dose and usual schedules:	135–200 mg/m^2 days 1–10 q 28 days, 100 mg/m^2 daily × 35
	Toxicity:	Leukopenia, thrombocytopenia, gastrointestinal (nausea and vomiting)
	Major indications:	Melanoma, breast, head and neck
	Storage:	Room temperature

6.1.5	Generic name:	Ifosfamide (Holoxan, Iphosphamide, Mitoxana)
	Dosage:	1000–5000 mg/m^2 i.v. every 3 weeks 500–1000 mg/m^2/day × 5 days every 3 weeks
	Administration:	i.v. infusion i.v. bolus in at least 75 ml water Or N. saline + N. saline flush
	Precautions:	Ensure adequate hydration during and after therapy to maintain high urine output and minimize urothelial toxicity. Ideally, maintain i.v. infusion for 24–48 h. Use mesnum with high doses, or if previous cystistis
	Toxicity:	Haemorrhagic cytistis. Use mesnum and increase fluid intake Nausea and vomiting Alopecia Myelosuppression Phlebitis Sedation Nephrotoxicity
	Monitoring tests:	Full blood count
	Metabolism and excretion:	Activated by liver microsomal enzymes, Metabolites excreted in urine
	Storage:	Available in 1- and 3-g vials. Stable, when refrigerated, for 5 years. Diluted in at least 30 ml of water for injection. Stable, when diluted for 1 week at room

		temperature and 6 weeks under refrigeration. If diluted in common infusion vehicles stable for 7 days at room temperature but use within 8 h because no bacteriostatic properties
	Interaction:	Possibly potentiated by phenobarbital, phenytoin and chloralhydrate
6.1.6	Generic name:	Mechlorethamine (Mustagen, Mustine, HN_2, nitrogen mustard)
	Dosage:	2-6 mg/m^2 every 3-4 weeks (when used in combinations) 0.2-0.25 mg/ml topically
	Administration:	i.v. bolus into fast-running N. saline infusion
	Precaution:	Avoid extravasation Avoid contact with skin and eyes (wear gloves and goggles when preparing and injecting)
	Toxicity:	Tissue necrosis if extravasated Phlebitis Nausea and vomiting Myelosuppression (nadir at 9-14 days recovery 16-20 days) Alopecia Pulmonary fibrosis
	Monitoring tests:	Full blood count
	Metabolism and excretion:	Inactive metabolites excreted in the urine
	Storage:	Powder - 10-mg vials refrigerated Solution - only stable for a few minutes
6.1.7	Generic name:	Melphalan (Alkeran, L-phenylalanine mustard, L-PAM)
	Dosage:	5 mg/m^2/orally daily for 5 days, every 6 weeks. 15-40 mg/m^2 oral or i.v. every 6 weeks
	Administration:	Oral 2-mg, 5-mg tablets i.v. bolus + N. saline flush
	Precaution:	Oral - ensure given with food i.v. - dilute each 100-mg vial with 1 ml

		of propanol diluent (supplied) and then 9 ml of water for injection
	Toxicity:	Myelosuppression (nadir at 21–28 days) Nausea and vomiting Amenorrhoea Sterility Cystitis Mucositis
	Monitoring tests:	Full blood count
	Metabolism and excretion:	Mainly excreted in the urine as metabolites (consider dose reduction if renal impairment)
	Storage:	Available as 2-mg tablets or 100-mg vial for injection with diluent. Stable for 24 h after reconstitution. Tablets and injection stored away from direct sunlight at room temperature
6.1.8	Generic name:	Thiotepa (triethylenethiophosphoramide, TSPA)
	Dosage:	6 mg/m^2 i.v. weekly Or 20–60 mg intracavitary Or 1–10 mg/m^2 intrathecal (i.t.)
	Administration:	i.v. bolus + N. saline flush intracavitary, intrathecal
	Toxicity:	Myelosuppression Sterility Amenorrhoea Nausea and vomiting Local pain
	Monitoring tests:	Full blood count
	Metabolism and excretion:	85% is excreted in the urine
	Storage:	Powder – 15-mg vials, refrigerated Solution – refrigerated stable for days
	Interaction:	Neuromuscular blockers
6.1.9	Generic name:	Treosulfan (L-threitol 1,4-dimethane sulfonate)
	Dosage:	1 g daily in divided doses continuously for 1 month and then alternate months if used as a single agent

Administration:	Oral 250-mg capsules
Toxicity:	Myelosuppression (nadir 2–3 weeks, of each course) Nausea and vomiting Abdominal pain Skin rash Alopecia Stomatitis (especially if capsule chewed)
Monitoring tests:	Full blood count
Storage:	Room temperature

6.2 Antimitotics

6.2.1	Generic name:	Etoposide (VP-16-213, Vepesid)
	Dosage:	i.v. 200 mg/m^2 weekly Or 60–100 mg/m^2 daily × 5 – every 3–4 weeks Oral twice i.v. dosage
	Administration:	i.v. infusion in 250–500 ml N.saline (NOT 5% dextrose) over 30–45 min Oral 100-mg capsules
	Precaution:	Avoid extravasation Avoid rapid infusion Do not dilute in 5% dextrose
	Toxicity:	Myelosuppression (nadir at 2 weeks, recovery by 3 weeks) Alopecia Nausea and vomiting (oral capsules + + +) Hypotension (occurs only with rapid infusion)
	Monitoring tests:	Full blood count
	Metabolism and excretion:	Mainly excreted in urine, partly in bile
	Storage:	Intact vials: room temperature. Avoid light, 3 years Capsules: room temperature, 2 years

6.2.2	Generic name:	Teniposide (VM-26)
	Dosage:	100–130 mg/m^2 weekly Or 30–60 mg/m^2 daily × 5 every 3–4 weeks
	Administration:	i.v. infusion in 250–500 ml N. saline (NOT 5% dextrose) over 30–40 min
	Precaution:	Avoid extravasation Avoid rapid infusion Do not dilute in 5% dextrose
	Toxicity:	Myelosuppression (nadir 3–10 days, recovery 7–14 days) Nausea and vomiting Alopecia Hypotension (occurs only with rapid infusion)
	Metabolism and excretion:	Mainly excreted in urine
	Storage:	Intact vials – room temperature, 4 years Solution – 6 h at room temperature in N. saline
6.2.3	Generic name:	Vinblastine (Velbe)
	Dosage:	6–10 mg/m^2 (every 2–3 weeks)
	Administration:	i.v. bolus in 10–20 ml N. saline + flush with N. saline
	Precaution:	Avoid extravasation
	Toxicity:	Myelosuppression (moderate to severe, nadir at 1 week, recovery 2–3 weeks) Tissue necrosis Neuropathy Phlebitis Constipation Alopecia SIADH (inappropriate ADH secretion) Muscle pain (especially jaw pain) Nausea and vomiting Mucositis
	Monitoring tests:	Full blood count
	Metabolism and excretion:	Liver and kidney
	Storage:	Dry – refrigerated, away from light

		Solution - refrigerated away from light 4 weeks
6.2.4	Generic name:	Vincristine (Oncovin)
	Dosage:	Adults 0.4-1.4 mg/m^2 (maximum 2 mg or 1.5 mg age > 65 yrs) Children up to 2 mg/m^2
	Administration:	i.v. bolus in 10-20 m N. saline + flush with N. saline
	Precaution:	Avoid extravasation
	Toxicity:	Neuropathy + + + + (may be dose-limiting) Tissue necrosis Alopecia Constipation (can be severe) Phlebitis Muscle pain (especially jaw pain) SIADH Nausea and vomiting Myelosuppression Mucositis Seizures Full blood count
	Metabolism and excretion:	Liver and kidney
	Storage:	Dry - refrigerated, away from light, 6 months Solution - refrigerated, away from light, 2 weeks
	Interaction:	Isoniazid, pyridoxine
6.2.5	Generic name:	Vindesine (Eldesine)
	Dosage:	Adults 3-4 mg/m^2 weekly Children 4-5 mg/m^2 weekly
	Administration:	i.v. bolus in 10-20 ml N. saline + flush with N-saline
	Precaution:	Avoid extravasation
	Toxicity:	Myelosuppression (moderate to severe, nadir at day 3-5, recovery by day 6-8) Tissue necrosis Neuropathy Alopecia

	Phlebitis Constipation Nausea and vomiting
Monitoring tests:	Full blood count
Metabolism and excretion:	Liver and kidney
Storage:	Dry - refrigerated, 1-2 years Solution - refrigerated, 2 weeks

6.3 Antimetabolites

6.3.1

Generic name:	5-Azacytidine (NSC - 102816)
Dosage:	100-200 mg/m^2 biweekly i.v. 150-400 mg/m^2 $\times 5$ every 21 days or preferably as a continuous infusion
Administration:	i.v. bolus + N.saline flush Continuous i.v. infusion in lactated Ringer's solution Subcutaneously
Toxicity:	Myelosuppression Nausea and vomiting (less with infusions) Diarrhoea Hepatotoxicity (coma +) consider omitting or reducing dose if severe impairment of liver function Neuromuscular Fever Hypotension Skin rash Rhabdomyolysis Hypophosphataemia
Monitoring tests:	Full blood count and liver function tests
Storage:	Undiluted drug is stable for 2 years if refrigerated. Supplied in 100-mg vials. Reconstitute with 19.9 ml of saline for injection (DO NOT use 5% dextrose in water). Stable for 30 min. If an infusion is to be used, reconstitute in lactated Ringer's solution where it is stable for 4 h.

	Interaction:	Pyrazofurin
6.3.2	Generic name:	Cytosine Arabinoside (Cytosar, ara-C, cytarabine)
	Dosage:	30–200 mg/m^2 i.v. or i.m. or s.c. daily for 1–7 days every 2–4 weeks 50 mg/m^2 i.t. once or twice a week
	Administration:	i.v. bolus + N. saline flush i.m. s.c. – 0.5 ml of diluent i.t.
	Precaution:	Reduce dose if severe liver dysfunction
	Toxicity:	Myelosuppression (nadir at 5–12 days, recovery 14–16 days) Nausea and vomiting Mucositis Diarrhoea Facial flushing Abdominal pain
	Monitoring tests:	Full blood count
	Metabolism and excretion:	Metabolized in the liver to uracil arabinoside 90% excreted in the urine as this inactive metabolite
	Storage:	Powder – 100-mg vials, refrigerated Solution – refrigerated, 48 h
6.3.3	Generic name:	5-Fluorouracil (5-FU)
	Dosage:	500–1000 mg/m^2 i.v. or orally weekly
	Administration:	i.v. bolus + N. saline flush Topical use as an ointment
	Toxicity:	Myelosuppression Pigmentation Nausea and vomiting Phlebitis Mucositis Diarrhoea Alopecia Skin rash Cerebellar ataxia Malabsorption Ocular
	Monitoring tests:	Full blood count

	Metabolism and excretion:	Enterohepatic circulation. Only 15% excreted by the kidney
	Storage:	Stable at room temperature. May precipitate if refrigerated Supplied in 250-mg vials (5 ml) and as an ointment
	Interaction:	Methotrexate
6.3.4	Generic name:	6-Mercaptourine (6-MP, Purinethol)
	Dosage:	50–75 mg/m² daily continuous treatment
	Administration:	Oral 2-mg tablet
	Precaution:	Allopurinol blocks metabolism. Reduce dose by at least 50% if given concurrently with allopurinol
	Toxicity:	Myelosuppression Nausea and vomiting Liver dysfunction Mucositis Skin rash Alopecia
	Monitoring tests:	Full blood count, liver function tests, check if patient is taking allopurinol
	Metabolism and excretion:	Oxidation liver to inactive form. 50% excreted in the urine in 24 h (consider dose reduction for renal impairment)
	Storage:	Tablets stable at room temperature
	Interaction:	Allopurinol
6.3.5	Generic name:	Methotrexate (amethopterin)
	Dosage:	Oral 25–50 mg/m² twice weekly i. v. 25–50 mg/m² twice weekly High dose i. v. with folinic acid rescue > 200 mg/m² every 1–3 weeks i. t. 5–12 mg once or twice weekly
	Precautions:	Modify dose if renal impairment Folinic acid rescue must be given if dose > 200 mg/m² May accumulate in effusions and cause prolonged toxicity. Drainage essential before giving high dose
	Administration:	Oral 2.5-mg, 10-mg tablets

		i. v. bolus + N. saline flush or infusion i. t. Intracavitary
	Toxicity:	Myelosuppression (nadir 7–10 days, recovery 14–16 days) Mucositis Nausea and vomiting (high dose) Diarrhoea Skin rash Cerebral atrophy Renal dysfunction (high dose) Alopecia Pneumonitis Malabsorption Ocular Liver dysfunction Osteoporosis
	Monitoring tests:	Full blood count, liver function tests, renal function. Methotrexate levels if using high dose
	Metabolism and excretion:	75% excreted unchanged in urine in first 5 h Consider dose reduction if renal impairment and only use high dose if renal function normal
	Storage:	Tablets: room temperature Powder: 500-mg vials - room temperature Solution: 5-mg, 50-mg, vials - room temperature, opened vials and reconstituted solution refrigerated 24 h
	Interaction:	5-Fluorouracil, alcohol, aspirin, cephalothin, corticosteroids, hypoglycaemic agents, probenecid, sulphonamides
6.3.6	Generic name:	Thioguanine (6-TG, 6-thioguanine)
	Dosage:	100 mg/m^2 orally twice daily 100–300 mg/m^2 i. v. infusion
	Administration:	Oral 40-mg tablets i. v. bolus in 50–150 ml N. saline + N. saline flush

Precaution:	Reduce dose if abnormal liver or renal function
Toxicity:	Myelosuppression (nadir 10-12 days, recovery 16-18 days) Diarrhoea Nausea and vomiting Liver toxicity (consider dose reduction if liver function abnormal) Renal toxicity (consider dose reduction if abnormal renal function)
Monitoring tests:	Full blood count and liver and renal function tests
Metabolims and excretion:	Rapidly enters purine pathways. Metabolites excreted primarily via the kidney
Storage:	Tablets - room temperature Powder - intact vial refrigerated, 4 years Solution - refrigerated, 24 h
Interaction:	Does NOT interact with allopurinol

6.4 Antibiotics

6.4.1

Generic name:	Actinomycin D (dactinomycin, Cosmegen, Lyovac)
Dosage:	0.015 mg/kg/day for 3-5 days (every 3-4 weeks). Usual maximum daily dose 0.6 $mg/m^2/day$
Administration:	i.v. bolus into fast-running N. saline infusion
Precaution:	Avoid extravasation
Toxicity:	Tissue necrosis Phlebitis Nausea and vomiting Myelosuppression (nadir at 10-14 days; recovery 16-20 days) Mucositis Alopecia Radiation recall
Monitoring tests:	Full blood count and liver function tests
Metabolism and excretion:	50%-90% excreted in the bile, 10%-20% in the urine (consider dose reduction for liver function impairment)

	Storage:	Powder – 500-μg vials, refrigerated, away from light Solution – refrigerated, 24 h
6.4.2	Generic name:	Adriamycin (doxorubicin, 14-hydroxy-daunomycin)
	Dosage:	1–2 mg/kg or 40–70/mg/m^2, usually given as a single intravenous injection once every 3 weeks. Total dose should not exceed 450 mg/m^2
	Administration:	i.v. bolus into fast-running N. saline infusion
	Precaution:	Avoid extravasation Avoid skin contact (wear gloves and goggles when preparing and injecting) Dose reduction if abnormal liver function (see below)
	Toxicity:	Tissue necrosis Phlebitis Complete alopecia Nausea and vomiting Myelosuppression (nadir at 9–14 days, recovery 16–20 days) Mucositis Pigmentation Urine appears red for up to 24 h after injection Nail changes Pyrexia/rigors Cardiomyopathy – increasing incidence at total doses of greater than 450 mg/m^2 Ocular Radiation recall Encephalopathy
	Monitoring test:	Full blood count and liver function tests Check cumulative dose does not exceed 450 mg/m^2
	Metabolism and excretion:	Enterohepatic: consider dose reduction or omission if liver function tests abnormal (bilirubin 20–50 μmol/l 50% reduction, 50 μmol/l 75% reduction)

	Storage:	Powder - 10-mg, 50-mg vials refrigerated Solution - refrigerated, away from light, 48 h
	Interaction:	Actinomycin, azathioprine, 6-mercaptopurine, mithramycin, barbiturates, hypoglycaemic agents
6.4.3	Generic name:	Bleomycin (Blenoxane)
	Dosage:	15 mg/m^2 i. m. once a week Or 15-30 mg/m^2 i. v. infusion daily for 5 days Or 1 mg/day s. c. continuous Total dose should not exceed 250 mg
	Administration:	i. v. bolus in 5-10 ml water or N. saline i. m. (dissolved in 0.5-1 ml of 1% lignocaine)
	Precaution:	Check total dose is less than 250 mg Avoid high-concentration oxygen administration
	Toxicity:	Erythema and pigmentation of skin Pyrexia/rigors (starts 3-6 h; may be prevented with antihistamines or corticosteroids) Hyperkeratosis Pneumonitis and pulmonary fibrosis (dose-limiting exacerbated by oxygen administration) Nail changes Alopecia Radiation recall Phlebitis Mucositis Nausea and Vomiting
	Monitoring tests:	Clinical examination of the respiratory system and chest x-ray. If lung function tests are used, carbon monoxide transfer is the most sensitive indicator of pulmonary toxicity
	Metabolism and excretion:	Renal excretion

	Storage:	Powder - 3-mg, 15-mg ampoules, room temperature Solution - stable 1 month refrigerated
6.4.4	Generic name:	Daunorubicin (rubidomycin, daunomycin, Cerubidin)
	Dosage:	1-3 mg/kg or 50-100 mg/m^2 given as a single injection once every 3 weeks Total dose should not exceed 600 mg/m^2
	Administration:	i.v. bolus into fast-running N. saline infusion
	Precaution:	Avoid extravasation Avoid skin contact (wear gloves and gogles when preparing and injecting) Reduce dose if abnormal liver function (see below)
	Toxicity:	Alopecia Tissue necrosis Phlebitis Nausea and vomiting Myelosuppression (nadir at 9-14 days, recovery 16-21 days) Red urine for up to 24 h after administration Mucositis Cardiomyopathy - increasing risk after total dose of 450-550 mg/m^2
	Monitoring tests:	Full blood count and liver function tests. Check total dose
	Metabolism and excretion:	Enterohepatic. If bilirubin 20-50 μmol/l, 50% dose reduction; >50 μmol/l, 75% dose reduction
	Storage:	Powder - 20-mg vials, refrigerated, away from light Solution - refrigerated, 24 h
	Interaction:	Azathioprine, 6-mercaptopurine, mithramycin, barbiturates
6.4.5	Generic name:	Mithramycin (Mithracin)
	Dosage:	1.0-1.5 mg/m^2/day for 5-10 days. May be repeated 3-4 days later, if necessary

		Hypercalcaemia; 25 μg/kg every 10–14 days
	Administration:	i.v. infusion over 20–30 min
	Toxicity:	Nausea and vomiting Hypocalcaemia Phlebitis Pyrexia Coagulopathy Myelosuppression Drowsiness Hepatic
	Monitoring tests:	Full blood count, calcium, coagulation screen if indicated
	Metabolism and excretion:	40% excreted in the urine within 15 h Consider dose reduction if renal function impaired
	Storage:	Powder – 2.5-mg vials – refrigerated Solution – only stable for a few minutes
	Interaction:	Actinomycin, Adriamycin
6.4.6	Generic name:	Mitomycin C (Mutamycin)
	Dosage:	20–25 mg/m^2 i.v. every 3–6 weeks
	Administration:	i.v. bolus + N. saline flush
	Precaution:	May cause severe phlebitis and pain at the site of injection Prolonged myelosuppression
	Toxicity:	Myelosuppression (nadir at 3–4 weeks, recovery by 6–8 weeks) Phlebitis and pain Nausea and vomiting Anorexia Mucositis Diarrhoea Alopecia
	Monitoring tests:	Full blood count and renal function
	Metabolism and excretion:	Metabolized primarily in the liver About 10% excreted unchanged in the urine
	Storage:	Powder – 5-mg vials – room temperature Solution – only stable for a few minutes

6.5 Nitrosoureas

6.5.1	Generic name:	Carmustine (BCNU)
	Dosage:	Up to 200 mg/m^2 i. v. every 6-8 weeks
	Administration:	i.v. infusion over 15-45 min in 100-250 ml 5% dextrose Flush with N. saline
	Precaution:	Follow carefully the manufacturer's instructions for making solutions. Dissolve the powder in each vial in 3 ml of absolute alcohol followed by 27 ml sterile water. Discard any vials with oily deposit indicating overheating and decomposition
	Toxicity:	Tissue necrosis Nausea and vomiting (severe lasts 6-8 h) Phlebitis + + + (pain at injection site and up the vein - try infusion 5 ml 0.5% lignocaine) Myelosuppression (moderate to severe - nadir at 3-4 weeks, recovery by 5-7 weeks) Facial flushing (lasts up to 2 h) Hepatic (transient elevation of enzymes)
	Monitoring tests:	Full blood count
	Storage:	Dry - refrigerated up to 2 years. Never store at > 27 °C Solution - use as soon as possible, do not store
	Metabolism and excretion:	Rapid biotransformation - slow urinary excretion of metabolites. Crosses to CSF
	Interaction:	Cimetidine
6.5.2	Generic name:	Lomustine (CCNU)
	Dosage:	100-130 mg/m^2 every 6 weeks
	Administration:	Oral 100-mg, 50-mg, 10-mg capsules
	Precaution:	Avoid giving more often than 6-weekly because of prolonged myelosuppression
	Toxicity:	Myelosuppression (moderate to severe,

		nadir at 3–5 weeks, recovery by 6–10 weeks)
		Nausea and vomiting (can be severe, lasts 2–6 h)
		Alopecia
		Mucositis
		Pulmonary fibrosis
	Monitoring tests:	Full blood count
	Metabolism and excretion:	Liver metabolism and renal clearance Fat-soluble, crosses to CSF
	Storage:	Room temperature, 2 years
	Interaction:	
6.5.3	Generic name:	Streptozotocin (streptozocin)
	Dosage:	1.0–1.5 g/m^2 weekly × 4 – repeat at 8 weeks
		Or 0.5–1.0 g/m^2 daily × 5 – repeat every 4–6 weeks
	Administration:	i.v. infusion in 100–200 mg 5% dextrose over 10–15 min
		i.v. infusion in 500 ml 5% dextrose over 6 h
		i.v. bolus
	Precaution:	Avoid extravasation
		Acute hypoglycaemia can be induced by release of insulin from damaged islet cells, especially in treatment of insulinoma
		Ensure adequate hydration
	Toxicity:	Tissue necrosis
		Nausea and vomiting
		Renal failure (may be a transient rise in blood urea, or tubule damage and Fanconi's syndrome)
		Phlebitis (pain at injection site with too rapid infusion)
		Myelosuppression (mainly anaemia)
		Hypoglycaemia (see above)
		Hyperglycaemia (may occur after long-term use)
	Monitoring tests:	Full blood count urea and electrolytes, blood and urine glucose

Metabolism and excretion:	Liver metabolism and renal clearance
Storage:	Refrigerated 3 years
Interaction:	Phenytoin

6.6 Miscellaneous

6.6.1

Generic name:	Asparaginase (colaspase, Crasnitin)
Dosage:	Variable, e.g. - 20000 U/m^2 i.v. weekly 4000 U/m^2 i.v. daily × 14
Administration:	i.v. infusion over > 30 min i.m. injection in < 2 ml N. saline
Precaution:	To prevent acute anaphylactic reactions skin test with 0.1 ml solution (20 IU) before each course Observe for at least 1 h after injection
Toxicity:	Pyrexia and rigors Hypersensitivity (usually mild and controlled by antihistamines) Hepatic (usually transient elevation of enzymes) Encephalopathy (occasionally coma) Hyperglycaemia Nausea and vomiting Renal dysfunction Myelosuppression
Monitoring tests:	Full blood count, liver function tests
Metabolism and excretion:	
Storage:	Dry - refrigerated - 4 years. Room temperature - 2 years Solution - refrigerated - 3 weeks
Interaction:	Vincristine, hypoglycaemic agents, prednisone

6.6.2

Generic name:	Cisplatin (Cis-platinum, Cis-DDP, Neoplatin)
Dosage:	50-120 mg/m^2 i.v. every 3-4 weeks Or 15-20 mg/m^2 daily × 5
Administration:	i.v. infusion in 1-2 l N. saline or 5% dextrose, at a rate of 1 mg/min
Precaution:	Check renal function (serum creatinine,

		or creatinine clearance) before each course Establish diuresis of >150 ml/h before administration, and maintain for 6 h after - keep up i.v. fluids until oral fluids tolerated Use mannitol (NOT loop diuretics) to enhance diuresis
	Toxicity:	Nausea and vomiting (severe lasts 12-24 h) Ototoxicity Myelosuppression (nadir at 3 weeks, recovery by 4 weeks) Renal failure (check renal function, ensure diuresis) Diarrhoea Hypomagnesaemia (very common biochemically, rarely symptomatic) Hypocalcaemia (rarely symptomatic) Neuropathy Fits
	Monitoring tests:	Full blood count, urea and electrolytes, creatinine clearance, audiometry
	Metabolism and excretion:	Excretion mainly renal (reduce dose or omit if renal function impaired)
	Storage:	Dry - refrigerated, away from light, 2 years Solution - room temperature 24 h
	Interaction:	Cephalothin, loop diuretics, gentamicin
6.6.3	Generic name:	Dacarbazine (DTIC, imidazole carboxamide)
	Dosage:	2-4.5 mg/kg daily × 10 } every 3-4 weeks Or 250 mg/m^2 daily × 5 } every 3-4 weeks Or 850 mg/m^2 } every 3-4 weeks
	Administration:	i.v. bolus in 10 ml N. saline over 1 min with N. saline flush i.v. infusion in 100-200 ml 5% dextrose or N. saline over 15-30 min with flush
	Precaution:	Avoid exposure to light Avoid extravasation

	Toxicity:	Myelosuppression (nadir at 3-4 weeks) Nausea and vomiting (severe, 1-12 h) Phlebitis Pyrexia/rigors (especially after large single dose, starts c.day 7, lasts 7-21 days) Tissue necrosis
	Monitoring tests:	Full blood count
	Metabolism and excretion:	Mainly hepatic
	Storage:	Dry - refrigerated, away from light, 4 months Solution - 200-500 ml N.saline or 5% dextrose, avoid exposure to light, use as soon as possible
6.6.4	Generic name:	Hydroxyurea (Hydrea)
	Dosage:	20-30 mg/kg continuously according to blood count or 80 mg/kg every 3rd day
	Administration:	Oral 500-mg capsules
	Precaution:	Hygroscopic, keep bottles tightly closed
	Toxicity:	Myelosuppression (nadir at 10 days) Nausea and vomiting (usually mild) Mucositis Pigmentation Nail changes
	Monitoring tests:	Full blood count
	Metabolism and excretion:	Mainly renal
	Storage:	Room temperature. Tightly closed bottles with dessiccant
	Interaction:	Alcohol, anti-emetics, barbiturates, CNS depressants, narcotic analgesics
6.6.5	Generic name:	Mitotane (o,p-DDD)
	Dosage:	1.0-2.5 g four times daily continuously
	Administration:	Oral 500-mg tablets
	Precaution:	Steroid replacement if total dose more than 3 g/day Discontinue in the event of intercurrent infection, trauma, etc.
	Toxicity:	Nausea and vomiting

		Adrenal insufficiency (ensure adequate replacement) Sedation
	Monitoring tests:	Urea and electrolytes, lying and standing blood pressure
	Metabolism and excretion:	Excreted in the urine as metabolites. Urinary metabolites detectable for many months
	Storage:	Room temperature
6.6.6	Generic name:	Procarbazine (Natulan)
	Dosage:	In combinations 100 mg/m^2 daily for 14 days every 4 weeks
	Administration:	Oral 50-mg capsules
	Precaution:	Avoid tyramine-containing foods because of weak monoamine oxidase (MAO) inhibition
	Toxicity:	Myelosuppression (mild to moderate, nadir at 4 weeks, recovery by 6 weeks) Nausea and vomiting (initially but less as therapy continues) Neuropathy Rash Mucositis Pulmonary fibrosis Encephelopathy
	Monitoring tests:	Full blood count
	Metabolism and excretion:	Liver and renal clearance
	Storage:	Room temperature
	Interaction:	Tyramine-containing foods, anti-histamines, alcohol, hypoglycaemic agents
6.6.7	Generic name:	Razoxane (Razoxin, ICRF 159)
	Dosage:	Variable, e. g. 150–500 mg/m^2 daily × 3–5 every 4 weeks Or 125 mg b.i.d. 3–5 days weekly Or 750 mg weekly
	Administration:	Oral 125-mg tablets
	Precaution:	Nil specific
	Toxicity:	Myelosuppression (nadir at 2 weeks, recovery by 3 weeks)

	Alopecia Nausea and vomiting Diarrhoea Mucositis Acneiform rash
Monitoring tests:	Full blood count
Metabolism and excretion:	Liver and renal clearance
Storage:	Room temperature, 2 years

6.7 Hormonal Agents

6.7.1	Generic name:	Aminoglutethimide (Orimeten)
	Dosage:	250 mg three or four times a day continous together with dexamethasone 2 mg three times a day or hydrocortisone 20 mg b.i.d.
	Administration:	Oral 250-mg tablets
	Precaution:	Simultaneous glucocorticoid administration essential Discontinue in the event of intercurrent infection, trauma etc. Increase dose slowly over 3-4 weeks when starting treatment, especially in elderly
	Toxicity:	Sedation (can be severe especially in elderly - introduce drug slowly) Rash (mild, usually transient even if drug continued) Adrenal insufficiency (ensure adequate glucocorticoid replacement - add fludrocortisone 0.1 mg alternate days if necessary)
	Monitoring tests:	Urea and electrolytes, blood pressure lying and standing
	Storage:	Room temperature
6.7.2	Generic name:	Androgens
	Drugs, dosage and administration:	Testosterone (Sustanon '250', 30-mg, 100-mg ampoules) 50-100 mg, three times per week i.m.

		Nandrolone phenylpropionate (Durabolin 25-mg ampoules, 25-mg, 50-mg syringes) 25–50 mg/week i.m. Nandrolone decanoate (Decadurabolin 25-mg, 50-mg syringes, 25-mg, 50-mg, 100-mg ampoules) 25–50 mg every 3 weeks i.m. Oxymethalone (Anapolon, 50-mg tablets) 50–100 mg/day oral Orostanolone (Masteril, 100-mg ampoules) 300 mg/week i.m. Fluoxymestrone (Ultrandren, 5-mg tablets) 30 mg/day oral
	Precautions:	Ensure i.m. injections not given i.v. or subcutaneously Contraindicated in severe renal failure or heart failure
	Toxicity:	Virilization Nausea and vomiting Oedema (mild) Intrahepatic cholestatic jaundice (testosterone and methyl derivatives only)
	Storage:	See manufacturer's literature for individual drugs
6.7.3	Generic name:	Oestrogens
	Drugs, dosage and administration:	Stilboestrol (0.1-mg, 0.5-mg, 1-mg, 25-mg, 100-mg tab lets) Breast carcinoma 10–20 mg/day oral Prostatic carcinoma 1–3 mg/day oral Ethinyloestradiol (Lynoral, 0.05-mg, 0.1-mg, 1-mg tablets) 1–3 mg/day oral Polyoestradiol phosphate (Estradurin, 40-mg vials) Prostatic carcinoma 40–80 mg/2–4 weeks i.m.

	Precautions:	Use with care in patients with heart failure
	Metabolism:	Liver
	Toxicity:	Feminization (e.g. gynaecomastia) Fluid retention Hypertension Nausea and vomiting Thrombosis
	Storage:	See manufacturer's literature for individual drugs
6.7.4	Generic name:	Progestogens
	Drugs, dosage and administration:	Medroxyprogesterone acetate (Provera - 100-mg tablets) 200-400 mg/day oral Gestronol hexanoate (Depostat, 400-mg ampoules) 200-400 mg/week i.m. Hydroxyprogesterone hexanoate (Proluton Depot, 250-mg and 500-mg syringes) 1 g/week i.m. Megestrol acetate (Megace - 40-mg tablets) 80-320 mg/day oral
	Precautions:	Ensure i.m. injections not given i.v. or subcutaneously Reduce dose if liver disease
	Toxicity:	Fluid retention
	Metabolism:	Liver
	Storage:	See manufacturer's literature for individual drugs
6.7.5	Generic name:	Tamoxifen (Nolvadex)
	Dosage:	10 mg b.i.d. continuously
	Administration:	Oral 10-mg tablets
	Precautions:	Avoid during pregnancy
	Toxicity:	Menopausal symptoms Nausea and vomiting Thrombocytopenia (transient)
	Metabolism and excretion:	Probable enterohepatic circulation of metabolites
	Storage:	Room temperature, avoid light

6.7.6	Generic name:	Antiandrogens
	Drugs, dosage and administration:	Cyproterone acetate (Androcur - 50-mg tablets) 100–200 mg/day oral
	Precautions:	Reduce dose if liver disease
	Toxicity:	Occasional gynaecomastia
	Storage:	Room temperature
6.7.7	Generic name:	Gonadotrophin-Releasing Hormone Analogues
	Drugs, dosage and administration:	Buserelin (Suprefact 5.5 mg vial and 0.1 mg each nasal spray) 0.5 mg subcutaneously three times a day for 7 days, then 0.4 mg intra-nasally three times a day Leuprolide (Lupron 14-mg vials) 1 mg/day subcutaneously
	Precautions:	Close observation of patients with vertebral metastases and/or urinary tract obstruction during the first weeks of treatment
	Toxicity:	Occasional worsening of symptoms during the first weeks of treatment due to transient testosterone level increase; hot flushes; occasional dizziness and nausea/vomiting
	Storage:	See manufacturer's literature for individual drugs

7 Planning of Chemotherapy, Monitoring of Effects and Side Effects, Drug-Dose Modifications

7.1 Factors to Be Considered in the Planning of Chemotherapy

1. Factors related to the cytotoxic drug regimen:
   Choice of drug
   Dose
   Route
   Schedule
   Single or combination
   Sequence
   Potential toxicities
   Potential interaction with other drugs
2. Factors related to the patient:
   Age, sex
   Socio-economic status
   Nutritional status
   Performance status
   Bone marrow reserve
   Pulmonary, renal, hepatic and cardiac function
   Associated diseases
   Possible individual drug metabolism
3. Factors related to the tumour:
   Histology, histological subtypes, grading
   Primary or metastatic
   Site of metastases
   Dimension of tumour mass (if possible cell kinetic characteristics)
   Presence of effusion (possible reservoir of drug activity)

7.2 Strategies for Cancer Chemotherapy

Remission induction: Intensive chemotherapy ± surgery or radiotherapy = visible large reduction in tumour burden

Consolidation:	Intensive chemotherapy in the absence of clinically detectable disease = presumed continuing reduction in tumour burden
Maintenance:	Continuous low-dose chemotherapy - much reduced toxicity = presumed control and/or elimination of residual tumour cells
Late intensification:	Further intensive chemotherapy given at a stage determined by observation of the natural history of treated primary disease to anticipate and prevent relapse = assumes residual disease and continuing sensitivity to chemotherapy

These therapeutic approaches are largely theoretical. The roles of maintenance chemotherapy and late intensification are under study in a variety of conditions and their values so far are not clearly proven. In acute lymphoblastic leukaemia (ALL) of childhood, however, maintenance chemotherapy does appear to significantly reduce the risk of relapse. What is so far unclear is the point at which it is safe to discontinue chemotherapy.

7.3 Essential Evaluation Procedures Before Starting Chemotherapy

With few exceptions, the chemotherapy of solid malignant tumours is not a curative treatment. When confronted with a cancer patient, the first question must be: "Is the cancer amenable to surgery, radiotherapy, hormonotherapy?"

1. Before starting treatment, it is necessary to:
   a) Obtain information on the patient's past and present history
   b) Carry out a complete clinical examination and relevant biological and radiological investigations
   c) Obtain a histological diagnosis
   d) Classify according to the staging system (see also Sects. 3.3 and 15.10)
2. When establishing the present history, the following points should be considered:
   a) Initial symptoms with particular attention to weakness, fever, pruritus, night sweats, loss of weight, visceral or bone pain, cough, digestive disorders and any symptoms suggesting sites of local infiltration
   b) Previous treatment (surgery, radiotherapy, chemotherapy) and results

3. The clinical examination should include:
   a) Performance status
   b) Weight and height (to permit calculation of body surface area in square metres)
   c) Complete physical examination with particular attention to the presence of liver enlargement, splenomegaly, abdominal masses, adenopathies, pleural and peritoneal effusion and signs of neurological deficit
   d) Centimetric measurement of tumour masses (see also Sect. 3.16)

   N.B. Disease-orientated check-up of organs and systems to detect possible metastatic involvement is essential.
4. The laboratory investigations should include:
   a) Complete blood count (haemoglobin, granulocytes, platelets)
   b) Bone marrow aspirate – in the case of blood count abnormalities and for staging certain diseases (in certain conditions trephine may be advisable, i.e. nodular lymphomas)
   c) Liver function tests
   d) Serum calcium
   e) Sedimentation rate
   f) Serum creatine – creatinine clearance
   g) Blood uric acid
   h) Further investigations according to requirements
5. The radiological examinations should include:
   a) Chest x-ray
   b) Bone survey (e.g. in myeloma and breast cancer, or where symptoms warrant)
   c) Other examinations according to requirements [e.g. lymphography, brain scan, computerized axial tomography (CAT) scan, etc.]

7.4 Contraindications for Chemotherapy

1. Absolute contraindications:
   a) Terminal disease (patients with very short life expectancy)
   b) Pregnancy (first trimester) unless interrupted
   c) Septicaemia
   d) Coma
2. Relative contraindications:
   a) Infants under 3 months
   b) Old age (in particular elderly patients with slow-growing tumours with low sensitivity to chemotherapy)
   c) Very low performance status (less than 40)

d) Severe organ failure (for certain drugs), e.g. kidney, heart, liver, bone marrow (however, organ failure may be reversed by chemotherapy when due to infiltration by a chemosensitive tumour)
e) Dementia
f) Inability of patient to attend clinic regularly
g) Lack of co-operation on part of patient
h) Tumour resistance to anti cancer chemotherapy
i) Lack of suitable support facilities

7.5 General Classification of Side Effects of Chemotherapy

1. Immediate:
   a) Anaphylactic shock
   b) Cardiac arrhythmia
   c) Pain at the site of injection
2. Early:
   a) Nausea, vomiting
   b) Fever
   c) Hypersensitivity reactions
   d) Flu-like syndrome
   e) Cystitis
3. Intermediate (within days):
   a) Bone-marrow depression
      - after 1–3 weeks (majority of myelodepressive drugs)
      - after 4–6 weeks (nitrosoureas)
   b) Stomatitis
   c) Diarrhoea
   d) Alopecia
   e) Peripheral neuropathy, loss of reflexes
   f) Paralytic ileus
   g) Renal toxicity
   h) Immunosuppression
4. Late (within months):
   a) Skin hyperpigmentation
   b) Inury to vital organs or system (heart-adriamycin; lung-bleomycin and busulfan; liver-methotrexate)
   c) Effects on reproductive capacity (amenorrhoea, decreased sperm concentration)
   d) Endocrinological changes (feminization, virilization, etc.)
   e) Carcinogenic effects

N. B. Absolute rejection in male patients and relative infertility in female patients follows MOPP chemotherapy for Hodgkin's disease. Some degree of recovery of fertility may follow other drug combinations.

7.6 Types of New Malignancies Encountered in Patients on Chemotherapy (Penn, modified)

Leukaemia
Non-Hodgkin lymphomas
Hodgkin's disease
Bladder cancer
Brain tumour
Sarcoma
Others (cervix, prostate, pancreas, colorectal, lung, vulva, floor of mouth, kidney, ovary and stomach carcinoma)

In Hodgkin's disease, the latent period before second malignancy appears to exceed 4 years (acute myelogenous leukaemia) but may extend to 10 years (non-Hodgkin lymphoma). The risk of second malignancy is significantly increased following combined-modality therapy (chemotherapy and radiotherapy). In the single-agent therapy of carcinoma of the ovary with chlorambucil, the risks appear dose-related – none occurring below a total dose of 800 mg.

7.7 Two Patterns of Bone Marrow Recovery, Rapid and Delayed, Following the Administration of Chemotherapeutic Agents (Bergsagel) (Fig. see p. 86)

7.8 Why is an Analysis of Delayed Side Effects Necessary?

1. Recognition of drugs which result in delayed toxicity → Parenchymal damage
2. Prolonged survival after chemotherapy → Increased duration of exposure to treatment with the chemotherapeutic agent
3. Wider use of adjuvant chemotherapy than in the past → Increase in the number of patients with no evidence of disease, who are exposed to chemotherapy

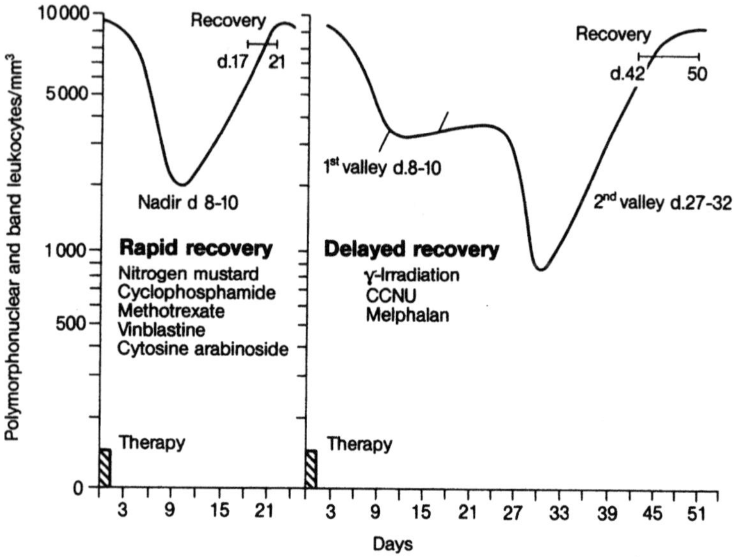

7.9 Side Effects of Conventional Agents That Should Be Monitored[a]

Target organ	Toxicity	Implicated drugs
Bone marrow	Leukopenia Thrombocytopenia	All drugs with the exception of steroids, bleomycin, L-asparaginase
Gastrointestinal tract	Stomatitis	Adriamycin, bleomycin, methotrexate, 5-fluorouracil, actinomycin
	Gastric ulcer	Corticosteroids
	Gastritis	All alkylating agents in higher dosages
	Diarrhoea	Methotrexate, 5-fluorouracil
	Paralytic ileus	Vincristine
Skin	Hyperpigmentation	Bleomycin, busulfan
	Alopecia	Adriamycin, cyclophosphamide, actinomycin D, vinblastine, vincristine
Nervous system	Paraesthesia, peripheral neuropathy	Vincristine, vinblastine, vindesine, *cis*-platinum
	Deafness	*Cis*-platinum
	Lethargy	L-Asparaginase

[a] See also individual drugs in Chap. 6.

Target organ	Toxicity	Implicated drugs
Heart	Cardiac failure (long-term)	Adriamycin, daunomycin, cyclophosphamide
	Hypertension (long-term)	Corticosteroids
Lungs	Fibrosis (long-term)	Bleomycin, busulfan, methotrexate, cyclophosphamide
Pancreas	Pancreatitis	L-Asparaginase
Uterus	Uterine bleeding	Oestrogens
Bladder	Cystitis	Cyclophosphamide, iphosphamide
Liver	Abnormal liver function (fibrosis)	Methotrexate, cytosine arabinoside, L-asparaginase, mithramycin
Kidney	Abnormal kidney function (tubule necrosis)	Methotrexate, *cis*-platinum, mithramycin

7.10 Drugs Used for the Control of Nausea and Vomiting

Corticosteroids (dexamethasone)
Metoclopramide (low dose or high dose)
Benzodiazepines (diazepam, lorazepam) - anticipatory vomiting
Cannabinoids (nabilone)
Phenothiazines (chlorpromazine, prochlorperazine)
Domperidone (dopamine antagonist)

7.11 Toxicity of Combined-Modality Treatments

Toxicity	Implicated treatment combinations
Bone marrow failure	Simultaneous use of myelosuppressive agents and irradiation which affects active marrow
Interstitial pneumonitis pulmonary fibrosis	High-dose cyclophosphamide, bleomycin (dose-related), bleomycin + cyclophosphamide, bleomycin + radiotherapy, cyclophosphamide + total-body irradiation, actinomycin D + vincristine + radiotherapy
Cardiotoxicity	MOPP + mantle radiotherapy, Adriamycin + radiotherapy to mediastinum
Oesophagitis	Razoxane (ICRF 159) + split radiotherapy (bronchial carcinoma)
Hepatitis	Actinomycin D + abdominal irradiation (childhood tumours)

Toxicity	Implicated treatment combinations
Neuropathy	Vincristine + procarbazine
Skin	Radiation + 5-fluorouracil or actinomycin D
Gut (paralytic ileus)	5-Fluorouracil together with or following abdominal irradiation, vincristine following abdominal radiation: increased incidence of paralytic ileus
Nephrotoxicity	*Cis*-platinum + abdominal irradiation

7.12 Dose Modifications

Standard doses may have to be reduced from the start or during the course of chemotherapy owing to decreased bone marrow reserve, impaired organ function or other toxicities. Under certain circumstances, doses may also be increased.

7.12.1 Circumstances Prohibiting Use of Certain Drugs or Necessitating 25%-30% Reduction in Initial Dose

Certain drugs should not be used at all or only at reduced dose levels under certain circumstances:

1. Extensive bone metastases or diffuse bone marrow infiltration: all myelotoxic agents
2. Previous heavy radio- or chemotherapy: all myelotoxic agents
3. Severe malnutrition: all antitumour agents
4. Impaired kidney function: methotrexate, *cis*-platinum
5. Impaired liver function: Adriamycin, methotrexate, actinomycin D, nitrosoureas
6. Impaired cardiac function (especially arrhythmia): Adriamycin, daunomycin

7.12.2 Suggested Dose Reduction Schedules During Chemotherapy of Solid Tumours

Grade	WBC/mm^3	Platelets	Next dose
0	4000	100000	100%
I	2500-4000	50000-100000	50%
II	<2500	<50000	0% (wait until bone marrow recovers)

7.12.3 Suggested Upward Dose Modifications in Chemotherapy of Solid Tumours

If, after two in three courses of chemotherapy with regular weekly blood counts, no haematological or other toxicity is observed, the dose of each drug *may* be increased by 20%-25%.

Further Reading

1. Abeloff MD (1979) Complications of Cancer. Diagnosis and Measurement. John Hopkins, Baltimore
2. Carter SK, Bakowski MT, Hellman K (1977) Chemotherapy of Cancer. John Wiley, London
3. Green JA, Macbeth FRM, Williams CJ, Whitehouse JMA (1983) Medical Oncology Pocket Consultant. Grant McIntyre, London
4. Mathé G, Oldham KK (1974) Complications of Cancer Chemotherapy. Springer-Verlag, Berlin

8 Hormone Treatment of Tumours

8.1 Hormone-Dependent Tumours

The administration of hormones or the suppression or antagonism of endogenous hormones may significantly inhibit the growth of certain malignant neoplasms (e.g. prostate, male and female breast and endometrium). Growth of tumours of the ovary, kidney and thyroid appear to be to some degree subject to hormonal influences; leukaemia and malignant lymphomas may also be influenced by corticosteroids.

Disease	Possible forms of additive, suppressive or antagonistic endocrine therapy
Breast cancer	*Additive* - oestrogens, androgens, progestational agents, corticosteroids *Suppressive* - oophorectomy, adrenalectomy, hypophysectomy, aminoglutethemide *Antagonistic* - antioestrogens
Prostatic cancer	*Additive* - oestrogens, corticosteroids, progestational agents *Suppressive* - orchidectomy, antiandrogens
Uterine adenocarcinoma	Progestational agents
Thyroid cancer	Thyroid hormones, hypophysectomy
Ovarian cancer	Progestational agents? oestrogens? testosterone?
Hypernephroma	Androgens? oestrogens? antioestrogens? progestins?
Chronic and acute lymphocytic leukaemia	Corticosteroids
Malignant lymphomas (especially non-Hodgkin lymphomas)	Corticosteroids

8.2 Hormone Receptors

Oestrogen and other hormone receptors consist of cytoplasmic and nuclear protein, which has great affinity for and binds specifically to the hormone. Oestrogen receptors are present only in tissues capable of responding to oestrogen. Some 60%–70% of all biopsies of breast cancer tissues demonstrate oestrogen receptors (= ER+).

Many aspects of oestrogen and other hormone receptor determinations and their correlation with the course of breast cancer and with responsiveness or unresponsiveness to hormonal and cytostatic therapy are still under study and partially controversial. However, the following statements can be made:

1. Most investigators class as ER+ tumours containing more than 10 fmol/mg cytosol protein.
2. Some 50%–60% of ER+ tumours respond to hormonal manipulation; ER− tumours respond to endocrine treatment in less than 10% of cases.
3. The response rate to hormonal therapies depends on the ER content, i.e. directly proportionate to the logarithmic increase in ER content.
4. ER positivity combined with positive progesterone receptors (PgR+) predicts a higher response rate to hormonal treatment than ER+ alone.
5. Data on the ability of ER to predict also the natural course and the aggressiveness of the disease are still controversial. Recent studies, however, indicate that ER positivity, at least during the first 3 years from surgery, is correlated with a higher relapse-free survival in comparison with ER negativity. However, it does not seem to predict the outcome of adjuvant chemotherapy (CMF) in patients with node-positive breast cancer. Data on the ability of ER to predict the response to cytotoxic agents in advanced breast cancer are still conflicting.
6. A new, simpler method to determine hormone receptors, using monoclonal antireceptor antibodies, is presently developing and will probably in the near future serve as the basis for a simple immunochemical and immunohistochemical assay.

8.3 Hormonal Compounds and Their Toxicity

1. Androgen Side Effects:
   Fluid retention
   Hirsutism
   Acne
   Hoarseness
   Clitoral hypertrophy
   Increased libido
   Possible cholestatic icterus
2. Oestrogen side effects:
   Nausea and vomiting

Fluid retention
Increased incidence of cardiovascular accidents
Nipple hyperpigmentation
Uterine bleeding
Signs of feminization in male patients: gynaecomastia, testicular atrophy, impotence

3. Progestin side effects:
Progesterone therapy is relatively free from side effects. High doses of medroxy-progesterone acetate may produce fluid retention, weight increase, Cushing's syndrome with hypertension and thrombophlebitis
4. Antioestrogen side effects:
These compounds are relatively free from side effects; however, they may occasionally produce:
Nausea
Vomiting
Hot flushes
Uterine bleeding
Fluid retention
5. Antiandrogen side effects:
Mammillary pain
Production of colostrum
6. Thyroid hormone side effects:
Clinical signs of hyperthyroidism:
Tachycardia
Fine tremor
Nervousness, emotional lability
Excessive sweating, heat intolerance
Increased basal metabolic rate

8.4 Uses of Corticosteroids in Medical Oncology

8.4.1 Antitumour Activity of Corticosteroids

Malignant disease	Use of corticosteroids
Acute leukaemia	Acute lymphoblastic leukaemia, particularly in children, is responsive to corticosteroids
Chronic lymphocytic leukaemia	Corticosteroids may successfully control chronic lymphocytic leukaemia
Multiple myeloma	Corticosteroids are an integral part of combination chemotherapy for multiple myeloma

Malignant disease	Use of corticosteroids
Malignant lymphomas	Corticosteroids are an essential part of multiagent chemotherapy for malignant lymphomas
Breast cancer	Corticosteroids may form part of combination chemotherapy for breast cancer: improved haematological tolerance

8.4.2 Major Indications for Corticosteroid Therapy in Some Complications of the Neoplastic Diseases

Complication of neoplastic disease	Use of corticosteroids
Hypercalcaemia	In about 70% of patients, corticosteroid administration is followed by rapid decrease in serum calcium
Brain metastases	In about 60% of patients, corticosteroid administration is followed by transient improvement in the signs of increased intracranial pressure
Haemolytic anaemia in malignant lymphomas and in chronic lymphocytic leukaemia Non-infectious fever	Corticosteroids are also indicated in these conditions

8.5 Side Effects of Corticosteroids

Target metabolism or system	Clinical toxicity
Carbohydrate metabolism	Rise in blood sugar, diabetes induction
Protein metabolism	Muscle wasting, osteoporosis, skin atrophy and stria
Mineral and water metabolism	Increased sodium retention, potassium loss, increased calcium excretion in urine
Haematopoietic system	Reduction in circulating lymphocytes, increase in circulating neutrophils
Gastrointestinal system	Delayed healing of gastric ulcers and gastric haemorrhage
Cardiovascular system	Hypertension
Nervous system	Anxiety, depression, psychoses

Further Reading

Allegra JC, Simon R, Lippman MC (1979) The association between steroid hormone receptor status and the disease free interval in breast cancer. In: Adjuvant therapy of cancer, Vol. II, Salmon SE, Jones SE (Eds.). Grune & Stratton, New York

Bonadonna G, Valagussa P, Tancini G, Di Fronzo G (1980) Estrogen-receptor status and response to chemotherapy in early and advanced breast cancer. Cancer Chemotherapy and Pharmacology, 4: 37

Carter SK (1979) The dilemma of estrogen receptors and the response rate to cytotoxic chemotherapy. A problem of comparability analysis. Cancer Clinical Trials, 2: 49

Clarysee A, Kenis Y, Mathe G (1976) Hormonal agents used in the treatment of cancer. In: Cancer Chemotherapy, Springer-Verlag, Berlin

Jensen EV (1973) Estrogen binding and clinical response of breast cancer. In: Cancer Medicine. Ed. by Holland JF, Frei E, (Eds). Lea & Febiger, Philadelphia

Lippman ME, Allegra JC, Thompson EB, Barlock A, Green L, Huff KK, Hoan MTD, Aiken SC, Warren R (1978) The relation between estrogen receptors and response rate to cytotoxic chemotherapy in metastatic breast cancer. N. England J Med, 298: 1233

McGuire WC, Carbone PP, Vollmer EP (Eds) (1975) Estrogen Receptors in Human Breast Cancer. North Holland Publishing Company, Amsterdam

Riedman MA, Hoffman PG, and Jones HW (1978) The clinical value of hormone receptor assays in malignant disease. Cancer Treat. Reviews 5: 185

Stoll BA (Ed) (1981) Hormonal Management of Endocrine Related Cancer. Lloyd-Luke LTD., London

Stoll BA (Ed) (1982) Endocrine Relationships in Breast Cancer. William Heinemann Med Books LTD, London

Talley RW (1973) Corticosteroids. In: Cancer Medicine, Holland JF, Frei E, (Eds). Lea & Febiger, Philadelphia

9 Human Tumour Immunobiology

9.1 Theoretical Basis of Human Tumour Immunology

Tumour cells in man must be immunologically "different" from normal cells and the human immune system must be able to "recognize" this difference. It has been demonstrated that:

1. Human tumour cells possess tumour-associated antigens (TAA) not present in normal tissues.
2. Mononuclear cells from patients bearing tumours are capable of destroying autologous tumour cells in in vitro experiments.
3. Plasma or serum from the tumour-bearing patient blocks the ability of that patient's mononuclear cells to destroy autologous tumour cells.

9.2 Clinical Evidence of Host Resistance Against Human Tumours

1. Spontaneous regressions of tumour growth.
2. Recurrence after long remission (sometimes associated with "stress").
3. Transplantation experiments: low "take" of autologous tumour cells.
4. Histology: cellular reactions against tumour (lymphocytic and plasmacytic infiltration).
5. Immune deficiency may be associated with an increased incidence of malignancy.

9.2.1 Organ Transplant Recipients

Malignant tumours arising in organ homograft recipients reported to the Denver Registry (Penn and Starzl)

Type of tumour	No. of patients
Epithelial	74
Mesenchymal	48
Total	122

The overall chance of developing a de novo malignancy in a patient receiving immunosuppressive therapy is 5%-6%.

9.2.2 Congenital Immunodeficient States

The increased incidence of lymphomas in patients with immunological deficiency diseases (Doll and Kinlen)

	Ataxia-telangiectasia	Wiskott-Aldrich syndrome	Chédiak-Higashi syndrome
No. of cases	200	90	50
No. of patients with malignant disease (usually of reticular endothelial system)	14 (7%)	11 (12%)	11 (22%)

9.2.3 Patients Receiving Chemotherapy for Malignant Disease

Tumour patients with impaired delayed hypersensitivity have a poorer prognosis than those with normal skin reactivity.

Delayed hypersensitivity responses and prognosis in 100 patients with potentially operable malignant disease (Eilber and Norton)

Subjects	Positive dinitro-chlorobenzene (DNCB)	Battery skin tests (positive to one or more)
Normal	>95%	>95%
Inoperable or with early recurrence	7% (2/29)	21% (6/29)
Disease-free at 6 months	92% (50/54)	55% (26/47)

9.2.4 Concept of Immune Surveillance

The immune system is constantly destroying malignantly transformed cells, and clinical tumour represents a failure of this system.

1. Specific immune reactivity by the host against malignant cells:
   In vitro tests

2. Immunotherapy:
   Some studies show promising results
   There is no definite evidence in man implicating specific immune reactions as a mediator of host resistance against tumours. Other non-immunological factors may well be of greater importance. There are serious difficulties in accepting the attractive concept that the host is protected from the development of new tumours by an immunosurveillance mechanism, since not all models of immunodepression result in increased neoplasia.

9.2.5 Interferon

Since their discovery in 1957, the interferons have been extensively studied. Their activity in modifying the growth of certain cells led to the US National Cancer Institute trials of synthesized interferon inducers in 1974. However, although interferon was induced in some of these patients, no tumour responses were seen.

A variety of interferons have now been produced and are under phase I and phase II study. So far, the number of patients treated is small (200–300) and many of the data are as yet not evaluated. However, sporadic responses have been reported in osteogenic sarcoma, nodular lymphoma, myeloma, breast cancer and melanoma. Side effects of interferon administration are fever, malaise, fatigue, neutropenia, thrombocytopenia, alopecia and arthralgias.

At the present time the anticancer activity of the interferons is the subject of intensive investigation in a number of centres. The enthusiastic claims made for antitumour activity by the media contrast severely with the responses reported by responsible observers and lend emphasis to the need for objective study.

9.3 Methods of Measuring Specific Immune Activity

Several in vitro and in vivo tests have been described purporting to demonstrate the existence of immune reactions in man specifically directed against the patient's own tumour cells. Unfortunately, it is still impossible to make a definitive statement that these autologous reactions are directed against specific antigens at the tumour cell surface, which are not present on corresponding normal cells.

1. Specific immune activity in vitro:

Antibody	Immunofluorescence Complement-dependent cytotoxicity Growth inhibition tests Mortality inhibition tests Cell-dependent antibody Miscellaneous
Cell-mediated	Cytotoxicity Growth inhibition Lymphokine production Leukocyte migration inhibition Lymphocyte blastogenesis

2. Specific immune activity in vivo:
Delayed hypersensitivity to tumour cells, tumour cell membranes or antigen preparation

9.4 Antigens Associated with Tumour Cells Which Could Prove Useful in Tumour Detection or Immunotherapy

1. Normal tissue components in the tumour cells:
   a) Associated with adult tissues
      Membrane (e.g. HLA antigens)
      Intracellular (polypeptide hormones)
   b) Embryonic
      Membrane (e.g. carcinoembryonic antigen)
      Intracellular (e.g. Regan isoenzyme, alpha-foetoprotein)
2. Virus-mediated antigens (passenger viruses or possibly causative agents)
3. Tumour-specific antigens: - Membrane
   - Intracellular
4. Immunorestorative agents:
   Many patients with malignancy have decreased circulating T-cells. Materials that are capable of restoring T-cell numbers to normal have been used in immunotherapy.
   Thymosin fraction 5, a family of mildly acidic polypeptides, is capable of increasing initially decreased T-cell markers in the blood of cancer patients. Cohen et al. have shown that the addition of thymosin to chemotherapy for small-cell lung cancer prolongs remission compared to surgery alone.
   Levamisole, an anti-helminthic drug, has also been shown to increase T-cell numbers in cancer patients. This material has been used as adjuvant to surgery in non-oat cell lung cancer (Amery et al.) and as an adjuvant

to chemotherapy in multiple myeloma. In both these studies, duration of disease-free survival was improved in levamisole-treated patients. Both thymosin and levamisole studies will require confirmation.

9.4.5 Immunologically Active Cell Products

Much interest has recently been developed in the use of human interferon in the therapy of cancer. Crude preparations (0.1% interferon) of human leukocyte interferon have been used in the therapy of multiple myeloma and breast cancer. Interferon is known to have a direct antiproliferative effect that can result in tumour cell death and also is an immunomodulating agent which increases T-cell cytotoxicity, natural-killer-cell cytotoxicity and antibody-dependent cellular cytotoxicity. The initial results in interferon trials are the following:

1. Multiple myeloma –	Dosage:	$3–6 \times 10^6$ units qd $\times$ 6 months
	Patients:	14 (9 untreated) (24%)
	Results:	Regression in 4/11 evaluable patients
		Osserman
2. Breast cancer –	Dosage:	$3–9 \times 10^6$ units qd $\times$ 42 days
	Patients:	23 (no prior treatment)
	Results:	Partial regression (PR) 5/23 (22%)
	Duration of PR:	14–121 days
		Borden et al.

9.5 Possible Approaches to Immunotherapy

9.5.1 Non-Specific Active Immunotherapy

Depends on concept that the tumour-bearing patient has a suppressed latent immune responsiveness against his tumour. Non-specific stimulation of the cellular immune system by predominantly bacterial products such as BCG (Calmette-Guerin bacillus) *C. parvum* and MER (the methanol extracted residue of BCG) is used to increase this latent immunity.

BCG is most commonly used and has been evaluated as:

1. Injection directly into tumour nodules
2. As adjuvant immunotherapy after patients have been rendered free of all clinically apparent disease

When BCG is directly injected into small cutaneous melanoma nodules, 60%–90% of tumours will regress. 5%–10% of uninjected nodules will regress also. The local injection of BCG is purely for local control.

The tumour cells may be destroyed non-specifically secondary to an intense inflammatory response.

BCG has been used as an adjuvant to chemotherapy (acute myeloblastic and acute lymphoblastic leukaemia, ovarian cancer) and to surgery (melanoma). Initial reports in all four tumours showed benefit. Further controlled studies have failed to confirm this benefit.

9.5.2 Adoptive Transfer of Informational Materials

Both immune RNA and transfer factor ribonucleoproteins extracted from lymphoid cells have been used in attempts at immunotherapy in man. There have been no positive results confirmed with these materials.

9.5.3 Specific Active Immunization

Tumour cells treated in various ways to increase antigenicity have been used in the immunotherapy of human cancer. Bekesi and Holland have reported improved remission duration in patients with AML receiving therapy with neuraminidase-treated allogenic leukaemia cells in addition to maintenance chemotherapy. Stewart and Hollinshead reported 90% disease-free survival at 3 years post-surgery in resected stage I non-oat cell lung cancer patients receiving three injections of an allogenic lung cancer antigen preparation with complete Freund's adjuvant. Both these studies need confirmation.

The toxicity of interferon was generally mild but did include nausea, malaise, alopecia and leukopenia. Much more thorough evaluation of interferon will be necessary to define the role of this material in the therapy of cancer.

9.6 Possible Reasons for the Failure of Immunotherapy

1. Tumour antigen too weak
2. Tumour antigen covered or not released from the tumour cell surface
3. Loss of tumour antigen - deletion - modulation
4. Specific tolerance to tumour antigen (antigen excess)
5. Tumour inaccessibility - immune cells and antibody fail to enter the tumour
6. Inhibition of immune reactivity - target cell blocking (antigen-antibody complexes)
   - effector cell inhibitor (antigen)

7. Immunological enhancement - antibody - cell-mediated
8. Failure of the normal immune system

9.7 Summary of Role of Immunotherapy in Human Cancer

Immunotherapy, in general, has no well-defined place in the treatment of human cancer. Of the many hundreds of studies utilizing such therapy, a clear advantage of unequivocally positive results has been rare, although a small increase in survival or remission duration has been shown in some studies involving relatively few patients. As noted previously, the positive studies require confirmation. It is clear that immunotherapy should still be thought of as purely a research treatment and cannot be recommended as standard therapy for any malignancy.

Further Reading

Gale RP (1980) Autologous bone-marrow transplantations in patients with cancer. J Am Med Assoc 236: 540-542
Hersch EM, Mavligit GM, Gutterman JU (1976) J Am Med Assoc 236: 1739-1742
Lobuglio AF (1980) Clinical Immunotherapy. Marcel Dekker, New York
MacDonald JS (1976) The immunobiology of colorectal cancer. Semin Oncol 3: 421-432
Oettgen HF (1977) Immunotherapy of cancer. N Engl J Med 297: 484-491
Sikora K (1980) Does interferon cure cancer? Brit Med J 281: 855-858
Stevenson GT, Laurence DJR (1975) The Immune Response to Human Tumours in Man. UICC Technical Report Series, Vol 22. UICC, Geneva
Terry WD, Windhorst D (Eds). (1978) Immunotherapy of Cancer: Present Status of Trials in Man. Raven Press, New York
Waldmann TA, et al (1978) Disorders of suppressor immunoregulatory cells in the pathogenesis of immunodeficiency and auto-immunity. Ann Intern Med 88: 226-235

10 Education and Psychological Support of the Patient

10.1 Psychological Impact of Cancer

Implied meaning that the patient attaches to the word "cancer":

1. Pain
2. Mutilation
3. Hospitalization
4. Debts, inability to care for his own family
5. Loss of sexual attractiveness
6. Possible death

10.2 Psychological Problems of Cancer

1. The physician's attitude to cancer
2. The patient's attitude to cancer
3. The doctor-patient relationship
4. The family attitude to cancer
5. The nurse's attitude to cancer

N. B. The special problems of the terminal care are dealt with in Chap. 11.

10.3 Attitude of the Physician Caring for the Patient

1. The pessimistic attitude is mostly related to lack of information in the field of clinical oncology.
2. Pessimism of the physician is psychologically dangerous for the patient.
3. Physicians specifically caring for cancer patients usually develop an "aggressive but optimistic" attitude, since they have experienced a number of cases in which "aggressive" treatment has produced long-term cure.
4. The physician caring for cancer patients should also be competent in offering emotional support. This can be perceived by his attitude towards the patient and his disease. Many of these elements of trust are non-verbal and developed over time, but they begin with the very first contact.

10.4 Patient's Attitudes

1. The patient's attitudes to cancer vary considerably in different parts of the world depending on cultural, ethnic, social, economic and educational factors.
2. The most important attitude is fear: initially a period of denial of the facts should be considered as a protective psychological mechanism.
3. The unique mechanism of coping of any patient should be understood by the clinical oncologist in order to develop reasonable ways of responding.
4. The patient's attitudes should be influenced by the goal of developing a therapeutic alliance with the physician.

10.5 Telling the Diagnosis

1. "Telling" or "not-telling" the diagnosis is a false dilemma.
2. The problem is "How" and "When" to inform the patient.

10.6 How to Inform the Patient

1. In the course of history-taking the physician should explore how the patient has handled past emotional crises and what his philosophical approach to life is.
2. It is not necessary to tell the patient the whole truth in all situations.
3. A deliberate lie should not be told.
4. The hopeful side should always be stressed.
5. Terms should be used which the patient can understand - not medical jargon.
6. The discussion should be unhurried and in privacy; repeated interviews may be necessary (plan more than one meeting).
7. Honesty does not mean cruelty.
8. The patient must feel the commitment of the physician to provide him with continuing care.
9. The physician should observe as well as listen to the patient during the interview.
10. The physician should be aware that in spite of all the above recommendations, maladaptive reactions do occur.

10.7 Using Booklets to Inform the Patient about Chemotherapy

Information given by the medical oncologist to the patient may be complemented and enriched by special booklets designed to meet the following questions:

1. What is chemotherapy?
2. How do the drugs work?
3. How are treatments given?
4. What is the length of treatment?
5. Which are the short-term side effects?
6. Which are the long-term side effects?

10.8 Questions Frequently Asked by Patients Receiving Chemotherapy and Answers, as Reproduced from the Chemotherapy Booklet of the Georgia Oncology Hematology Clinic

Q. How long will I be taking drugs?

A. Each case is different. The drugs are administered until the full effect on the cancer is seen. Some people take a drug for several weeks, others for months, and some for years. Depending on the tumour type it may be necessary to give several drugs in combination.

Q. Should I do anything different while taking drugs? Rest, eat more, eat less?

A. In general we advise that you use good common sense. When you are tired ... rest, if you feel like being active then do so. Many patients on chemotherapy carry on with their usual jobs without difficulty. Some patients require more rest than others. With regard to diet, we suggest that you try to maintain ideal body weight and eat foods which you like. If any special diets are required, we will let you know.

Q. Should I be taking vitamins or shots to build up?

A. Each case is different. Most patients who are eating regular meals do not require vitamins. If you need them, we will prescribe them.

Q. What medicines or drugs should I avoid while on chemotherapy?

A. Do not take any medicines unless they have been prescribed by your doctor. Do not use aspirin or any products containing aspirin such as Bufferin, Anacin, Stanback, cold capsules, etc. If your are having pain use Tylenol which can be purchased at any drugstore without a prescription. Use two or three tablets every four hours for pain.

Q. Can I drink alcohol while taking chemotherapy?

A. We do not object to the occasional use of alcohol beverages, i. e. one or two cocktails at a party or at dinner. Excessive use of alcohol may interfere with bone marrow or liver function.

Q. Can I smoke?

A. Smoking is a strong factor which contributes to the cause of cancer, especially in the lung, mouth, throat and esophagus. Patients who have one tumour are at a greater risk for developing a second tumour. For their own protection as well as the protection of others, we prefer that all of our patients not smoke.

Q. While taking chemotherapy should I be exposed to other people who are known to have minor infections such as colds and flu?

A. In general, we feel that people who are known to have an infection such as cold or flu should avoid contact with patients undergoing chemotherapy. Special care should be taken to avoid contact with people known to have active chicken pox since this can develop into a serious infection in patients on chemotherapy.

Q. Will cancer drugs make me sterile?

A. Many patients, male and female, do become sterile while being treated with cancer drugs, while others do not. Each case is different and depends on several factors including the patient's age, type of tumour, dose and type of drug. If you do become sterile there is no way of knowing whether this is permanent or temporary. Some patients have had return of normal reproductive function while others have not.

Q. Should I avoid sexual relations while on chemotherapy?

A. There is no medical reason to avoid sexual relations while taking these drugs.

Q. Is it possible to become pregnant while on chemotherapy?

A. Yes, it is possible. Although many people will become sterile while on therapy, there are patients who have become pregnant while receiving these medicines. We do not advise that patients attempt to have children while receiving these drugs because of the possible risk to the unborn fetus. If you are a woman and you cease having menstrual periods, be sure to let us know.

Q. How soon after chemotherapy is stopped should I try to have children?

A. Each case is different and requires individual counselling regarding this question.

Q. What should I do if dental work is needed?

A. Have your dentist call us prior to performing any work on your teeth.

Q. Will other forms of therapy such as surgery, radiotherapy and immunotherapy be considered in my case?

A. Each patient's case will be treated individually so that he is assured of the most advanced, up-to-date therapy which is possible. If surgery or radiotherapy is necessary, we will obtain appropriate consultation with experts in these areas.

Q. Are these cancer drugs experimental and am I being used as a guinea pig?

A. The majority of cancer drugs used today have been available for several years. At times, we will use drugs obtained from the National Cancer Institute which are not available for general use and are listed as investigational drugs. If an investigational drug is deemed necessary in your case, we will discuss the benefits and risks with you. If you agree to its use, we will ask you to sign a form demonstrating that you understand and agree to being treated with the drug.

Q. Can I have a permanent?

A. Yes.

10.9 Assisting the Patient to live with Cancer (Hersh 1982)

1. The process for assisting the patient to live with cancer begins with informing him of his diagnosis.
2. Physicians must be concerned with the patient's autonomy. This involves participation in self-care, medical treatments, and maintaining self in the roles held prior to illness (student, parent, spouse, lover, bread-winner).
3. Problems in psychological and social adjustment should be identified and attended to as soon as possible.
4. Maintain your awareness of the tremendous potential cancer patients have for feeling lonely and isolated from others.
5. Monitor the status of each patient's support system: family; friends; workschool; community; religious involvement.
6. Encourage the use of support system, including appropriate and available self-help groups as well as telephone networking of patients.
7. Use speciality consultation and special resources when they can improve the patient's quality of life.

10.10 Indications for Psychiatric Consultation (Holland)

1. Diagnosis and explanation of mental symptoms
2. Management of concurrent or complicating psychiatric illness
3. Emotional disturbance in response to illness or medical management
4. Evaluation of depression and suicidal risk
5. Use of psychopharmacologic drugs

Further Reading

Holland J (1982) Psychologic Aspects of Cancer. In: Cancer Medicine, Holland JF and Frei III, E (Eds), Lee & Febiger, Philadelphia

Hersh SP (1982) Psychological Aspects of Patients with Cancer. In: Cancer Principles and Practice of Oncology, De Vita VT, Helmann SH and Rosemberg SA (Eds), JB Lippincott Company, Philadelphia-Toronto

Psychosocial Aspects (1982) In: UICC Manual of Clinical Oncology, Springer-Verlag, Berlin

11 Pain Control and Terminal Care

11.1 Available Methods of Pain Palliation in Advanced Cancer

Radiotherapy
Chemotherapy
Analgesic therapy
Interruption of neural pathways

11.2 Sequence of Application of Methods of Pain Palliation

1. Usually, best palliation is derived from tumour-specific therapy.
2. If a pain is not controlled by tumour-specific therapy, and the pain is diffuse, use:
   a) Non-narcotic analgesics
   b) Weak narcotic analgesics
   c) Strong narcotic analgesics
3. If pain is localized and not palliated by tumour-specific therapy, use interruption of neural pathways.

11.3 General Principles of Pain Palliation in Advanced Disease

In diseases where effective hormone or chemotherapy is available, pain is usually well-controlled by these modalities.

Where pain persists despite hormone or chemotherapy, these modalities should be supplemented by radiotherapy for local pain control.

In diseases where hormone and chemotherapy have limited effects, radiotherapy (with or without hormone or chemotherapy) should be used first to control pain.

As a general principle, localized pain is better controlled by radiotherapy and generalized pain by hormone or chemotherapy – where the latter are effective.

11.4 Most Important Occurrences of Pain in Neoplastic Disease

1. Bone metastases
2. Infiltration of nerves, nervous plexuses and other nerve structures

11.5 Different Levels of Interruption of Neural Pathways in the Management of Pain

Level of interruption	Procedure
Peripheral	Analgesic nerve blocks, blocks of the autonomous nervous system, subarachnoid neurolytic blocks
Spinal	Percutaneous and surgical rhizotomy Percutaneous and surgical cordotomy
Central	Thalamotomy Hypophysectomy Leukotomy

11.6 General Strategy of Pain Relief in Advanced Cancer (from Twycross)

11.6.1 Aim

To keep the patient both free of pain and fully alert

11.6.2 Assessment

1. Treatment varies according to the cause of the pain; use body chart to record sites of pain and their probable mechanism.
2. Because a person has cancer, it does not mean that the malignant process is necessarily the cause of the pain.

11.6.3 Choice of Analgesics

1. Establish a simple, practical analgesic "league table":
   a) Non-narcotic - aspirin (alternative, acetominophen)
   b) Weak narcotic - codeine (alternative, D-propoxyphene)
   c) Strong narcotic - morphine (alternative, papaveretum, diamorphine)
2. Avoid pentazocine, meperidine and dextromoramide (Palfium)

3. Methadone should be used with caution, particularly in the elderly and debilitated.
4. The use of a narcotic analgesic is dictated by intensity of pain and not by brevity of prognosis.
   "Morphine exists to be given, not merely to be withheld".

11.6.4 Use of Analgesics

1. Oral medication is normally possible. When injections are necessary, use freeze-dried ampoules of diamorphine.
2. Persistent pain requires preventive therapy. This means that analgesics should be given regularly and prophylactically: "as required" medication is both irrational and inhumane.
3. Doses should be determined on an individual basis; the right dose is that which gives relief for at least 3, preferably 4 or more hours.
4. Adjuvant medication is the rule rather than the exception. Laxatives are almost always necessary, an anti-emetic commonly so.
5. If very anxious, an anxiolytic such as diazepam should be tried; if depressed, an antidepressive.
6. The perception of pain requires both attention and consciousness. Diversional therapy - people to talk to, activities to attend, etc. - is of great value.
7. Tolerance is not usually a practical problem.
8. Rightly used, psychological dependence (addiction) does not occur.
9. Physical dependence does not prevent the downward adjustment of the dose of a narcotic analgesic should the pain ameliorate.
10. Neither diamorphine nor morphine is the panacea for terminal pain. Their use does not guarantee automatic success, particularly if the psychological component of pain is ignored.

11.6.5 Reassessment

1. Relief of pain should be assessed in relation to comfort achieved:
   a) During the night
   b) In the daytime at rest
   c) On movement
2. Reassessment remains a continuing necessity; old pains may get worse and new ones may develop.

11.7 Relative Potency of Analgesics (from Houde)

11.7.1 Relative Potencies of Analgesics Commonly Employed for severe Pain, Expressed in Terms of the Intramuscular (i.m.) and Oral (p.o.) Doses Approximately Equivalent in Total Effect to a 10-mg i.m. Dose of Morphine

	i.m. (mg)	p.o. (mg)	Major differences from morphine
Oxymorphone (Numorphan)	1	6	None
Hydromorphone (Dilaudid)	1.5	7.5	Shorter-acting
Levorphanol (Levo-Dromoran)	2	4	Relatively high p.o. to i.m. potency
Phenazocaine (Prinadol)	3	15	None
Metopon	3	18	None
Heroin	4		Shorter-acting
Dextromoramide (Palfium)	7.5	10	High p.o. to i.m. potency
Piminodine (Alvodine)	7.5		None
Methadone (Dolophine)	10	20	Relatively high p.o. to i.m. potency
Morphine	10	60	
Oxycodone	15	30	Shorter-acting. Relative high p.o. to i.m. potency
Dipipanone (Pipadone)	20		None
Methotrimeprazine (Levoprome, Nozinan)	20		Phenothiazine - unlike morphine
Anileridine (Leritine)	30	50	Relatively high p.o. to i.m. potency
Alphaprodine (Nisentil)	45		Very short-acting
Pentazocine (Talwin)	60	180	Narcotic antagonist analgesic
Meperidine (pethidine, Demerol)	75	300	None
Codeine	130	200	Relatively high p.o. to i.m. potency; relatively more toxic in higher doses
Dextroproxyphene (Darvon)	240		Similar to codeine, but more toxic in high doses

11.7.2 Relative Potencies of Analgesics Employed Orally for Less Severe Pain, Expressed in Terms of Doses Approximately Equivalent in Total Effect to 650 mg of Aspirin

	p.o. (mg)	Salient features
Pentazocine (Talwin)	30	Weak narcotic - narcotic antagonist, high analgesic potential, a low addiction liability
Codeine	32	Weak narcotic, high analgesic potential, relatively low addiction liability
Meperidine (Demerol)	50	Narcotic, high analgesic potential, high addiction liability
Propoxyphene (Darvon)	65	Weak narcotic, low analgesic potential, low addiction liability
Aminopyrine (Pyramidon)	600	Non-narcotic, low analgesic potential, no addiction liability, risk of agranulocytosis
Aspirin (ASA)	650	Non-narcotic, anti-inflammatory, low analgesic potential, no addiction liability or tolerance
Phenacetin (acetonphenetidin)	650	Similar to aspirin but with limited anti-inflammatory properties
Acetaminophen (paracetamol)	650	Similar to phenacetin, less potential renal toxicity
Sodium salicylate	1000	Similar to aspirin

11.8 Effective Doses of Non-Narcotic Analgesics for Control of Cancer Pain (from Gerbershaghen)

Generic name	Dose (mg)	Interval of administration during day
Acetylsalicylic acid	750–1250	q 3 h
Salicylamide	750–1000	q 3 h
Phenacetin	400– 600	q 3 h
Paracetamol	600– 800	q 3 h
Acetylaminosalol	400– 800	q 3 h
Phenazon	500–1000	q 3 h
Propyphenazon	450– 800	q 3 h
4-Aminophenazon	450– 800	q 3 h
Aminophenazon	450– 800	q 3 h
Noramidopyrine methansulfonatesodium (metamizol)	750–1000	q 3 h
Mofebutazon (monophenylbutazon)	200– 400	q 4 h
Phenylbutazon	200– 400	q 4 h
Oxyphenbutazone	100– 200	q 4 h

Generic name	Dose (mg)	Interval of administration during day
Mefanamic acid	500	q 3 h
Flufenamic acid	200	q 4 h
Indomethacin	50- 70	q 4 h
Benzydamin	100	q 4 h
Ibufenac		q 4 h
Ibuprofen	200- 400	q 3 h
Naproxen	250- 500	q 3-4 h
Niflumic acid	250- 500	q 3-4 h
Bumadizon	220	q 4 h
Alclofenac	500-1000	q 4 h
Nefopam	60- 120	q 3 h

11.9 The Brompton Cocktail (From Twycross)

Composition of a morphine-cocaine elixir used at the Brompton Hospital since 1952:

Morphine hydrochloride	¼ grain	(15 mg)
Cocaine hydrochloride	⅙ grain	(10 mg)
Alcohol 90%	30 minims	(2 ml)
Syrup	60 minims	(4 ml)
Chloroform water to	½ fl. oz.	(15 ml)

In recent years diamorphine (diacetylmorphine, heroin) has commonly been used instead of morphine as the analgesic component, now generally known as the Brompton Cocktail.

11.10 Use of the Brompton Cocktail in Cancer Pain Compared with the Use of Injected Morphine for Acute Severe Pain (from Twycross)

	Brompton cocktail (cancer pain)	Injected morphine (acute pain)
Aim	Pain relief	Pain relief
Sedation	Usually undesirable	Often desirable
Desired duration of effect	As long as possible	2-4 h
Timing	Every 4 h regularly (in anticipation)	Every 2-6 h as required (on demand)
Dose	Individually determined (5-100 mg)	Usually standard (10 mg)
Route	By mouth	Injection
Adjuvant medication	Common	Uncommon

11.11 Terminal Care

There is a general understanding that terminal care refers to the management of patients in whom the advent of death is felt to be certain and not too far off and for whom medical effort has turned away from therapy and become concentrated on the relief of symptoms and the support of both patients and family (Holford). When patients enter what is thought to be the terminal stage of malignant disease, the emphasis in treatment is on the control of distressing symptoms.

11.12 "Cure" and "Care" System (Modified from Saunders 1978)

It is imperative to recognize the moment when active treatment is becoming irrelevant to the needs of a particular patient and this should be switched from the "cure" to the "care" system as shown diagrammatically below. The aims of the two are, however, not mutually exclusive: effective control of symptoms may accompany or revive the prospect of further treatment.

"Cure system"		"Care system"
Investigation and Treatment, elimination and control of tumour	⟶ ⟵	Assessment and investigations only if relevant to control of symptom of uncontrollable tumour

11.13 Overlap of the "Cure" and "Care" Systems (from Saunders 1978)

Terminal care is a facet of oncology concerned with the control of symptoms instead of with the control of tumour. As diagrammatically shown below there is an increasing overlap between these two parts of the total discipline.

Active palliative care	⟵ ⟶ Overlap place of decision	Terminal care

11.14 Factors to Be Assessed in Fach Individual Patient to Determine if the Time for Terminal Care Has Been Reached

1. Symptomatology
2. Evidence for advanced, progressing disease
3. Inability to treat the disease by conventional chemotherapy or failure to respond to new anticancer agents
4. Psychological attitude of the patient

N.B. Continued assessment is the key to appropriate care. A second opinion may be necessary.

11.15 Medical and Psychosocial Aspects of Terminal Care - Main Guidelines of Intervention

1. Avoid unnecessary diagnostic and therapeutic procedures.
2. Prescribe drugs only to relieve distressing symptoms.
3. Give pain medication to cover entire 24 h.
4. Favour religious belief of everybody.
5. Switch from home to hospital admission and vice versa on the basis of the changing requirements and taking into account the economic and family environment.
6. Assist family to give to the relatives the necessary elements of information.
7. Require the co-operation of well-trained nurses and social assistants.

Further Reading

1. Bonica JJ, Ventafridda V (Eds) (1979) Advances in Pain Research and Therapy. International Symposium on Pain of Advanced Cancer. Raven Press, New York
2. Saunders CM (1978) The Management of Terminal Disease. Edward Arnold, London

12 Organization of Cancer Treatment

12.1 Organizational Problems

Data recording and documentation
Interdisciplinary co-ordination and co-operation
Personnel training
Appropriate organization for cancer treatment within the general hospital
Multi-institutional co-operation for randomized clinical trials

12.2 Interdisciplinary Organization of an Oncological Centre Located Within a General Hospital

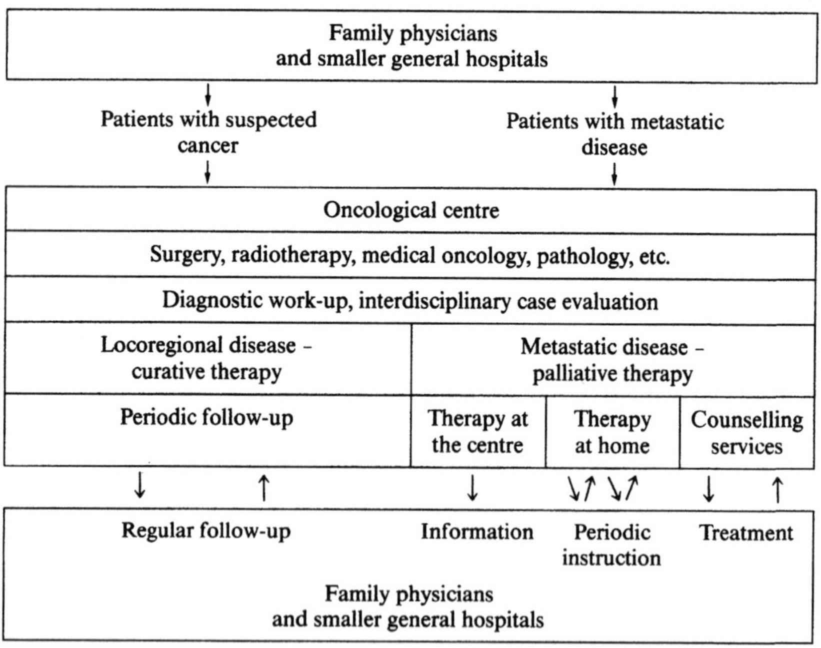

12.3 Organization of Medical Oncology in a General Hospital

12.3.1 Medical Ward for Hospitalized Patients

1. Special ward for all medically treated cancer patients:
   Advantage: facilitates organization, documentation and specific aspects of cytostatic treatment
2. Hospitalization on a general medical ward with special attendance of medical oncologists and oncology nurses:
   Advantage: may improve non-specialized general medical care and supportive care; probably decreases psychological burden for patients and staff

12.3.2 "Five-Day" Special Ward

Open from Monday to Friday for short-term hospitalization (with reduced nursing staff) for:
1. Diagnostic procedures, e.g. lumbar puncture, laparoscopy, biopsies, etc.
2. Special therapeutic procedures, e.g. infusion chemotherapy, other heavy chemotherapy (*cis*-platinum, etc.), blood transfusions, etc.

12.3.3 Outpatient Clinics

Main functions:
1. Initial work-up and evaluation of newly referred patients or of patients referred after interdisciplinary evaluation
2. Application of all forms of hormonal and cytostatic treatment and supportive medical care on an ambulatory basis
3. Information and communication with family physician, family members etc.; handling of socio-economic and psychological aspects
4. Documentation and evaluation of routine chemotherapy or protocol study chemotherapy

12.4 Organization of the Outpatient Medical Oncology Clinic

12.4.1 Necessary Staff

1. Medical staff, consultants for the different specialities
2. Specially trained oncology nurses
3. Assistant nurses
4. Secretarial staff, data managers

12.4.2 Necessary Room Facilities

1. Waiting room for patients
2. Office for patient admissions and appointments
3. Offices for medical and nursing staff; secretarial staff
4. Examination and treatment rooms: approximately one for every eight patients per day
5. Specially equipped room for head and neck (HN) and GYN examinations; emergency room with emergency equipment
6. Centrally located room for storage of drugs and preparation of the various forms of chemotherapy
7. Archive room for documentation and evaluation of all diagnostic and therapeutic procedures and storage of all documents

12.4.3 Basic Procedures for Ambulatory Patients

12.4.3.1 Before Patient Visits Outpatient Clinic

1. The compilation of all documentation relevant to previous diagnostic and therapeutic procedures performed:
   Histology reports
   Operative reports
   Data on previous radio- and/or chemotherapy
   x-Ray documents, etc.
2. Assignment of the patient to the physician responsible for the outpatient care
3. Preparation of all necessary laboratory and radiological examinations planned for the outpatient clinic visit
4. Outline of therapy plan

12.4.3.2 During Outpatient Clinic Visit

Admission

↓

Patient sent for planned laboratory and radiological examination

↓

Waiting room
(until above results are available)

↓

Examining room

- Physical examination
- Information of the patient
- Definitive establishment of plan of therapy
- Written drug order with mode of application to the oncology nurse
- Application of specific therapy by the oncology nurse
- Establishment of the next appointment and written order for necessary laboratory or other examinations during next visit

↓

12.5 Special Qualifications for an Oncology Nurse

1. Special training in basic pharmacology, toxicities and the different forms of application of cytostatic drugs and hormones
2. Special training in basic medical aspects of the different forms of cancer, their course and treatment
3. Special training in socio-economic and psychological aspects of cancer
4. Experience in treatment evaluation and documentation

12.6 Organization of Interinstitutional Interdisciplinary Co-operation in Clinical Cancer Research

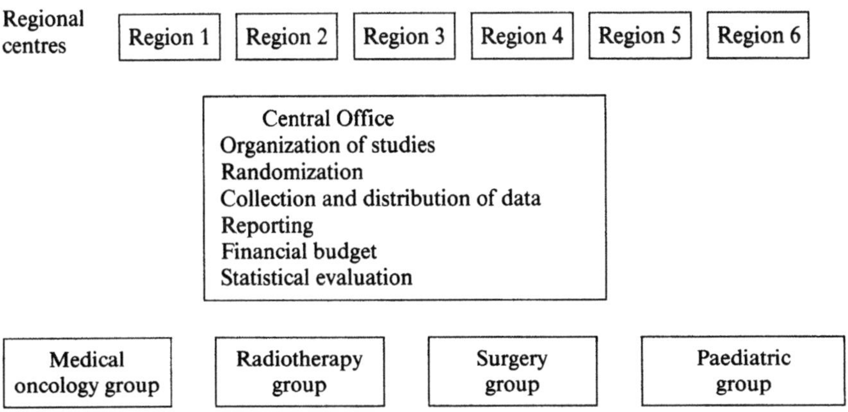

Stages in the organization of co-operative studies:
1. Study of propositions coming from members
2. Establishment of mutually approved protocol, and nomination of study chairman and the team of interested participants
3. Standardized documents for each patient: follow-up sheet - measurement sheet - summary sheet
4. Intermediate evaluation of all documents twice per year
5. Final statistical evaluation

Further Reading

Barckley V (Ed) (1980) Basic Concepts in Cancer Nursing. UICC Technical Report Series, Vol 39. UICC, Geneva

Comittee on international collaborative activities (1980) Guidelines for Developing a Comprehensive Cancer Centre, Second Edition. UICC Technical Report Series, Vol 53. UICC, Geneva

Committee on international collaborative activities (1978) International Second Edition. UICC Technical Report Series, Vol 33. UICC, Geneva

Germain C (1979) The Cancer Unit - An Ethnography. Nursing Resources, Inc, Wakefield

Guidelines for Cancer Care - Organization - Personnel - Facilities. Commission on Cancer, American College of Surgeons, Chicago, no date

Handbook on the Organization and Management of Cancer Centers. Association of American Cancer Institutes, 1979. Available from Fox Chase Cancer Center, Philadelphia

Tiffany R (1978) Cancer Nursing, Vol. 1. - Medical. Faber & Faber, London

Tiffany R (1978) Oncology for Nurses and Health Care Professionals Vol 2: Care and support. Allen & Unwin, London

Part II

Management of Adult Malignancies by Site

13 Acute Leukaemia

13.1 Incidence and Age Distribution

13.1.1 Incidence

Acute myelogenous leukaemia (AML): 2–3 per 100000
Acute lymphoblastic leukaemia (ALL): 2–3 per 100000

13.1.2 Age Distribution

		AML		*ALL*
Adults	approx.	85%	approx.	15%
Children	approx.	18%	approx.	82%

AML affects all age groups, but has an increasing incidence with age. ALL affects mainly children, with a peak incidence between the 2nd and 4th year of age, and an increasing incidence after 65 years.

Both forms of acute leukaemia are slightly more frequent in male patients than in female patients.

13.2 Aetiology

1. Genetic factors:
   a) Identical twins during first 5 years
   b) Patients with trisomy 21 (Down's syndrome)
   c) Other chromosomal defects
2. Congenital immunodeficiencies:
   See also Sect. 9.2.2
3. Ionizing irradiation:
   a) cf. Experience in Hiroshima and Nagasaki
   b) Irradiation for M. Bechterew or Hodgkin's disease (especially when combined with chemotherapy)
4. Chemical agents:

a) Benzene
b) Chloramphenicol
c) Phenylbutazone
d) Hexachlorocyclohexane
e) Chlorophenotane (DDT)
f) Lindane, etc.
g) Cytotoxic drugs, especially alkylating agents
5. Viral agents:
Proof in man is lacking

13.3 Main Prognostic Factors in Acute Leukaemia

1. Age: better prognosis in the younger age group.
2. Total cell burden as expressed by total WBC and total blast cells.
3. Number of organs involved: lymph nodes, mediastinal mass, liver, spleen, etc.; CNS-leukaemia (CNS β_2-microglobulin↑).
4. Presence or absence of infectious complications at the start of therapy.
5. Presence or absence of specific chromosomal abnormalities, insufficient metaphases and karyotypic instability: with such abnormalities, prognosis is poorer (e.g. Down's syndrome).
6. Preceding haematological disorder or secondary acute leukaemia: poorer prognosis.
7. *For ALL, in addition:* immunological characteristics: non-B-, non-T-ALL better than pre-B-ALL and T-ALL better than B-cell ALL better than pre-T-cell ALL. The latter is often associated with a mediastinal mass; *Ph*[1] chromosome in ALL predicts shorter remission duration.
WBC $> 100 \times 10^9$/l and age < 1 or > 10 years: poor prognosis
WBC $< 20 \times 10^9$/l and age 2–6 years: good prognosis
All others: intermediate prognosis

13.4 Main Clinical Features of Acute Leukaemia

1. General fatigue, pallor, loss of appetite
2. Anaemia
3. Haemorrhage: petechiae, bleeding, disseminated intravascular coagulation (promyelocytic leukaemia)
4. Infection
5. Enlarged lymph nodes, mediastinal mass, spleen, liver

6. Bone pain due to periostal infiltration: especially in L1 lymphoblastic leukaemia
7. Gum hypertrophy and skin infiltration (myelomonocytic and monoblastic leukaemia)

13.5 Classification of Acute Leukaemia

13.5.1 French-American-British (FAB) Classification of ALL[a] (Benett et al. 1976)

Cytological features	L1	L2	L3 Burkitt-like
Cell size	Small cells predominate	Large, heterogenous in size	Large and homogenous
Nuclear chromatin	Homogenous in any one case	Variable - heterogenous in any one case	Finely stippled and homogenous
Nuclear shape	Regular, occasional clefting or indentation	Irregular; clefting and indentation common	Regular - oval to round
Nucleoli	Not visible, or small and inconspicuous	One or more present, often large	Prominent; one or more vesicular
Amount of cytoplasm	Scanty	Variable; often moderately abundant	Moderately abundant
Basophilia of cytoplasm	Slight or moderate, rarely intense	Variable; deep in some	Very deep
Cytoplasmic vacuolation	Variable	Variable	Often prominent

[a] L1 corresponds to ALL in children; L2 to ALL in adults; and L3 is a poor-risk form of ALL.

13.5.2 FAB Classification of AML

M_1, myeloblastic leukaemia without maturation
M_2, myeloblastic leukaemia with different degrees of maturation
M_3, hypergranular promyelocytic leukaemia
M_4, myelomonocytic leukaemia
M_5, monoblastic leukaemia
M_6, erythroleukaemia
These classifications have limited prognostic and therapeutic implications.

13.6 Classification of ALL by Immunological Markers

13.6.1 Immunological Markers and Their Determination

Surface immunoglobulins (sIg)	By polyvalent and monospecific antisera
T-cells by E-rosettes	By sheep erythrocytes (SRBC)
Common ALL antigen (CALLA)	I_5 monoclonal antibody
T-cell antigen (T-Ag)	By T101 and OKT11 antisera
Ia-antigen (Ia)	By BA-4 and SC-4460 antisera
Terminal deoxynucleotidyl transferase (TdT)	By biochemical determination of special staining

13.6.2 Markers for the Main Immunological Types of ALL

All types	%	Markers						
		TdT	CALLA	Ia	T-Ag	SRBC	sIg	cIgM
CALLA	75%	+	+	+	–	–	–	–
Null-ALL		+	–	+	–	–	–	–
Pre-B-ALL	25%	+	+	+	–	–	–	+
T-ALL		+	–	–	+	+	–	–
Pre-T-ALL		+	+/–	–	+	–	–	–
B-ALL		–	–	+	–	–	+	–
Undifferentiated ALL		+	–	–	–	–	–	–

13.7 Cytochemical Differentiation for Four Leukaemic Cell Types

Reaction	Lymphoblast	Myeloblast	Monoblast	Erythroblast
Periodic-acid-Schiff (PAS)	Coarse granules or blocks may be present. Cytoplasmic background negative	Usually negative. Occasional cytoplasmic tinge with or without superimposed fine granules	Some negative; some show cytoplasmic tinge with fine granules	Variable. Early blasts may show strong granular or diffuse staining. Usually diffuse in later forms
Sudan black	Negative	Localized or heavy overall positivity. Auer rods positive	Usually positive with discrete scattered granules	Negative
Peroxide	Negative	Usually positive. Auer rods positive	Usually negative	Negative

Reaction	Lymphoblast	Myeloblast	Monoblast	Erythroblast
Aryl sulphatase	Nuclear staining usually present	Negative nuclear staining	Negative nuclear staining	Negative nuclear staining
Esterases α-naphthyl acetate	Negative (normal lymphocytes occasionally positive)	Negative	Strongly positive	Variable. Occasional strong positivity
Naphthol acetate	Occasional weak granular positivity	Occasional positivity not inhibited by NaF	Strong positivity	Some positivity
Naphthol chloroacetate	Negative	Usually positive. Auer rods positive	Negative	Negative
Acid phosphatase	Weak/moderate positivity. Positive in T-blasts	Strongly positive	Strongly positive	Positive paranuclear activity
Phosphorylase	Very strong positivity	Moderately positive	Strongly positive	Variable, occasionally strong positive in early forms
Dehydrogenases	Intramitochondrial enzymes normal, extramitochondrial increased. Quantitive tests	No difference from normal No discrimination value	As for myeloblast	As for myeloblast

13.8 General Strategy for the Chemotherapy of Acute Leukaemia

Treatment	*Possible result*	*Definition*
1. Remission Induction	Disease eradication	Complete remission
- Maximum tolerated chemotherapy	Disease reduction	Partial remission
- Maximum supportive care (see under sec. 4.8.–4.15)	No change or progression	Failure
2. Intensification		
- Additional intensive chemotherapy after complete remission	Prolonged remission or survival	
- CNS-prophylaxis in ALL	More cures	
3. Maintenance Therapy		
Optimal duration unknown ALL: 2–3 years AML: 2 years?	Prolongs remission duration and survival in AML probably only in patients not cured by induction therapy	

13.9 Assessment of Remission in Acute Leukaemia

For complete remission (CR), the patient should have no symptoms referable to leukaemia and be clinically free from apparent disease. The bone marrow cellularity should be normal with blasts amounting to less than 5% nucleated count and no obviously leukaemic blasts seen; Hb > 12 g/100 ml not maintained by transfusion; WBC > 3000/µl with a normal differential count and granulocytes numbering more than 2000/µl and a platelet count 100000/µl. The cerebrospinal fluid examination should be normal. (Exact definition of CR see below).

N. B. The achievement of a CR is the essential first step for long survival and potential cure.

There is no generally agreed definition of a partial remission in patients with acute Leukaemia.

The definition of partial remission is of less value in acute leukaemia, since there is nearly always a reduction of tumour cell mass in the face of chemotherapy and its precise documentation has less prognostic significance than the documentation of complete remission.

13.9.1 Assessment of Partial Remission in Acute Leukaemia

Assessment of partial remission is essential during remission induction to monitor treatment. More detailed assessment is given in the following tables.

	Marrow ratings (M)				
	M4	M3	M2	M1	M0
1. Leukaemic cells					
ALL % blast cells	> 50%	25%–50%	5%–25%	< 5%	No leukaemic cells
% blasts + lymphocytes	–	70%	70%	< 40%	
AML % blast cells	> 50%	25%–50%	5%–25%	< 5%	No leukaemic cells
% blasts + promyelocytes	> 55%	30%–55%	10%–30%	< 10%	
2. % Erythroid elements			> 10%	> 15%	> 15%
% Granulocytic elements			> 15%	> 25%	> 25%

	Haemogram ratings (H)				
	H4	H3	H2	H1	H0
1. Blast	> 20%	5%–20%	5%	0%	0%
2. Platelets	< 25 000	25 000–49 000	50 000–90 000	100 000–199 000	> 200 000
3. Neutrophilic					
Granulocytes < 4 years	< 500	> 500	> 750	> 1000	> 2000
Granulocytes > 4 years	< 500	> 500	> 1000	> 2000	> 3500
4. Haemoglobin					
(Adults) Male patients	< 7g%	7g%–8.9g%	> 9g%	> 12g%	> 14g%
(Adults) Female patients	< 7g%	7g%–8.9g%	> 9g%	> 11g%	> 13g%

	Ratings of physical findings (P)				
	P_4	P_3	P_2	P_1	P_0
1. Liver	Below umbilicus	> 5 cm↓ costal margin	< 5 cm↓ costal margin	Normal size	Normal size + biopsy
2. Spleen	Below umbilicus	> 2 cm↓ costal margin	< 2 cm↓ costal margin	Normal size	Normal size + biopsy
3. Lymph nodes	> 5 cm or generalized > 2 cm	2–5 cm	< 2 cm	Normal size	Normal size + biopsy
4. Haemorrhage	Severe	Moderate	Mild	None	None
5. Infection	Severe	Moderate	Mild	None	None
	Ratings of symptoms (S)				
	S_4	S_3	S_2	S_1	S_0
Organ symptoms	Severe > 50% in bed	Moderate < 50% in bed	Mild	None Normal activity	None Normal activity
	Disease status				
	D	C	B	A	α
	Rating 4 in 1 or more categories	Rating 3 in 1 or more categories	Rating 2 in 1 or more categories	Rating 1 in 1 or more categories	Rating 0 in all categories

13.10 Improvement in Prognosis for Acute Leukaemia Patients with Modern Treatment

Treatment	*ALL (Childhood)*	*ALL (Adult)*	*AML*
Supportive treatment only	No or rare remissions Median survival = 3.5 months	No remissions Median survival = 2 months	No remissions Median survival = 2 months
Modern treatment	Remission rate > 95% > 50% remain in first remission at 5 years	Remission rate > 75% Median survival = 2 years 20% alive at 5 years	Remission rate 50%–75% Median survival = 2 years 10% alive at 5 years

I. Acute Lymphoblastic Leukaemia[1]

13.11 Major Drugs Effective in Acute Lymphoblastic Leukaemia

Remission rate: 50% for childhood ALL when used singly:
Vincristine
Prednisone
L-Asparaginase
Remission rate: 30% when used singly:
Daunorubicin
Cyclophosphamide
Methotrexate
Cytosine arabinoside (ara-C)

13.12 Recommended Treatment Schedule for Acute Lymphocytic Leukaemia

13.12.1 Remission Induction

a) Vincristine 1.8 mg/m^2 i.v. weekly (max. 2 mg): 3–5 doses
b) Prednisone 40 mg/m^2 daily p.o. for 3 weeks, then taper
c) Asparaginase 500 IU/kg/days i.v., starting on day 22 or after last dose of vincristine

[1] See also Chap. 35, "Childhood Acute Lymphocytic Leukaemia".

N. B. For high-risk ALL patients (Pre-B-cell ALL, B-cell ALL, T-cell ALL or L3) or common ALL with bad prognostic features or when patients do not achieve a complete remission after 4 weeks and for all adult patients:

add danurobicin 45 mg/m^2 i.v. weekly for the first 3 weeks (some forms may even need additional ara-C and daunomycin).

13.12.2 CNS Prophylaxis

This follows remission induction or first course of maintenance therapy.

a) Whole-skull irradiation, 2400 rads in 10–15 fractions (3 weeks): may produce structural CNS changes
b) Three to five intrathecal doses of methotrexate 12 mg/m^2 (max dose 15 mg)

13.12.3 Maintenance Therapy

This should last for at least 2 years and consist of:

a) Vincristine/prednisone reinduction every 3 months, with the same dosage as during induction, but with only 2 doses of vincristine and 2 weeks of full-dose prednisone
b) 6-Mercaptopurine p.o. and methotrexate p.o. between reinduction courses, e.g.:

– 6-Mercaptopurine 200 mg/m^2 per day for 5 days – Methotrexate 7.5 mg/m^2 per day for 5 days	three courses every 2 weeks between vincristine/prednisone reinduction courses

For high-risk ALL (to which nearly all adult ALL cases belong, independent of immunological type) even more intensive and prolonged treatment programmes, including cyclophosphamide, intermediate high-dose methotrexate with citrovorum factor and three–four alternating maintenance schedules over 2 years should be considered.

II. Acute Myelogenous Leukaemia

13.13 Therapeutic Strategy for Acute Myelogenous Leukaemia

Initial management

For patients

Over 60 years of age
with no complications
or with hypoplastic acute
myelogenous leukaemia

↓

Observe disease pro-
gression or complications
of haemorrhage or infection

↘ Intensive chemotherapy (REMISSION INDUCTION)

All other cases

Allopurinol 200 mg b.i.d.

↓

Improve clinical state:
- Adequate fluids
- Clear infection
- Control haemorrhage
- Return haemoglobin to normal

↓

Clinical state satisfactory

↙ Intensive chemotherapy (REMISSION INDUCTION)

Pre-treatment procedures

↓

Intensive chemotherapy
(REMISSION INDUCTION)

N.B. If there is 50% blast infiltration of the marrow, some authorities advise a conservative approach until there is evidence of progressive disease.

Prior to chemotherapy	check	- Clinical condition (especially renal and hepatic function)
	check	- Drugs to be used
		- Correct dosage
		- Route of administration
		- Treatment schedule
During and after treatment	control	- Haemorrhage } urgently
		- Infection } urgently
	check	- Response to chemotherapy

13.14 Strategy for Remission Maintenance in Acute Myelogenous Leukaemia

Possible alternative for remission maintenance	Comment
No treatment	Risk of early relapse
Intermittent chemotherapy	Many combinations used Median complete remission duration for combinations of two or three drugs is about 40 weeks Possible agents: daunorubicin (max. total dose 550 mg/m^2), ara-C, 6-thioguanine, cyclophosphamide, 6-mercaptopurine
Other: (including immunotherapy)	No proven value
Heterologous bone marrow transplantation in first remission	30%-50% long-term survivors in younger age group

13.15 Single Drugs Active in Acute Myelogenous Leukaemia

1. Ara-C:
   a) Used for first remission induction.
   b) Continuous infusion better than bolus injection.
   c) Seven days' continuous infusion better than 5 days.
2. Anthracyclines:
   a) Daunorubicin:
      - Used for first remission induction combined with ara-C.
      - Usually given for 3 days during first remission induction course.
   b) Adriamycin
3. 6-Thioguanine:
   a) May be used in first remission induction in addition to ara-C and daunorubicin, or later for remission maintenance.
   b) Usually given during 5 days orally every 12 h.
4. Vinca alkaloids:
   a) Vincristine:
      - May be added during first remission induction, together with prednisone, or used in maintenance phase.
   b) Vindesine:
      - May be used in second remission induction.
      - Continuous infusion for 5 days seems to produce better results than bolus injection.

c) Vinblastine:
   - May be used in second remission induction regimens.

5. Amsacrine (m-AMSA):
   a) Used in second remission induction regimens (or first induction in AML with bad prognostic features?).
   b) Given in 1-h infusions for 5 days.
6. Etoposide (VP-16-213):
   a) Used in second remission induction regimens.
   b) Given by continuous infusion for 5 days or daily i.v. for 3-5 days.

13.16 Drug Combinations Effective in Acute Myelogenous Leukaemia

Drug combinations are more effective than single agents in remission induction in AML. Of the many combinations used, the most successful use an anthracycline (e.g. daunorubicin), ara-C and thioguanine. The more modern combinations have a high remission rate following a single course. During the last 5-10 years there has been a gradual increase in the proportion of long-term survivors with no evidence of disease. These results are attributed to a more intensive approach to remission induction and to intensification of subsequent chemotherapy.

13.17 Recommended Therapy for Acute Myelogenous Leukaemia

13.17.1 Induction Therapy

Ara-C: 100 mg/m^2 for 7 days, given in a continuous infusion
Daunorubicin: 45 mg/m^2/day 1, 2 and 3 i.v.

If over 5% leukaemic cells persist in marrow on day 14, repeat ara-C for 5 days and daunorubicin for two doses.

If on day 14, marrow is hypocellular or aplastic without or with less than 5% leukaemic cells: wait, and repeat marrow after another week.

13.17.2 Maintenance Therapy: Optimal Duration Unknown (2-3 years?)

After achieving disease status α or A with more than 2000 granulocytes and more than 100000 platelets:
Treatment cycles every 4 weeks during 2-3 years with:

1. Ara-C: 100 mg/m^2 s.c. q 12 h × 10 doses (5 days)
2. Alternate with these 5-day courses of ara-C:
   - 6-Thioguanine 100 mg/m^2 p.o. q 12 h × 10 doses (5 days) on maintenance course 1, 5, 9, 13, etc.
   - Vincristine 2 mg/day 1 plus prednisone 40 mg/m^2/day × 5 days on maintenance courses 2, 4, 6, 8, 10, etc. (every other course)
   - Daunorubicin 45 mg/m^2 i.v. day 1 + 2 (two doses) on maintenance courses 3, 7, 11, 15 etc. (maximum total dose 450 mg/m^2)

13.17.3 Reinduction Therapy after Relapse:

High dose Ara-C and m-Amsa may be useful drugs in relapsing AML or a primary therapy in poor risk AML.

13.18 Bone Marrow Transplantation in Acute Leukaemia

Experimental procedure, which should be considered in the following situations:
1. When an identical twin is available as donor: heterologous bone marrow transplantation is indicated in first complete remission.
2. In patients of the younger age group in first remission of acute leukaemia, when an HLA-matched sibling is available as donor: heterologous bone marrow transplantation should be considered.

13.18.1 Sequences of the Procedure

1. Total-body irradiation + aggressive chemotherapy for eradication of all residual leukaemic cells (and normal bone marrow stem cells)
2. Infusion of the donor's marrow
3. Intensive supportive care, until recovery from total aplasia occurs by the donor's marrow
4. Immunosuppressive measures for the prevention of graft-versus-host disease (GVHD), due to minor histocompatibility differences:
   - Methotrexate
   - Anti-thymocyte globulin
   - Cyclosporin A
   - Acyclovir?
   - Monoclonal anti-T-cell antibodies?
   - Hyperalimentation

13.18.2 Complications of Bone Marrow Transplantation

a) Mortality by GVHD: is decreasing from 50% to 30%, acute or chronic
b) Mortality by opportunistic infection due to immunological incompetence after transplantation:
   - Gram-negative bacteria, fungi (especially *Candida*)
   - Pneumocystis carinii pneumonia
   - Cytomegalovirus infection
   - Other "idiopathic" or opportunistic infections

13.18.3 Results

30%-50% long-term survivors, when bone marrow transplantation is performed in first remission of AML or first and second remission or early relapse of ALL

Further Reading

1. Aisenberg AC (1981) Current concepts in immunology: cell-surface markers in lymphoproliferative disease. New Engl J Med 304: 331
2. Benett JM et al (1976) Proposal for the classification of the acute leukaemias. Brit J Haematol 33: 451-458
3. Bloomfield CD (1980) Treatment of adult acute nonlymphocytic leukemia - 1980. Ann Intern Med 93: 133
4. Ellison RR (1975) Management of acute leukaemia in adults. Medical and Paediatric Oncology 1: 149-158
5. Gale RP (1979) Advances in the treatment of acute myelogenous leukemia. N Engl J Med 300: 1189-1199
6. Gee TS, Haghbin M, Dowling MD, et al (1976) Acute lymphoblastic leukaemia in adults and children. Cancer 37: 1251-1264
7. McCredie KB, Freireich EJ (1975) Acute leukemia: Chemotherapy and management. In: Greenspan EM (ed) Clinical cancer chemotherapy. Raven Press, New York
8. Prognostic factors in acute leukemia. Seminars in Oncology 3: 199-325, 1976
9. Whittacker JA (1980) Immunotherapy in the treatment of acute leukemia. Brit J Haemat 45: 187

14 Chronic Leukaemia

14.1 Epidemiology and Aetiology of Chronic Leukaemias

Few statistical data concerning incidence and mortality of the chronic leukaemias are available because these are rarely separated from other leukaemias.

Chronic myelocytic leukaemia (CML) accounts for about one-third to one-fourth of the acute leukaemias with about 12 cases per million individuals. It is slightly more frequent in male than in female patients. The incidence steadily increases with age and reaches 30 cases per million in people over 60 years.

The incidence of chronic lymphocytic leukaemia (CLL) increases from less than 5 per 100000 under the age of 50 years, to more than 20 per 100000 over the age of 60 years, where it is the commonest type of leukaemia. Men are affected twice as often as women, which is the highest male-to-female ratio of all leukaemias.

Exposure to radiation (Hiroshima, Nagasaki, etc.) and chronic exposure to benzene and other chemicals play a role in the appearance of some CML, but not of CLL. Familial factors with possible genetic predisposition seem to be involved in some cases of both forms of chronic leukaemias. CLL is associated with other lymphomas and "auto-immune disorders", CML with genetic factors (Ph^1 chromosome, von Recklinghausen's disease, immune suppression, etc.).

I. CLL

14.2 Clinical Staging of CLL and Survival by Stage (Rai et al. 1975)

Stage		Median survival in months
0	Lymphocytosis only (> 5000/μl blood associated with diffuse lymphocytic infiltration of marrow	> 150
1	Lymphocytosis + lymphadenopathy	101
2	Lymphocytosis + liver and/or splenic enlargement	71
3	Lymphocytosis + anaemia (< 11 g/100 ml) with or without liver, spleen or lymph node enlargement	19
4	Lymphocytosis + thrombocytopenia (< 100000/μl) with or without liver, spleen or lymph node enlargement	19

N. B. If the patient changes stage, the prognosis appears to alter to that of the new stage, from the date of change.

14.3 Definition and Clinical Features of CLL

1. A peripheral blood lymphocytosis of greater than 5000 lymphocytes/μl
2. Diffuse infiltration (greater than 40%) of the marrow with small lymphocytes. Associated features of the disease include:
   a) Lymphadenopathy
   b) Splenomegaly
   c) Hepatomegaly
   d) Other organ infiltration (e. g. lung, pleura, bone, skin, etc.)
   e) Anaemia (haemolytic)
   f) Thrombocytopenia
   g) Increased infection risk and incidence
   h) Hypogammaglobulinaemia
   i) Monoclonal gammopathy (e.g. macroglobulinaemia with hyperviscosity syndrome)
   j) T-cell CLL: hepatosplenomegaly without lymphadenopathy, neutropenia, skin infiltration; abnormal karyotype with pattern of 45 chromosomes. Refractory to therapy: median survival < 1 year
   k) Abnormal karyotypes are frequent, especially an extra chromosome 12

14.4 Investigations for CLL

Haemoglobin
WBC
Differential WBC
Reticulocyte count
Sedimentation rate
Bone marrow examination
Serum immunoglobulins
Blood urea
Uric acid
Calcium
Serum protein and electrophoresis
Chest x-ray
Liver function tests

14.5 Therapeutic Strategy for CLL

14.5.1 Indications for Treatment

Patients with asymptomatic, stable or slowly progressive disease (stages 0+1) may be left untreated and can do well for several years without treatment. There is no evidence that treating these patients when they are asymptomatic leads to longer survival. Several studies are in progress concerning this topic.

Progressive lymphadenopathy or splenomegaly, anaemia, thrombocytopenia and symptoms due to pressure from deposits require treatment (stages 2–4).

14.5.2 Treatment

Is essentially palliative and improves signs and symptoms of the disease, but does not fundamentally change the course of the disease.

1. Chemotherapy. Chlorambucil is the drug most commonly used (4–8 mg/ m^2 p.o. daily for induction). Some authorities prefer to use an intermittent schedule.

Prednisone (40 mg/day initially) is useful for its lympholytic effect and for symptomatic therapy. It is useful in patients with anaemia and thrombocytopenia (stages 3 and 4), but the dose should be reduced after a short course since maintenance therapy can be attended by serious side effects.

Combination chemotherapy has been used with some success in resistant cases and the chlorambucil + vincristine + prednisone (CVP) regimen (see Sect. 15.47) has proved useful in this regard. Other second-line single-agent therapy includes other alkylating agents and streptonigrin. Phase-dependent agents are not, in general, very effective in this disease.

2. Radiotherapy. Local radiotherapy for symptomatic local disease may be useful.

Extracorporeal irradiation of circulating lymphocytes has been used to reduce lymphocytosis and reduce lymphoid-cell masses, but this therapy does not have any real advantage over more conventional forms of treatment.

Other forms of therapy such as antilymphocyte serum and lymphocytophoresis have been used, but these are still experimental. Splenectomy may be helpful if the spleen is causing troublesome symptoms or in patients with hypersplenism.

14.6 Hairy Cell Leukaemia (Leukaemic Reticuloendotheliosis)

a) Massive splenomegaly, absence of lymphadenopathy.
b) Leukocytosis, later pancytopenia and marrow hypoplasia.
c) Marrow infiltration by atypical cells with prominent cytoplasmic projections (hairy cells) and B-cell characteristics.
d) Hairy cells contain tartrate-resistant isoenzyme 5 of acid phosphatase; they may lack reverse transcriptase activity (typical for all other leukaemic cells).

Therapy: Usually resistant to chemotherapy. Interferons promising.
Splenectomy: often results in an increase of WBC, platelets and haemoglobin.

II. Chronic Myeloproliferative Disease

14.7 Myeloproliferative Disease

Dameshek introduced the concept of "myeloproliferative disease" to describe proliferative disorders of bone marrow cells. The concept is a useful one since it is helpful in describing the interrelationship between different members of the group and variants which may occur.

14.7.1 Classification of Chronic Myeloproliferative Disease

Chronic granulocytic leukaemia
- *Ph*[1]-positive: 88%
- *Ph*[1]-negative: 12%: higher age, poorer prognosis

Polycythaemia rubra vera
Essential haemorrhagic thrombocythaemia
Primary myelofibrosis

14.7.2 Clonal Origin of Blood Cells

CML and other myeloproliferative disorders are probably diseases of a multipotential stem cell.

14.8 Chronic Myelocytic Leukaemia

Leukocytosis (WBC frequently $>50\,000/\mu l$).
"Shift-to-the-left" in the blood differential with a small percentage of blast cells and greatly increased numbers of myelocytes and more mature granulocytes. Basophils, eosinophils and their precursors are usually present in increased numbers and may be prominent.
Initial thrombocythaemia is a frequent occurrence.
Hypercellular bone marrow with increased numbers of megakaryocytes and increased granulopoiesis.
Philadelphia chromosome present in red cell, white cell and platelet precursor cells.
Leukocyte alkaline phosphatase absent or low.
Serum B_{12} and B_{12}-binding proteins greatly elevated.

14.9 Distinguishing Features Between Chronic Myelocytic Leukaemia and Myelofibrosis

Distinguishing features	*In chronic myelocytic leukaemia*	*In myelofibrosis*
Ph[1] chromosome	Usually present	Absent
Myelofibrosis	Little or none	Present
Osteosclerosis	Absent	May be present
Red cell morphology	Normal or only slightly abnormal	Anisocytosis prominent and tear drop poikilocytes
Nucleated red cells	Small numbers	Often numerous
WBC	Frequently >50000 µl	Rarely >50000/µl
Leukocyte alkaline phosphatase	Absent or reduced	Normal or increased
Serum B_{12} and B_{12}-binding proteins	Markedly elevated	Normal or slightly elevated

14.10 Course of Chronic Myelocytic Leukaemia

1. Chronic Phase. Months to years (median 36-44 months): this phase is responsive to busulfan.

2. Terminal Phase. Usually blast crisis. Lasts in most cases only 2-3 months until death. Resistant to busulfan. Myeloid blastic phase responds poorly to treatment
Treatment: lymphoid blastic phase may respond to vincristine and prednisone.

14.11 Premonitory Signs of Terminal Phase and/or Blast Crisis in Chronic Myelocytic Leukaemia

1. Fever of unknown origin - often accompanied by weight loss
2. Rapidly increasing organ infiltration in a patient previously well-controlled with chemotherapy:
   a) Rapid increase in spleen size
   b) Lymphadenopathy
   c) Osteolytic bone lesions
   d) Skin infiltration
3. Haemoglobin <9.0 g/100 ml in the absence of haemorrhage

4. Haemoglobin <10.5 g/100 ml, WBC $>30000/\mu l$ and platelet count $<100000/\mu l$ occurring together
5. Falling platelet count
6. Myeloblasts and promyelocytes in the blood $>25\%$
7. Increasing aneuploidy, on chromosomal analysis

14.12 Ph¹-Positive Leukaemia: Surface Marker and Enzymatic Characteristic

	Ia	ALL Antigen	TdT	E	SmIg
Chronic phase	–	–	–	–	–
Blastic phase (myeloid)	+	–	–	–	–
Blastic phase (lymphoid)	+	+	+	–	–
*Ph*¹-positive acute lymphoblastic leukaemia	+	+	+	–	–

TdT, terminal deoxynucleotidyl transferase; E, sheep red cell rosettes; SmIg, surface membrane immunoglobulin

14.13 Treatment and Prognosis of Chronic Myelocytic Leukaemia

14.13.1 Treatment

Busulphan is the most extensively studied agent in chronic myelocytic leukaemia and no other agent has been shown to be superior. The most effective dose schedule is 4 mg/day orally with weekly blood counts. Allopurinol should be given in addition (300 mg daily orally), to prevent hyperuricaemia. Treatment should be interrupted when the leukocyte count reaches 10000/µl. It is wise to reduce the dose if the fall in leukocyte count is rapid, since prolonged myelosuppression may ensue with this agent. The drug is potentially dangerous in patients with platelet counts below 100000/µl. Maintenance doses of 2–4 mg/day may be continued intermittently keeping the leukocyte count at 10000–20000/µl. Dibromomannitol and hydroxyurea may prove useful in patients no longer responsive to busulphan.

Radiotherapy may be useful in reducing splenomegaly and will also lower the leukocyte count. Chemotherapy is more effective in the long term.

Splenectomy in CML is controversial but it may be useful in patients with hypersplenism or in patients with prolonged pancytopenia following chemotherapy. Prophylactic splenectomy may be of advantage in preventing the painful consequences of massive splenomegaly, but it does not alter survival.

Recent clinical studies suggest, that recombinant α-interferon is a very procesising new therapy for CML.

The role of immunotherapy and leukophoresis remains experimental. Chemotherapy for *blast crisis* is unsatisfactory and the median survival is only a few months. Remissions are relatively infrequent and there is no one recommended form of chemotherapy.

There is evidence that there are at least two forms of blast crisis - the lymphoid and myeloid forms which may be distinguished on morphological and biochemical criteria. Vincristine and prednisone may be of value in the former. Lymphoid blast crisis occurs in 20%-30% and has L1 characteristics.

14.13.2 Prognosis

The median survival is about 3 years and has not changed since the introduction of busulphan.

14.14 Polycythaemia Rubra Vera

Clinical features:

1. Headache and fullness in the head.
2. Dizziness, tinnitus.
3. Fatigue.
4. Pruritus.
5. Plethoric appearance - injected mucous membranes.
6. Symptoms related to arterial insufficiency - coronary, cerebral and peripheral.
7. Venous thrombosis.
8. Abdominal pain - associated with splenomegaly, splenic infarction, mesenteric thrombosis, dyspepsia, flatulence, duodenal ulceration.
9. Gastrointestinal haemorrhage.
10. Effects of hyperuricaemia - gout, renal failure, renal stones, tophaceous deposits.
11. Hypertension may be present.

N.B. Diagnostic features: total red cell volume >36 ml/kg (male patients); >32 ml/kg (female patients). Arterial oxygen saturation >92%, splenomegaly

14.15 Differential Diagnosis of Polycythaemia

1. Relative dehydration or redistribution of body fluids.
2. Polycythaemia rubra vera.
3. Secondary polycythaemia (associated with increased erythropoietin).
4. Hypoxia - due to chronic respiratory failure, congenital cyanotic heart disease or altitude.
5. Tumour - Renal carcinoma, nephroblastoma
   - Uterine fibroma
   - Posterior cerebral fossa tumours, e.g. cerebellar haemangioblastoma
   - Hepatoma
   - Androgen-secreting tumours
   - Bronchial carcinoma
   - Phaeochromocytoma
6. Haemoglobinopathy - with Hb having high avidity for O_2 (e.g. Hb.Ypsi).
7. Benign familial polycythaemia (some haemoglobinopathies may be included here).

14.16 Distinguishing Features Between Polycythaemia Rubra Vera and Secondary Polycythaemia

Distinguishing features	Polycythaemia rubra vera	Secondary polycythaemia
Pruritus	Common	Absent
Splenomegaly	Common	Usually absent
WBC	Frequently increased	Usually normal
Platelet count	Frequently increased	Normal
Leukocyte alkaline phosphatase	Frequently increased	Normal in the absence of infection
Serum B_{12}	Moderately increased	Normal
B_{12}-binding proteins	Moderately increased	Normal

14.17 Differential Diagnosis of Myelofibrosis

Primary:	Acute	
	Chronic	
Secondary:	Intoxication	Fluorosis
		Benzene poisoning
	Malignant infiltration of marrow	Metastases (e.g. carcinoma of breast, prostate)
		Hodgkin's disease
		Secondary to other chronic myeloproliferative disorders
	Chronic infection	Tuberculosis
		Syphilis
	Renal osteodystrophy with osteosclerosis	
	Irradiation	
	Marble bone disease	
	Mastocytosis with generalized osteosclerosis, hepatosplenomegaly and urticaria pigmentosa	

14.18 Polycythaemia Rubra Vera

14.18.1 Treatment

1. Venesection. Venesection is of value in reducing the packed cell volume and helping viscosity problems associated with polycythaemia. The effect is, however, usually short-lived and recurrent venesection may result in iron deficiency.

2. Radioactive Phosphorus, ^{32}P. 5–10 mCi ^{32}P as a single i.v. injection is useful in the control of a high platelet count and, to a lesser exent, the polycythaemia. Remissions may last 2–3 years following a single dose. Doses may be repeated but are not recommended within 6 months. With repeated injections, there is an increasing risk of developing leukaemia.

Allopurinol should be used in addition to prevent hyperuricaemia.

3. Chemotherapy. Chemotherapy using oral alkylating agents such as busulphan may also be useful in controlling the polycythaemia and high platelet count.

14.18.2 Prognosis

The median survival is about 13 years.

Further Reading

1. Hugueley CM Jr (1978) Treatment of chronic lymphocytic leukaemia. Cancer Treat Review 4: 261-273
2. Liepman MK (1980) The chronic leukaemias. Med Clin N Amer 64: 705
3. Rai KR, Sawitsky A, Cronkite EP, et al (1975) Clinical staging of chronic lymphocytic leukaemia. Blood 46: 219
4. Spiers ASD (1976) The treatment of chronic granulocytic leukaemia. Brit J Haematol 32: 291
5. Symposium on leukaemia (1976) Archives Int Med 136: 1375

15 Malignant Lymphomas

I. Hodgkin's Disease

15.1 Incidence and Epidemiology

Marked variation from country to country, ranging from 1/100000 in rural Poland to 9.1/100000 in the non-Jewish population of Israel

15.2 Aetiology and Risk Factors

15.2.1 Aetiology

Aetiology is unknown.

15.2.2 Host Factors

1. *Sex.* M/F changes as a function of age but male incidence greater than female.
2. *Age.* Incidence remains constant after peak in 3rd decade in developed countries.
3. *Genetic Predisposition.* Controversial. Recent familial studies suggest that this is minimal; there is some association with several HLA antigens.

15.2.3 Environmental Factors

Insufficient evidence is available to imply an association.

15.3 Histopathological Classification of Hodgkin's Disease

Rye	*Distinctive features*	*Relative frequency %*
Lymphocyte predominance (LP)	Abundant stroma of mature lymphocytes and/or histiocytes; no necrosis; Reed-Sternberg cells may be sparse	10–15
Nodular sclerosis (NS)	Nodules of lymphoid tissue, partially or completely separated by bands of doubly refractile collagen of variable width; atypical Reed-Sternberg cells in clear spaces ("lacunae") in the lymphoid nodules	30–70
Mixed cellularity (MC)	Usually numerous Reed-Sternberg and atypical mononuclear cells with a pleomorphic admixture of plasma cells, oesinophils, lymphocytes and fibroblasts; foci of necrosis commonly seen	20–40
Lymphocyte depletion (LD)	Reed-Sternberg and malignant mononuclear cells usually, though not always, numerous; marked paucity of lymphocytes; diffuse fibrosis and necrosis may be present	5–15

15.4 Main Clinical Presentations in Hodgkin's Disease

Superficial adenopathy in $\geqslant$80% of cases
Mediastinal adenopathy in ~50% of cases
Fever, night sweats, weight loss, pruritus in ~40% of cases

15.5 Anatomical Lymph Node Regions to be Used for Staging Definition in Hodgkin's Disease (and Non-Hodgkin Lymphomas)

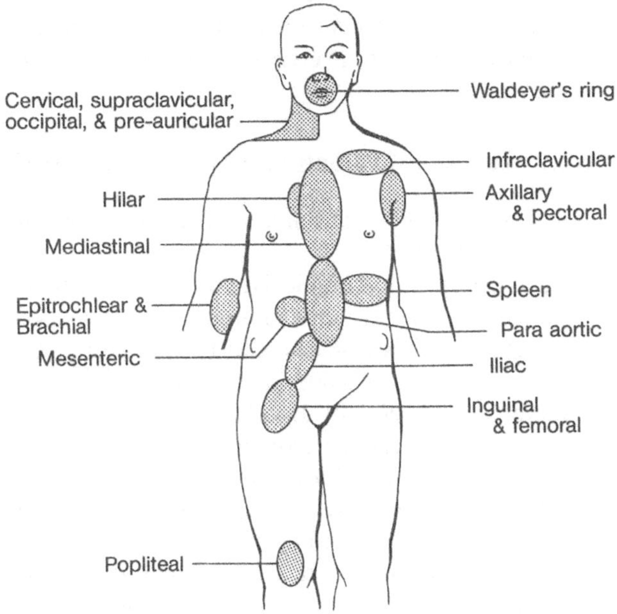

15.6 Staging Procedures

15.6.1 Required Evaluation procedures for 'Clinical Staging'

1. Detailed history with special attention to systemic symptoms outlined above
2. Complete physical examination with attention to lymphadenopathy, including epitrochlear nodes, Waldeyer's ring, hepatomegaly or splenomegaly, bone tenderness
3. Adequate surgical biopsy, reviewed by an experienced haemopathologist
4. Radiological studies:
   a) Chest x-ray (postero-anterior and lateral views) with mediastinal tomography
   b) Bilateral lower extremity lymphangiograms
5. Laboratory studies:

a) Complete blood count, platelet count, erythrocyte sedimentation rate
b) Evaluation of liver function to include at least serum alkaline phosphatase level and serum electrophoresis
c) Evaluation of renal function to include urinalysis, blood urea nitrogen (BUN), serum creatinine, serum uric acid, serum electrolytes (Na, Cl, K, Ca, P)

15.6.2 Required Evaluation Procedures for 'Pathological Staging'

1. Core needle biopsy of bone marrow from posterior iliac crest. Biopsy should be bilateral.
2. Laparoscopy with multiple liver biopsies (4 to 6) if bone marrow is normal and no other distant extranodal lesions are present. Laparoscopy is indicated in clinical stages (CS) IB, IIA and IIIB if the treatment programme consists of combined radiotherapy-chemotherapy; in obese, elderly and emotionally unstable patients as well as in patients with other systemic diseases (cardiovascular, renal, etc.).
3. Staging laparotomy with splenectomy, needle and wedge biopsy of liver, and biopsies of para-aortic, mesenteric, portal, and splenic hilar lymph nodes is indicated after negative bone marrow biopsy in cases with CS I–II (A and B) and IIIA if therapeutic decisions will depend on the identification of occult abdominal involvement, particularly splenic involvement.
4. Cytological examination of any effusion.

15.7 Results of Staging Laparotomy in Hodgkin's Disease

Spleen:	Positive in 30%–35% at laparotomy (only one-third of positive cases detected from laparoscopy)
Liver:	Positive in 2%–6% at laparotomy (almost equivalent percentage at laparoscopy)
Occult retroperitoneal lymph nodes:	Positive in 2%–5%
Coeliac and hepatic hilar lymph nodes:	Positive in 10%–12%
Mesenteric lymph nodes:	Positive in 2%–4%

15.8 Technique and Advantages of Laparoscopy

15.8.1 Technique

1. Sedation with diazepam and local anaesthesia with Xylocaine.
2. Insertion of a Veress needle into the left lower quadrant of the abdomen and creation of pneumoperitoneum (2–3 l CO_2).
3. Insertion of trocar 1–2 cm above the umbilicus in the midline. In patients with prior abdominal surgery, the trocar is placed laterally on the right side.
4. Examination through Wolf cold light endoscope.
5. Liver biopsies (four to six) with Tru-cut needle. Wedge biopsy of liver carried out with Palmer forceps.
6. Spleen biopsies (one to three) with Tru-cut needle can be obtained in selected patients.

15.8.2 Advantages

1. Detects liver involvement in most patients with hepatic infiltration.
2. Detects spleen involvement in approximately one-third of patients with splenic infiltration, especially when tumour nodules are present on the surface.
3. Can be easily repeated to assess the status of remission when liver is involved before chemotherapy.
4. Can be performed under local anaesthesia; operating room is not required; the procedure is usually completed in 20–30 min.
5. Produces minimal morbidity, and recovery is rapid (12–24 h).
6. Reduces costs and hospital stay.

15.9 Required Evaluation Procedures Under Certain Conditions

1. Whole-lung tomography, if abnormality on chest x-ray
2. Intravenous pyelogram if bulky retroperitoneal lymph nodes are present
3. If indicated, appropriate bone x-rays in areas of suspected abnormality
4. Skeletal scintigrams in presence of bone pain and/or tenderness, or elevated serum alkaline phosphatase and/or elevated serum calcium and negative skeletal survey plus bone marrow biopsy
5. Whole-body gallium-67 scintigram
6. Abdominal computed tomography or abdominal sonography
7. Lung or bone biopsy in presence of equivocal x-ray findings
8. Determination of serum iron and iron-binding capacity

15.10 Staging

15.10.1 Ann Arbor Modification of the Rye Staging System for Hodgkin's Disease (1971)

Stage	*Description*
Stage I	Involvement of a single lymph node region (I) or of a single extralymphatic organ or site (I_E)
Stage II	Involvement of two or more lymph node regions on the same side of the diaphragm (II) or localized involvement of a single extralymphatic organ or site and of one or more lymph node regions on the same side of the diaphragm (II_E). Optional recommendation: number of node regions involved indicated by subscript, e.g. $II_{(3)}$
Stage III	Involvement of lymph node regions on both sides of the diaphragm (III), which may also be accompanied by localized involvement of extralymphatic organ or site (III_E) or by involvement of the spleen (III_S), or both (III_{SE})
Stage IV	Multiple or disseminated involvement of one or more extralymphatic organs or tissue with or without associated lymph node enlargement. The reason for classifying the patient as being in Stage IV should be identified further by defining site symbols

Subclassification:

A – denotes no specific symptoms

B – denotes specific symptoms as follows

1. Unexplained body weight loss of more than 10% over a 6-month period
2. Unexplained recurrent fever with temperature above 38 °C
3. Night sweats

15.10.1.1 Splenic and Hepatic Involvement in Clinical Staging as Defined in the Ann Arbor Classification

Involvement	*Definition*
Splenic	Either palpable enlargement confirmed by radiographic or radioisotopic studies on an isotopic scan showing marked filling defects. 50% of clinically enlarged spleens are not involved histologically; 50% of normal-sized spleens are involved histologically
Hepatic	An enlarged liver and at least an abnormal serum alkaline phosphatase value, two different liver function test abnormalities, or an abnormal liver scan and one abnormal liver function test

15.11 Ann Arbor Pathological Stage Distribution of Previously Untreated Patients with Hodgkin's Disease

Ann Arbor stage	Percentage of cases
I	10-15
II	45-50 (A 30-40; B 15-20)
III	28-30
IV	10-12

15.12 Percentage Rate of Systemic Symptoms Related to Stage in 349 Consecutive Untreated Patients with Hodgkin's Disease Admitted to the Istituto Nazionale Tumori of Milan from 1962 to 1972

Systemic symptoms	Stage				
	I (84)	II (127)	III (122)	IV (16)	Total (349)
No	93	65	47	12.5	63
Yes	7	35	53	87.5	37

15.13 Radiation Therapy Fields in Hodgkin's Disease [and Non-Hodgkin Lymphomas (modified from Kaplan and Rosenberg)]

1. Mantle. Encompasses mediastinal, hilar, and bilateral supraclavicular, infraclavicular, cervical, and axillary node chains, with lead shields shaped to lungs, heart, and spinal cord (after 2000 rads).

2. Inverted-Y. Encompasses splenic or splenic pedicle, para-aortic, iliac, inguinal, and femoral node chains, with lead shields for rectum and bladder, iliac and upper femoral bone marrow, and "gap" at junction with mantle field; or

3. Spade. Encompasses splenic or splenic pedicle, para-aortic and common iliac node chains with double-thickness lead shields for gonads and pelvic structures; or

4. Para-Aortic/Hepatic. Encompasses splenic hilar and para-aortic node chains and entire right lobe of liver (through 50% transmission lead block), usually joined across another "gap" by a separate pelvic field.

5. Pelvic Field. Encompasses external iliac, inguinal, and femoral node chains, with lead shields for rectum and bladder, iliac and upper femoral bone marrow.

6. "Waldeyer". For HD opposed lateral fields, encompassing preauricular nodes and lymphatic tissues of Waldeyer's ring when clinically involved or when adenopathy is present in high cervical nodes. In patients with non-Hodgkin lymphoma primary in Waldeyer's ring, larger fields must always be employed to broadly encompass both the extranodal sites to include the base of skull as well as the entire cervical regions.

7. Abdominal Bath. Full-thickness lead blocks protect the right hepatic lobe during the initial 1500-rad whole abdominal treatment (through anterior-posterior opposed fields). Horizontal decubitus (cross-table) lateral fields are then used to bring the para-aortic and mesenteric lymph node radiation doses to 3000 rads, followed by an additional 1400 rads through wide anterior-posterior ports, for a total central abdominal dose of 4400 rads.

15.14 Main Conventional Radiation Fields for Hodgkin's Disease

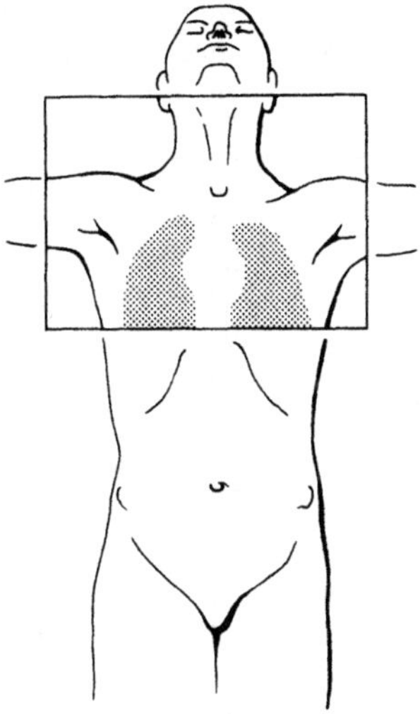

A Mantle

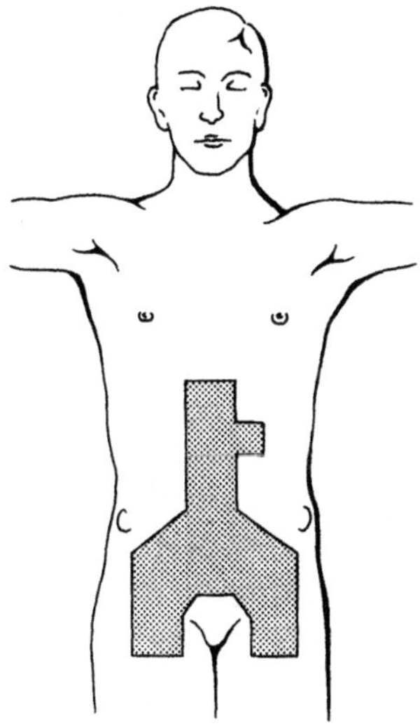

B Inverted "Y"

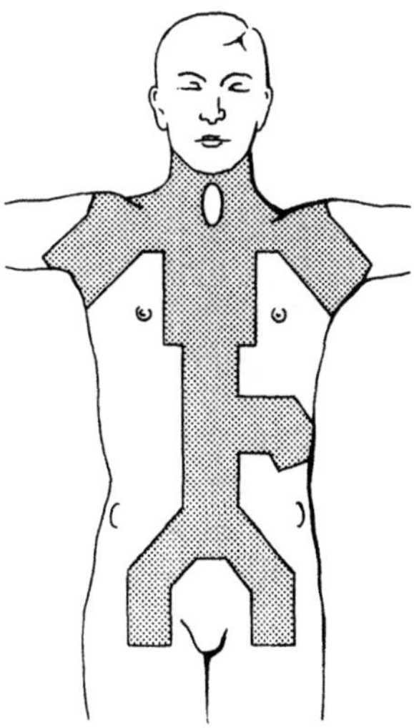

C Total nodal irradiation (TNI)

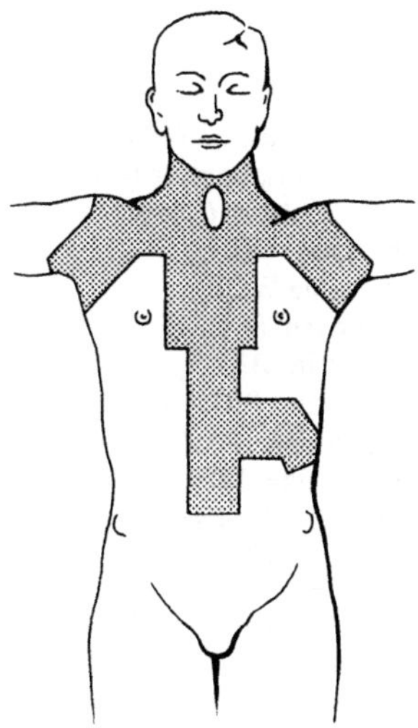

D Subtotal nodal irradiation (STNI)

15.15 Examples of 5-Year Relapse-Free Survival and Overall Survival in Hodgkin's Disease after Extensive Radiotherapy

Institution	Pathological stage	No. of cases	Type of radiotherapy	Relapse-free survival (%)	Survival (%)
Stanford	IA-IIA	87	TNI	70	84
	IB-IIB	53	TNI	79	89
	IIIA	60	TNI	67	81
	IIIB	44	TNI	7	44
Harvard	IA	38	STNI	97	100
	IIA	80	STNI	80	93
	IIB	11	STNI/TNI	82	91
	IIIA	37	TNI	51	82
	IIIB	7	TNI	43	-
Milan	IA	49	Mantle/STNI	73	85
	IIA	48	Mantle/STNI	62	78
Royal Marsden	I-II	78	Mantle/STNI	80	-
Yale	IIIA	48	TNI	35	80
Memorial	IIIA	78	TNI	78	89
	IIIB	29	TNI	48	80

15.16 Single Agents Effective in Hodgkin's Disease

Single drugs	Response rate
Nitrogen mustard (HN_2), cyclophosphamide (CTX), chlorambucil (CHL)	70%-80%
Vinblastine (VBL)	70%-80%
Vincristine (VCR)	40%-60%
Adriamycin (ADM)	60%-75%
Bleomycin (BLM)	45%-60%
Prednisone (PRD), prednisolone	40%-65%
Procarbazine (PCZ)	40%-80%
Dacarbazine (DTIC)	56%
Carmustine (BCNU)	40%-50%
Lomustine (CCNU)	50%-65%

Complete remission (CR) in only 10%-20% of cases.

15.17 Combinations Effective in Hodgkin's Disease

Combination	No. of patients	CR (%)[a]
HN_2-VCR-PCZ-PRD (MOPP)	1189	68
HN_2-VBL-PCZ-PRD (MVPP)	227	69
CTX-VCR-PCZ-PRD (COPP)	102	66
CTX-VBL-PCZ-PRD (CVPP)	114	64
CHL-VBL-PCZ-PRD (CHLVPP)	118	69
BCNU-CTX-VBL-PRD (BCVP)	25	52
ADM-BLM-VBL-DTIC (ABVD)	35	72
HN_2-ADM-BLM-VCR-PRD (MABOP)	56	63
BLM-HN_2-VCR-PCZ-PRD (B-MOPP)	156	82
BCNU-CTX-VLB-PCZ-PRD (BCVPP)	115	68

[a] Approx. 60% of complete responders after MOPP remain in CR at least 5 and 10 years.

15.18 CR Following MOPP Chemotherapy in Patients Relapsing After Radiotherapy

Institution	Patients	CR (%)
Stanford	60	62
Stanford	41	51
Southwest Oncology Group (SWOG)	31	74
NCI	27	70
NCI	21	76
Harvard	12	73
Total	192	65

15.19 Response to ABVD in Refractory Hodgkin's Disease (Bonadonna and Santoro)

Reference	No. of patients	Response rate (%)	
		CR	Overall
Santoro	54	59	72
Krikorian	27	22	37
Case	24	4	63
Amiel	22	32	32
Bauters	21	43	77
Vicente	15	33	87
Sutcliffe	11	0	46.5
Clamon	9	0	11
Rossof	3	0	100
Total	186	32	57.5

15.20 Recommended Drug Combination Schedules for Hodgkin's Disease

15.20.1 First-Line Chemotherapy

1. Outline of MOPP schedule (one cycle)

Drugs (mg/m^2)	Days				
	1	8	14		28
HN_2[a]	6	6			
VCR	1.4	1.4		No	
PCZ	100 ⟶	⟶	⟶	Therapy	
PRD[b]	40 ⟶	⟶	⟶		

[a] Cytoxan or chlorambucil can be used as an alternative.
[b] Given on cycles 1 and 4.

2. Outline of MVPP schedule (one cycle)

Drugs (mg/m²)	Days 1	8	14		42
HN₂[a]	6	6			
VBL	6	6		No	
PCZ	100 ⟶	⟶	⟶	Therapy	
PRD[b]	40 ⟶	⟶	⟶		

[a] Also as MOPP.
[b] Also as MOPP.

15.20.2 Second-Line Chemotherapy

MOPP salvage regimen (ABVD schedule – one cycle)

Drugs (mg/m²)	Days 1	14		28
ADM	25	25		
BLM	10	10	No	
VBL	6	6	Therapy	
DTIC	375	375		

15.20.3 Other Salvage Regimens

1. Outline of B-DOPA schedule (one cycle)

Drugs (mg/m²)	Days 1	2	3	4	5	6		22
BLM		4			4			
DTIC	150	150	150	150	150		No	
VCR	1.5				1.5		Therapy	
PRD	40					40		
ADM	60							

2. Outline of B-CAVe schedule (one cycle)

Drugs (mg/m²)	Days 1	28	35		43
BLM	2.5	2.5	2.5		
CCNU	100			No	
ADM	60			Therapy	
VBL	5				

3. Outline of BVDS schedule (one cycle)

Drugs (mg/m²)	Days 1	15		29
BLM		6		
VBL	6	6	No	
ADM	30		Therapy	
Streptozotocin	1500	1500		

4. Outline of CVB schedule (one cycle)

Drugs (mg/m²)	Days 1	8		29
CCNU	100			
VBL	5	5	No	
BLM	8-10	8-10	Therapy	

5. Outline of SCAB schedule (one cycle)

Drugs (mg/m²)	Days 1	2	3	4	5	8		29
Streptozotocin	500	500	500	500	500			
CCNU	100						No	
ADM	45						Therapy	
BLM	15					15		

15.21 Therapeutic Strategy of Hodgkin's Disease by Stage

Stage	Therapy
IA-IIA	STNI
IB-IIB	TNI or STNI + chemotherapy[a]
IIIA-IIISA	TNI or STNI + chemotherapy[a]
IIIB-IIISB	TNI + chemotherapy
IVA-IVB	Chemotherapy (MOPP or MOPP + ABVD)
Relapse after radiotherapy	Chemotherapy ± radiotherapy
MOPP resistance	Non-cross-resistant chemotherapy (ABVD or other second-line regimens)

[a] Although combined-modality treatment is not a fully established treatment modality, it should be tried in the case of patients with unfavourable prognosis.

15.22 Prognostic Factors in Hodgkin's Disease

1. Age. Survival significantly better in young compared to elderly patients.

2. Sex. Better prognosis of female patients.

3. Histopathology. In patients treated with combination chemotherapy, the nodular sclerosis seems correlated with the less favourable prognosis.

4. Stage. Survival is correlated to the anatomical extent of disease. Bulky disease in nodal and extranodal sites carries unfavourable prognosis.

5. Systemic Symptoms. They are associated with more unfavourable prognosis.

6. Complete Remission. Patients achieving CR live longer than those with partial remission (PR) or no remission (NR).

15.23 Main Long-Term Side Effects of Radiotherapy in Hodgkin's Disease

a) Radiation pneumonia
b) Growth retardation in children
c) Reduction in fertility only when pelvis irradiated (ovaries)

15.24 Complications of Chemotherapy and Combined Treatment in Hodgkin's Disease

1. For toxic signs related to the types of drugs included in the various regimens, see Chap. 6.
2. Long-term chemotherapy induces sterility in at least 50% of men and women. ABVD produces lower incidence of azospermia and prolonged amenorrhoea than MOPP. After MOPP-induced sterility, 10% of men and 40% of women regain fertility. Potency is not affected in the long term.
3. Total incidence of acute non-lymphoblastic leukaemia within 10 years ranges from 2% to 3%. The highest incidence occurs in patients treated with extensive radiotherapy and MOPP (4.5%–5%).

II. Non-Hodgkin Lymphomas

15.25 Incidence and Epidemiology

Incidence varies from 2 to 6/100000. Linear increase in rate from childhood to age 75 years.

15.26 Risk Factors

15.26.1 Host Factors

1. Sex. Male slightly higher than female patients. Childhood peak exists especially for Burkitt's lymphoma. Most childhood lymphomas have a diffuse histology.
2. Genetic Predisposition. Increased in families with immunological defects.

15.26.2 Environmental Factors, Drugs

Immunsuppressive therapy and diphenylhydantoin

15.27 Rappaport Histopathological Classification of Non-Hodgkin Lymphomas

Nodular pattern		Diffuse pattern	
NLWD	Lymphocytic well-differentiated	DLWD	Lymphocytic well-differentiated
NLPD	Lymphocytic poorly-differentiated	DLPD	Lymphocytic poorly-differentiated
NH	Histiocytic	DH	Histiocytic
NM	Mixed histiocytic-lymphocytic	DM	Mixed histiocytic-lymphocytic
		DU	Undifferentiated (non-Burkitt)

15.28 Working Formulation of Non-Hodgkin Lymphomas for Clinical Usage and Equivalent or Related Terms in the Rappaport and Kiel Classifications

Rappaport	Working formulation	Kiel
	Low Grade	
LWD	A. Small lymphocytic consistent with CLL, plasmacytoid	Lymphocytic (CLL) Lymphoplasmatic/lymphoplasmacytoid (LPL)
NLPD	B. Follicular, predominantly small cleaved cell, diffuse areas-sclerosis	Centroblastic-centrocytic (CB-CC) (small), follicular ± diffuse
NM	C. Follicular mixed, small cleaved and large cell, diffuse areas sclerosis	
	Intermediate Grade	
NH	D. Follicular, predominantly large cell, diffuse areas sclerosis	Centroblastic-centrocytic (CB-CC) (large), follicular ± diffuse
DLPD	E. Diffuse, small cleaved and large cell, sclerosis	Centrocytic CC (small)
DM	F. Diffuse mixed, small and large cell, sclerosis epitheloid cell component	Lymphoplasmacytic-cytoid, polymorphic (LPL, polym.) Centroblastic-centrocytic (CB-CC) (small), diffuse
DH	G. Diffuse large cell, cleaved cell, non-cleaved cell, sclerosis	Centroblastic-centrocytic (CB-CC) (large), diffuse Centrocytic (large) (CC-LG) Centroblastic (CB)
	High Grade	
DH	H. Large cell, immunoblastic plasmacytoid clear cell, polymorphous epitheloid cell component	Immunoblastic (IB) T-zone Lymphoepitheloid cell
LB	I. Lymphoblastic convoluted cell, nonconvoluted cell	Lymphoblastic (LB), convoluted cell type Lymphoblastic (LB), unclassified
Undifferentiated	J. Small non-cleaved cell, Burkitt's follicular areas	Lymphoblastic (LB) Burkitt-type and other B-lymphoblastic
	Miscellaneous	
	Composite	-
	Mycosis fungoides	mycosis fungoides
	Histiocytic	-
	Extramedullary plasmacytoma	Plasmacytic -
	Unclassifiable	-
	Other	

CLL, chronic lymphocytic leukaemia

15.29 Non-Hodgkin Lymphomas: Prognosis

Favourable	Unfavourable
1. Long natural history	1. Rapid disease progression
2. Middle-aged patients	2. Young and elderly patients
3. Disease confined to lymph nodes, marrow and liver	3. Extranodal disease - CNS, GI tract, bone, testis, leukaemia
4. Cytokinetic: low growth fraction	4. Cytokinetic: high growth fraction
5. B-lymphocyte markers	5. T-cell markers or null cell
6. Nodular histology	6. Diffuse histology
NLWD	DU (Burkitt's)
NLPD	DH (immunoblastic)
NM	DLPD (lymphoblastic)
DLWD	DM

15.30 Main Clinical Presentations in Non-Hodgkin Lymphomas: Sites of Individual Involvement

Lymph nodes
Extranodal sites
- Head and neck (Waldeyer's ring)
- Gastrointestinal tract (stomach, small bowel, ileocaecal region)
- Skin
- Bone
- Lung and pleura

N.B. Fever, night sweats, weight loss, pruritus in ~10% of cases.

15.31 Staging Evaluation Procedures for Non-Hodgkin Lymphomas

15.31.1 Required Evaluation Procedures for Clinical Staging

1. Detailed history
2. Complete physical examination with attention to lymphadenopathy, Waldeyer's ring, hepatomegaly, splenomegaly, bone tenderness
3. Adequate surgical biopsy, reviewed by histopathologist
4. Radiological studies: chest x-ray (postero-anterior and lateral views) with mediastinal tomography, bilateral lower-extremity lymphangiogram
5. Laboratory studies:

a) Complete blood counts, platelet count, erythrocyte sedimentation rate
b) Evaluation of liver function to include at least serum alkaline phosphatase level and serum electrophoresis
c) Evaluation of renal function to include urinalysis, BUN, serum creatinine, serum uric acid, serum electrolytes (Na, Cl, K, Ca, P)

15.31.2 Required Evaluation Procedures for Pathological Staging

1. Bilateral bone marrow biopsy
2. Laparoscopy with multiple spleen and liver biopsies; laparotomy may be considered for those patients with apparently truly localized disease - stage I only
3. Skeletal survey (thoraco-lumbar vertebrae, pelvis, proximal extremities and areas of bone tenderness or pain)

15.31.3 Required Evaluation Procedures Under Certain Conditions

1. Intravenous pyelogram, if bulky retroperitoneal lymph nodes are present
2. Bone scan and skeletal survey (thoraco-lumbar vertebrae, pelvis, proximal extremities if areas of bone tenderness or pain are present
3. Abdominal computed tomography or ultrasonography of liver and abdomen
4. Determination of serum iron and iron-binding capacity

15.32 Staging Classification

The Ann Arbor Classification is also being adopted for the non-Hodgkin lymphomas. The clinical utility is less evident for the non-Hodgkin lymphomas because of the frequent difficulty of assigning to the four established stage designations all types of extranodal presentations and because of the fact that the survival of most patients with follicular lymphoma is prolonged even in advanced stages, while in patients with diffuse histology the survival tends to be comparatively short, even with nodal disease alone.

Splenic and hepatic involvement in clinical staging as defined in the Ann Arbor Classification is also used for non-Hodgkin lymphomas.

15.33 Results of Pathological Staging in Non-Hodgkin Lymphomas

Spleen: Positive in 24%-30% at laparoscopy
Liver: Positive in 20% at laparoscopy; laparotomy in patients with negative laparoscopy has shown liver involvement only in small number of patients
Bone marrow: Positive in 10% if one-needle marrow biopsy performed, in 20% of cases with bilateral biopsy

15.34 Ann Arbor Pathological Stage Distribution of Previously Untreated Patients with Non-Hodgkin Lymphomas

Non-Hodgkin Lymphomas (%)		
Stage	Follicular	Others
I	7-10	15-20
II	7-10	20-22
III	10-15	10-15
IV	66-70	45-55

15.35 Five-Year Survival in Early Stages of Non-Hodgkin Lymphomas Treated with Radiation Therapy

Author	Stage	Patients	Nodular (%)	Diffuse (%)
Fuller	I-II	226	65	26
Tubiana	I-II	123	55	36
Unnik	I-II	180	55	32
Peckham	I-II	51	78	50
Patchefksy	I-II	65	55	58
Milan	I-II	117	79	39

15.36 Single Agents Effective in Non-Hodgkin Lymphomas

Drugs	CR + PR (%)	
Chlorambucil	45-65	CR in only 10-20% of cases
Cyclophosphamide (CTX)	55-65	
Vincristine (VCR)	40-65	
Vinblastine (VLB)	20-35	
Adriamycin (ADM)	45-65	
Bleomycin (BLM)	35-45	
Methotrexate (MTX)	25-30	
Cytosine arabinoside (CA)	25-30	
BCNU, CCNU	20-35	
Procarbazine (PCZ)	30-50	
Prednisone (PRD)	20-80	
L-asparaginase	40	
Vindesine	30-40	
Etoposide (VP-16-213)	40	

15.37 Principal Combinations Effective in Stage III and IV Non-Hodgkin Lymphomas

C-MOPP	: CTX, VCR, PCZ, PRD
CHOP	: CTX, ADM, VCR, PRD
HOP	: ADM, VCR, PRD
BACOP	: BLM, ADM, VCR, CTX, PRD
CHOP-BLEO	: CTX, ADM, VCR, PRD, BLM
M-BACOD	: BACOP modified (DEX and MTX + CF)
COMA	: CTX, VCR, MTX, CA
COMLA	: CTX, VCR, MTX + CF, CA
CVP + ABP	: CTX, VCR, PRD + ADM, BLM, PRD
PRO MACE-MOPP	: CTX, ADM, VP-16-213, MTX + CF, PRD

CF, citrovorum factor; DEX, dexamethasone

15.38 Results Which Can be Achieved with Combination Chemotherapy in DLPD, DM, DU, NH Lymphomas

Subgroup	CR (%)	Tendency to recurrence
DLPD	44-68	Higher than DH
DM	50-71	
DU	40	Almost superimposable to DH
NH	50	Almost superimposable to DH

15.39 Prolonged Initial Remission in Patients with Nodular Mixed Lymphoma (Modified from De Vita)

Treatment	No. of patients	CR (%)	Median duration of CR (months)
C-MOPP	52		>72
CVP			22
Radiotherapy	17	75	8
Radiotherapy + C-MOPP	6		72

Of 27 patients relapsing from CR, 14 (52%) achieved a second CR with median survival from relapse = 5.5 years

15.40 Patients with Stage IV Non-Hodgkin Lymphomas Favourable Histologies. Results of the Controlled Stanford Study (1981)

Treatment	No. of patients	CR (%)	Median relapse-free survival (months)	Actuarial survival at 7 years
CVP	23	83	50	56%
CVP-TLI	20	65	50	60%
Single alkylating agents	20	65	50	78%

TLI, total lymphoid irradiation

15.41 Factors to be Considered for the Clinical Management of Non-Hodgkin Lymphomas with Favourable Histology

1. Most often they present as advanced disease.
2. The incidence of CR after single agents (alkylating agents) is generally not inferior to that induced by combination chemotherapy.
3. A pattern of continuous late recurrence follows unmaintained CR. Therefore, maintenance chemotherapy is indicated.
4. Prolonged chemotherapy of moderate intensity can induce long-term survival in PR_S.
5. NH can be probably cured by combination chemotherapy.

15.42 Results of Whole-Body Irradiation of Indolent Non-Hodgkin Lymphomas with Stage III and IV (modified from Portlock)

Author	No. of patients	CR (%)	Median duration of CR (months)	Actuarial survival (median in months)
Carabell	43	-	24	>96
Young	33	85	26	>26
Choi	31	84	24	>48
Thar	28	85	30	>48

15.43 No Initial Therapy in Stage III and IV Non-Hodgkin Lymphomas with Favourable Histologies (Portlock)

Therapy	No. of patients	Symptoms	Median time before treatment (months)	Actuarial survival at 48 months (%)
Withheld until required	44[a]	Relatively asymptomatic	31	77
Initial therapy	112	{ 67 Without 45 With	0	83

[a] Seven with spontaneous tumour regression.

15.44 Treatment Strategy in Non-Hodgkin Lymphomas

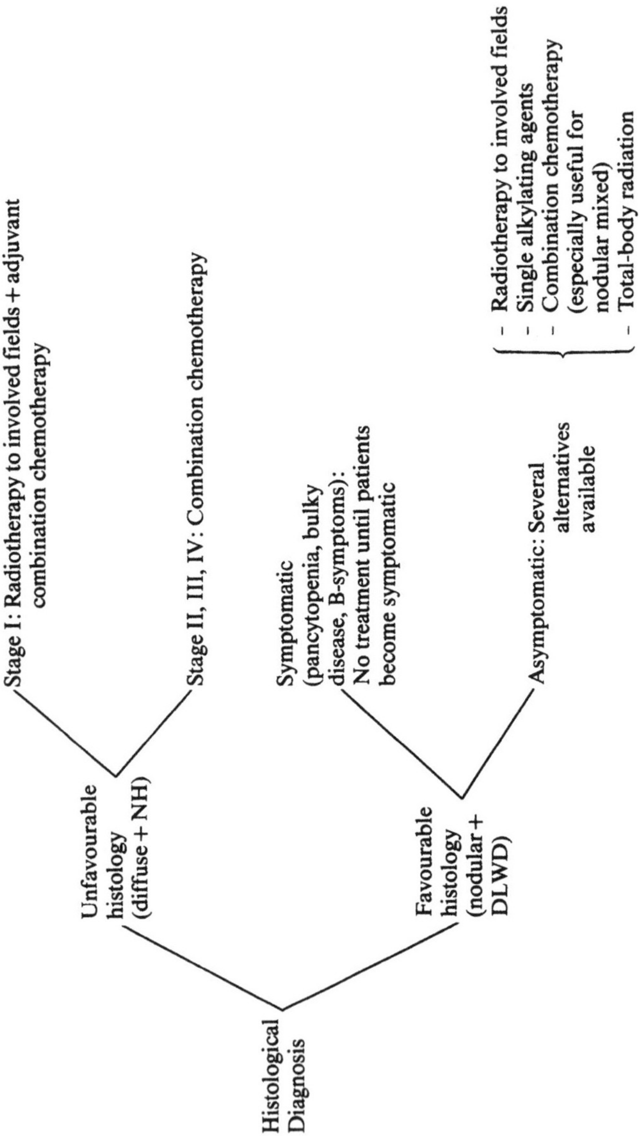

15.45 Burkitt's Lymphoma (see also Chap. 34)

The non-African variant of this disease is associated with a high incidence of CNS complications (particularly cranial nerve palsies) and poor prognosis. Treatment should be initiated immediately on diagnosis as for a poor-prognosis lymphoma.

15.46 Possible Retreatment of Patients with Stage III–IV Non-Hodgkin Lymphomas in Relapse After Initial CR

Unfavourable histology: 1. Same combination inducing: CR + PR ≥ 40%
2. Single (non-cross-resistant) agents chemotherapy: CR + PR ≥ 20%
Favourable histology: 1. CVP: CR 50%
2. Combinations including ADM + BLM: CR ~30%–50%

15.47 Recommended Drug Combinations in Non-Hodgkin Lymphomas

1. Outline of CVP
(one cycle)

Drugs and dosage	Days 1	2	3	4	5	5–20
CTX 400 mg/m^2 p.o. i.v.	↑	↑	↑	↑	↑	No therapy
VCR 1.4 mg/m^2 i.v.	↑					
PRD 100 mg/m^2 p.o. i.m.	↑	↑	↑	↑	↑	

2. Outline of C-MOPP
(one cycle)

Drugs and dosage	Days 1	2	3	4	5	6	7	8	9	10	11	12	13	14	14–28
CTX 650 mg/m^2 i.v.	↑							↑							No therapy
VCR 1.4 mg/m^2 i.v.	↑							↑							
PCZ 100 mg/m^2 p.o.	———	———	———	———	———	———	———	———	———	———	———	———	———	→	
PRD 40 mg/m^2 i.m.	———	———	———	———	———	———	———	———	———	———	———	———	———	→	

3. Outline of VAP

Drugs and dosage

VCR 1.4 mg/m^2 i.v. weekly
ADM 50 mg/m^2 i.v. every 2 weeks — Continued for 6–8 weeks
PRD 40 mg/m^2 daily for 2 weeks

4. Outline of ABP (one cycle)

Drugs and dosage	Days 1	2	3	4	5	6	7	8 – 20
ADM 60 mg/m² i.v.	↑							No therapy (days 8–20)
BLM 10 mg/m² i.v.	↑							↑ (day 8)
PRD 100 mg/m² p.o. i.m.	↑	↑	↑	↑	↑			

5. Outline of BACOP (one cycle)

Drugs and dosage	Days 1	8	14	15	22	28
ADM 25 mg/m² i.v.	↑	↑				
CTX 650 mg/m² i.v.	↑	↑				
VCR 1.4 mg/m² i.v.	↑	↑				
BLM 5 mg/m² i.v.				↑	↑	
PRD 60 mg/m² i.m.				———	———	——→

6. Outline of CHOP-BLM (one cycle)

Drugs and dosage	1	2	3	4	5 – 20
CTX 750 mg/m² i.v.	↑				No therapy (days 5–20)
ADM 50 mg/m² i.v.	↑				
VCR 2 mg (total dose)	↑				↑ (day 5)
PRD 100 mg (total dose)	↑	↑	↑	↑	↑ (day 5)
BLM 15 mg (total dose)	↑				

15.48 Special Problems and Their Treatment in Non-Hodgkin Lymphomas

CNS involvement - Meningeal: MTX 10 mg/m², CA 25 mg/m², Hydrocortisone 25 mg/m² i.t. every 4 days and/or Cranio-spinal irradiation (2400 rads) - Spinal cord compression: Radiotherapy or emergency laminectomy + radiotherapy	
Superior vena cava (SVC) syndrome	Combination chemotherapy + radiotherapy (3500–4000 rads) to the mediastinum
Pleural effusion	HN2 - 12 mg/m² or BLM 30 mg/m² or ADM 30 mg/m² i.pl. after maximum removal of pleural fluid
Acute renal failure from bilateral replacement of kidney tumour	Combination chemotherapy + radiotherapy (1000 rads) to one or both kidneys

15.49 Incidence of CNS Involvement of Non-Hodgkin Lymphomas in the Principal Case Series

No. of patients	CNS involvement (%)	Author
348	7	Law
52	29	Bunn
138	19	Longpre
1039	5	Herman
445	8.5	Young
292	11	Litam
592	9	Levit
111	17	INT, Milano
227	10.5	Mackintosh

15.50 Prognostic Factors in Non-Hodgkin Lymphomas

1. Age. Prognosis worse in children and in elderly patients.

2. Histopathology. Prognostic grouping (Rappaport nodular and diffuse; Kiel low-grade and high-grade; Working Formulation low-, intermediate- and high-grade) has a definitive value since it is correlated with survival.

3. Stage. Less important than in Hodgkin's disease. Extranodular disease more unfavourable in diffuse than in nodular. Bulky disease carries unfavourable prognosis.

4. Results of Treatment. Cure rate has been improving as result of treatment in selected subgroups such as stage III and IV diffuse histiocytic and stage I and II.

15.51 Second Neoplasms in Non-Hodgkin Lymphomas

1. The observed incidence of a second solid tumour is similar to the predicted one.
2. Second neoplasia (ANLL) in patients treated for NHL develops with a 10- to 37-fold increase over the predicted number.
3. Similarly to what is observed for Hodgkin's disease, the increase in the incidence of ANLL seems to be treatment-related.
4. The risk of developing ANLL is greater in patients treated with radio- and chemotherapy as opposed to those treated with chemotherapy alone (6% vs 1%).

15.52 Problems to Be Solved in Non-Hodgkin Lymphomas

1. Unfavourable histology:
   - Lack of achievement of CR (especially for DH) related to a probable survival <2 years
   - Lack of alternative drugs or combinations
   - Leukaemic evolution not controlled by chemotherapy
2. Favourable histology:
   - Pattern of continuous late recurrence
   - Uncertainty of present therapeutic strategy
3. Favourable and unfavourable histology:
   - Quality of life altered by combination chemotherapy
   - Risk of ANLL related to treatment

15.53 Needs and Perspectives in Non-Hodgkin Lymphomas

1. To be avoided:
   a) Risk of overtreatment in patients with indolent disease
   b) Risk of undertreatment in patients with rapidly growing (and potentially curable) disease
2. Need of a better clinical-pathological correlation (results of treatment-working formulation) to develop an improved modulation of treatment
3. Need of developing new non-cross-resistant drugs and/or combinations for an effective second-line therapy (chemo-sensitivity testing?)

Further Reading

Bonadonna G, Santoro A (1979) Current diagnosis and treatment of malignant lymphomas. Cancer Clinical Series. Published as an Educational Service. Bristol-Myers Company International Mission, New York

De Vita VT, Hellman S (1982) Hodgkin's disease and the non-Hodgkin's lymphomas in Cancer Principles and Practice of Oncology. De Vita VT, Hellman S, Rosenberg SA (eds) J.B. Lippincott Company, Philadelphia Toronto, pp 1331-1401

Golomb HM (1980) Non-Hodgkin Lymphoma. Seminars in Oncology, September 1980

Kaplan HS (1972) Hodgkin's Disease. Harvard University Press, Cambridge, Mass

Levy R, Kaplan HS (eds) (1978) Malignant Lymphoma. UICC Technical Report Series, Vol 7, UICC, Geneva

Mathé G, Seligmann M, Tubiana M (1978) Recent Results in Cancer Research - Lymphoid neoplasias I: Classification, Categorization, Natural History. Springer, Berlin Heidelberg New York

Mathé G, Seligmann M, Tubiana M (1978) Recent Results in Cancer Research - Lymphoid Neoplasias II: Clinical and Therapeutic Aspects. Springer, Berlin Heidelberg New York

Whitehouse JMA, Kay HEM (1979) CNS Complications of Malignant Disease. Macmillan Press, London

16 Multiple Myeloma

16.1 Incidence and Epidemiology

Incidence: 3/100000 - similar to that of Hodgkin's disease
Increased incidence in black population

16.2 Aetiology and Risk Factors

Host factors: M > F
Environmental factors - possible increase following exposure to radiation and certain chemicals
Highest rates in persons over 78-80 years of age, mean age 64 years at diagnosis

16.3 Classification of Disease Associated with M Proteins

Benign monoclonal gammopathy
Multiple myeloma
Waldenström's macroglobulinaemia
Plasma cell leukaemia
Heavy-chain disease

16.4 Immunoglobulin Molecule

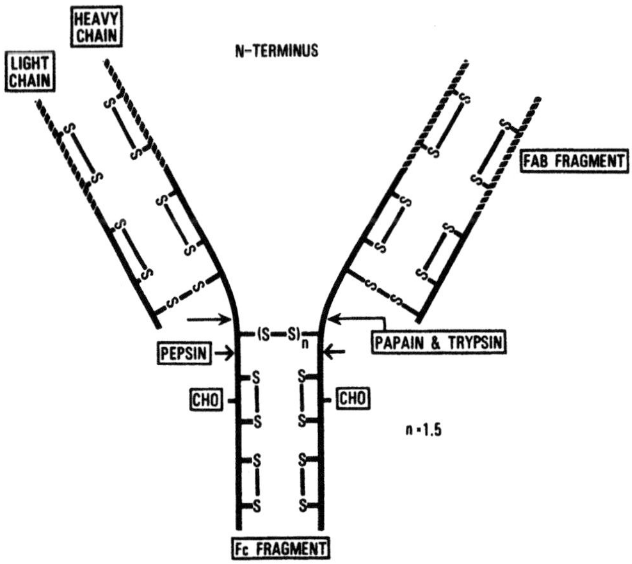

16.5 Results of Serum Immunoelectrophoresis in Myeloma Patients (Mayo Clin. Proc., Jan. 1975)

Immunoglobulin	No. (and percentage) of patients	
IgG	316	(59)
IgA	126	(23)
IgD	6	(1)
Negative (heavy chain)	89	(17)
Total	537	(100)
Light chain		
Kappa	320[a]	(60)
Lambda	158[a]	(30)
Negative	55	(10)
Total	533	(100)

[a] Includes Bence Jones proteinaemia.

16.6 Monoclonal Gammopathy

The diagnosis of myeloma can be difficult. An increase in plasma cells in the marrow can occur in diseases such as auto-immune disorders and chronic infection, and a serum monoclonal gammopathy may be associated with other lymphoid tumours or may even occur without apparent disease (benign monoclonal gammopathy).

Analysis of 400 cases of monoclonal gammopathy (Osserman and Takastuki)

	No. (and percentage) of cases	
Multiple myeloma	262	(65.5)
Heavy-chain disease	3	(0.8)
Waldenström's macroglobulinaemia	41	(10.2)
"Monoclonal gammopathy" associated with lymphomas	23	(5.8)
"Monoclonal gammopathy"		
a) With associated neoplasm	31	(7.8)
b) Without associated neoplasm	40	(10.0)

16.7 Relationship to Multiple Myeloma of Solitary Plasmacytoma of Bone and Extramedullary Plasmacytoma (Adapted from Crowing and Lindberg)

16.7.1 Plasma Cell tumours Originating in Skeletal (Multiple and Solitary) or Extramedullary Sites

	Number	Percentage
Plasma cell tumours of bone		
Multiple	856	93.2
Solitary	26	2.8
Extramedullary plasma cell tumours	37	4.0
Total	919	100.0

16.7.2 Sites of Extramedullary Plasma Cell Tumours

	Percentage
Upper air passages (tonsil, palate, nasal sinuses, naso-pharynx, nose, orbit)	76
Lymph nodes and spleen	6
Bronchial and lung	4
Skin and subcutaneous	3.5
Gastrointestinal tract	3
Thyroid	3
Testes	1
Other	3.5
Total	100.0

16.8 Main Clinical Features

1. Bone pain
2. Fatigue, loss of weight
3. Anaemia, fever
4. Manifestation caused by M proteins:
   a) Bleeding diathese
   b) Alteration of cerebral, renal, ocular blood flow, progressive heart failure (hyperviscosity syndrome)
5. Other symptoms related to complications (see sect. 16.10)

16.9 Diagnostic Criteria for Multiple Myeloma

1. Demonstration of focal or generalized increase in abnormal plasma cells in bone marrow or other tissue
2. Presence of serum or urinary myeloma protein often with an associated reduction of immunoglobin levels
3. Typical x-ray changes: lytic lesions of bone

Two of these three criteria are required for diagnosis.

16.10 Major Complications of Multiple Myeloma

1. Pathological fractures
2. Hypercalcaemia
3. Renal failure
4. Infection
5. Bone marrow suppression
6. Hyperuricaemia
7. Hyperviscosity syndrome (plasmapheresis may be used)
8. Amyloidosis

16.11 Diagnostic Procedures

1. Haematology:	Hb, WBC, platelets, differential, marrow aspiration
2. Biopsy:	Solitary lytic lesion, extramedullary plasmacytoma, skin nodules, enlarged lymph nodes
3. Biochemistry:	Calcium, blood urea nitrogen (BUN), creatinine, uric acid, alkaline phosphotase, blood sugar
4. Serum proteins:	Total serum protein, electrophoresis, M protein and albumin, M protein immunoelectrophoresis, quantitative immunoglobulin assay
5. Urine:	24-h urine protein, creatinine clearance, electrophoresis of concentrated urine, immunoelectrophoresis (light and/or heavy chain)
6. Radiology:	Skeletal survey
7. Myelogramm:	Only if indicated (neurological signs and symptoms of spinal cord or nerve root compression)
8. Special examinations:	Serum viscosity Cryoglobulins Plasma volume Rectal biopsy for amyloid

16.12 Staging of Multiple Myeloma (Salmon)

Stage[a]	Criteria	Cell mass
I	All of the following: 1. Hb >10 g/100 ml 2. Normal calcium (<12 mg/100 ml) 3. x-Ray picture normal or solitary lesion only 4. Low M protein production rate: - IgG <5 g/100 ml - IgA <3 g/100 ml - Light chains in urine <4 g/24 h	$<0.6 \times 10^{12}/m^2$ Low
II	Characteristics which fit neither stage I nor III	$0.6-1.20 \times 10^{12}/m^2$ Intermediate
III	One or more of the following: 1. Hb <8.5 g/100 ml 2. Calcium >12 mg/100 ml 3. Advanced lytic bone lesions 4. High M protein production - IgG >7 g/100/ml - IgA >5 g/100 ml - Light chains in urine >12 mg/24 h	$>1.20 \times 10^{12}/m^2$ High

[a] Stages I, II and III can be further subdivided into: A - serum creatinine <2.0 mg/100 ml, and B - serum creatinine >2.0 mg/100 ml.

16.13 Single Agents Effective in Multiple Myeloma (Modified from Clarysse et al. 1976)

Drug	No. of cases evaluated	Response (%)
Melphalan	499	42
Cyclophosphamide	413	29
Prednisone	39	49
6-Mercaptopurine	19	10
Carmustine (BCNU)	31	39
Procarbazine	33	15
Nitrogen mustard	9	11
Chlorambucil	15	33
Adriamycin	23	13

16.14 Results of Combination Chemotherapy for Plasma Cell Myeloma Obtained by the Southwest Oncology Group (SWOG) and the National Cancer Institute (NCI) (Modified from Bergsagel and Rieder 1982)

Drug	Group	No. evaluable	Response rate (%)	Median survial (months)
M	SWOG	54	24	18
MP	SWOG	139	48	21
	NCI	100	40	28
MP+PROC	SWOG	205	59	23
MAP	SWOG	67	46	21-26
CAP	SWOG	59	39	21-26
MCP	SWOG	74	47	21-26
MCBP	SWOG	70	49	~34
MP+PROC	SWOG	127	50	34
VMCP	SWOG	77	62	~34
VCAP	SWOG	74	57	~34

A, adriamycin; B, carmustine; C, cyclophosphamide; M, melphalan; P, prednisone; PROC, procarbazine; V, vincristine

16.15 Evaluation of Response to Treatment in Multiple Myeloma

Any of the following disease parameters may be used to evaluate response to treatment in multiple myeloma:

1. Serum myeloma protein (fall to 50% or less of initial level)
2. Palpable (or x-ray-visualized) plasmacytoma (reduction of 50% or more in the product of the two largest diameters)
3. Urinary myeloma protein (fall to 50% of a pre-treatment level >1.0 g/24 h or fall to less than 0.1 g/24 h of a pre-treatment level <1.0 g/24 h)
4. Definite radiographic evidence of skeletal healing
5. Myeloma cells in bone marrow aspirate (significant reduction)

N.B. Response in multiple myeloma is evaluated separately for each disease parameter present at the time of diagnosis.

16.16 How to Evaluate the Response to Treatment (Modified from Bergsagel and Rieder 1982)

1. Physical examination: weight, temperature, performance status, symptoms, and signs.

2. Haemoglobin, leukocytes, platelets and differential - once-weekly until an acceptable pattern of toxicity is established, then repeat only before each treatment.
3. Measure the M protein regularly, every 1 month to 2 months.
   a) Electrophoresis is more reliable than immunoglobulin assays if an M peak is visible.
   b) Urine protein-grams per 24 h. Measurement of the total protein excreted per 24 h is usually sufficient, with occasional checks of the electrophoresis pattern to determine the fraction of urinary light chains.
4. Serum calcium and BUN (or creatinine) checked regularly, with a frequency determined by the status of the patient. Check the serum calcium whenever the patient mentions nausea, vomiting, polydipsia, somnolence or confusion.
5. If the initial creatinine clearance was decreased, this test should be repeated to evaluate the response to treatment.
6. Bone roentgen films should be repeated to investigate the cause of new painful sites, skull roentgen films, at 6-month to 12-month intervals, help to assess skeletal healing.
7. Look for evidence of paraspinal mass whenever the patient complains of back pain. If a paraspinal mass is suspected, a myelogram should be done, do a cytospin on the CSF and look for myeloma cells.

16.17 Recommended Chemotherapy for Multiple Myeloma

A regimen comprising a single alkylating agent + prednisone, used intermittently, is the mainstay of treatment for multiple myeloma. There is no good evidence at present that combining more agents improves survival in myeloma, although there is some suggestion that this may be the case.

Melphalan	$10\ mg/m^2/day \times 4$	orally every 6 weeks
+		
Prednisone	$60\ mg/m^2/day \times 4$	
or		
Cyclophosphamide	$1000\ mg/m^2 \times$ i.v.	every 3–4 weeks
+		
Prednisone	$60\ mg/m^2/day \times 4$ 4 oral	

In resistant patients, BCNU, procarbazine, vincristine and Adriamycin may prove to be of value.

16.18 Prognostic Factors in Multiple Myeloma

1. Median survival is directly related to stage:
   Stage I - 61 months
   Stage II - 54 months
   Stage III A - 30 months
   Stage III B - 15 months
2. Median survival of responders to chemotherapy > to that of non-responders.
3. Slow-growing tumours have the best prognosis [growth rate assessed by (a) patient history; (b) M protein production rate; and (c) labelling index].
4. Production of only γ-chains is associated with poorer prognosis (median survival ~10 months).

16.19 Difference in Prognosis of Plasma Cell Tumours (Skeletal Multiple and Solitary and Extramedullary Sites) (Adapted from Crowing and Lindberg)

	Solitary bone plasmacytoma	Multiple myeloma	Extramedullary plasmacytomas
Number	114	250	325
Age (years) median	53	64	62
Median survival (months)	114	30	192

16.20 Plasma Cell Myeloma: Causes of Death

Cause	Number (%)
1. During the chronic phase:	
Progressive myeloma	38
Plus renal failure	24
Plus sepsis	33
Plus both	16
	111 (46)

Cause	Number (%)
2. During the acute terminal phase:	
Progressive myeloma	31
Plus renal failure	4
Plus sepsis	22
Plus both	5
	62 (26)
3. Acute leukaemia	12 (5)
4. Other causes	48 (20)
5. Unknown	7 (3)
Total	240 (100)

16.21 Therapeutic Strategy in Plasma Cell Neoplasms

1. Relative role of radiotherapy and chemotherapy:
   Radiotherapy - Solitary plasmacytoma
   - Extramedullary plasmacytoma
   - Spinal cord compression
   - Palliative treatment

   Chemotherapy - Multiple myeloma
   - Waldenström's macroglobulinaemia
   - Heavy-chain disease
   - Light-chain disease
2. Chemotherapy in multiple myeloma should be administered considering the following points:
   1. Alkylating agents have been improving the prognosis: survival of responders to that of non-responders.
   2. The addition of prednisone to intermittent courses of melphalan doubles the response rate.
   3. Combination chemotherapy with 3-4 drugs might prove to be superior to melphalan or melphalan prednisone.
   4. Patients with "asymptomatic", "stable", or "indolent", disease may not require treatment for intervals varying from a few months to more than 8 years.
   5. It may be possible to suspend treatment after a satisfactory remission has been induced.
3. Guidelines for treatment of Waldenström's macroglobulinaemia are very much the same as for multiple myeloma.

16.22 Problems Under Study and Future Prospects in Multiple Myeloma

1. Upper and lower half body irradiation has been used successfully, but has still to be considered as an experimental procedure.
2. Reduction of the number of neoplastic plasma cells has been improving survival; in the future, however, research should be directed at correcting the mechanism controlling the growth and differentiation of immunoglobulin-producing cells.

Further Reading

Bergsagel DE, Rieder WD (1982) "Plasma Cell Neoplasms, pp. 1439/ 1475. In: "Cancer Principles & Practice of Oncology, Ed by De Vita VT, Hellman S, Rosenberg SA, J. B. Lippincott Company, Philadelphia, Toronto
Clarysse A, Kenis Y, Mathé G (1976) Cancer chemotherapy - its role in the treatment strategy of hematologic malignancies and solid tumors. Springer, Berlin Heidelberg New York
Durie BMG, Salmon SE (1975) A clinical staging system for multiple myeloma. Correlation of measured myeloma cell mass with presenting clinical features. Cancer 36: 842-854
Hoffbrand AV, Brain MC, Hirsch J (1977) Recent Advances in Haematology, No 2. Churchill Livingstone, London
Waner NL, Potter M, Metcalf D (1974) (Eds) Multiple Myeloma and Related Immunoglobulin-producing Neoplasms. UICC Technical Report Series, Vol 13. UICC, Geneva

17 Breast Tumours

17.1 Incidence and Epidemiology

The most frequent form of cancer in women in the western world.
Every 10th–15th woman develops breast cancer.
The incidence is still increasing in women between 40 and 45 years.
The most frequent cause of death in women aged between 40 and 45 years.
Relative survival after 20 years of observation is about 30% for all stages (stage I: 53%; stage II: 18%).

17.2 Aetiology and Risk Factors

Far from being well-understood; nevertheless, numerous factors have been credited with a major or minor role in determining the onset of the tumour.

17.2.1 Genetic Predisposition

Increased incidence in women with mothers or sisters having breast cancer, especially if occurring bilaterally and/or at an early age. Increased incidence in phenotypic male patients with Klinefelter's syndrome. Some high-risk families have cancer of multiple site, including ovary, large-bowel and soft-tissue sarcomas.

17.2.2 Risk Factors

1. Nulliparae and late first pregnancy (older than 35 years).
2. Risk in single women is twice that in women who have married. Nuns present the highest incidence.
3. Obesity.
4. Benign breast lesions.

17.3 Pathological Classification

According to the revised WHO classification, malignant breast tumours include:

I Epithelial tumours
- Non invasive:
  a. Intraductal carcinoma
  b. Lobular carcinoma in situ
- Invasive:
  a. Invasive ductal carcinoma
  b. Invasive ductal carcinoma with a predominant intraductal component
  c. Invasive lobular carcinoma
  d. Mucinous carcinoma
  e. Medullary carcinoma
  f. Papillary carcinoma
  g. Tubular carcinoma
  h. Adenoid cystic carcinoma
  i. Secretory (juvenile)carcinoma
  j. Apocrine carcinoma
  k. Carcinoma with metaplasia
    i. Squamous type
    ii. Spindle-cell type
    iii. Cartilaginous and osseous type
    iv. Mixed type
  1. Others (e. g. signet ring)
- Paget's disease of the nipple

II Mixed connective tissue and epithelial tumours
Phyllodes tumour (cystosarcoma phyllodes)
Carcinosarcoma

III Miscellaneous tumours (malignant only)
Soft-tissue tumours
Skin tumours
Tumours of haematopoietic and lymphoid tissues

IV Unclassified tumours (malignant only)

17.4 Main Clinical Features

The course of disease is very variable. Metastases may occur early or late (after an interval of more than 5-10 years).

17.4.1 Five-Year Recurrence Rate (%) by Tumour Size and Level of Axillary Node Involvement in 1048 Patients (Fischer)

Axillary lymph node involvement	Tumour size 0.1–0.9 cm	Tumour size 2.0–3.9 cm	Tumour size >4.0 cm	Total
Negative	12	20	26	21
Positive (1–3)	40	46	56	49
Positive (>3)	66	71	88	81
Total	28	39	56	44

17.5 Diagnostic Procedures

1. Patient history:
   a) Date of first change in the breast
   b) Local and general symptoms, weight changes
   c) Menstrual status
   d) Familial history
2. Complete clinical examination:
   a) Loco-regional – Tumour size, mobility
      – Status of the regional nodes, mobility.
      – Skin changes
   b) General – Liver, lung, bone, etc.
3. Radiological examination
   a) Mammography (to assist diagnosis)
   b) Chest x-ray
   c) Bone scintigraphy
   d) Abdominal ultrasound or computerized axial tomographic (CAT)-scan (essential in stage III; if possible in all stages)
4. Laboratory examinations
   a) Erythrocyte sedimentation rate (ESR), platelets, haemoglobin, WBC, differential count
   b) Alkaline phosphatase, serum glutamic-oxaloacetic transaminase (SGOT), serum and urine calcium, blood urea nitrogen (BUN)
   c) Vaginal exfoliative cytology or quantitative oestrogen determination in women 1–3 years after menopause
   d) Determination of oestrogen receptor in tumour tissue
   e) Carcinoembryonic antigen (CEA) as tumour marker: 50%–80% positive (limited value)

17.6 Staging Classification

17.6.1 TNM Summary

T1 ≤2 cm
T2 >2–5 cm
T3 >5 cm
a) Without fixation fascia/muscle
b) With fixation fascia/muscle

T4 Extension to chest wall/skin:
a) Chest wall
b) Skin oedema (infiltration or ulceration)
c) Both

N1 Mobile axillary:
a) Not considered metastatic
b) Considered metastatic

N2 Fixed axillary
N3 Supraclavicular/oedema of arm
M0 No evidence of distant metastases
M1 Evidence of distant metastases
MX The minimum requirements to assess the presence of distant metastases cannot be met

17.6.2 Stage Grouping

Stage I	T1a, T1b	NO, N1a	MO
Stage II	T1a, T1b	N1b	MO
	T2a, T2b	NO, N1a	MO
	T2a, T2b	N1b	MO
Stage IIIa	T3a, T3b	NO, N1	MO
	T1a, b, T2a, b, T3a, b	N2	MO
Stage IIIb	T1a, b, T2a, b, T3a, b	N3	MO
	T4a, b, c	Any N	MO
Stage IV	Any T	Any N	M1

17.6.3 pTNM Post-Surgical Histopathological Classification (see page 192)

pTO	–	No evidence of tumour found on histological examination of specimen
pT1a–pT4c	–	Correspond to pre-treatment classification, but tumour found on histological examination
pNO	–	No evidence of invasion of regional lymph nodes
pN1–pN3	–	Evidence of invasion

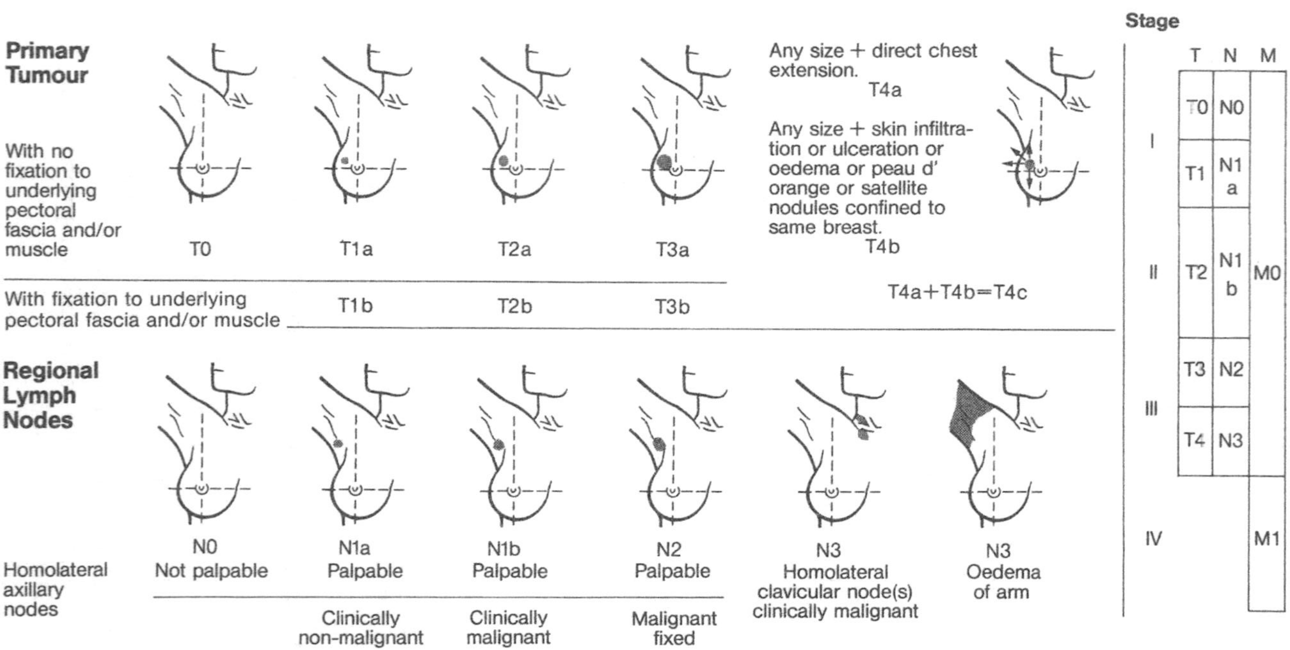

TNM Staging in breast cancer

T = Extent of primary tumour
N = Condition of regional lymph nodes
M = Absence or presence of metastases

The clinical classification may not be changed but information regarding the assessment of the regional lymph nodes may be added to the N category: thus

N– (minus) for nodes with no microscopic evidence of metastasis; or

N+ (plus) for microscopic evidence of metastasis.

By courtesy of Lederle Inc.

17.7 Prognostic Factors

17.7.1 Prognostic Factors in Non-Metastatic Breast Cancer (T1-3; NO-1; MO)

1. Size of the primary tumour
2. Number, site and size of positive axillary nodes
3. Skin involvement
4. Fixation of the primary tumour or of positive nodes
5. Histological typing (?), vascular invasion, signs of immunological reactions in lymph nodes
6. Degree of anaplasia (I-IV)
7. Age and menstrual status (?)
8. Delay in treatment
9. Pregnancy
10. Oestrogen receptor content

17.7.2 Prognostic Factors for Survival in Metastatic Breast Cancer (any T; any N; M1)

1. Disease-free interval between primary treatment and metastases
2. First site (S) and estimated extent of metastatic involvement:
   a) One organ site involved: soft-tissue, skeleton, lung, limited tumour mass
   b) Two organ sites involved, but no visceral metastases
   c) Two or three organ systems involved, with visceral metastases
3. Performance status: clinical signs and symptoms, such as weight loss, anaemia, elevation of alkaline phosphatase
4. Total tumour load
5. Immunological factors: interaction between host and tumour (lymphocyte infiltration, sinus histiocytosis)
6. Menstrual status
7. Response to previous hormonal treatment
8. CEA level
9. Oestrogen receptor (ER) content

17.8 Strategy of Management of Non-Metastatic Breast Cancer

17.8.1 Operable (Stages I and II; T1-3a; N1; MO)

1. Confirmation of diagnosis:
   a) Clinical evaluation.
   b) Mammography.
   c) Needle biopsy or open biopsy in preparation for mastectomy.
2. Therapy:
   a) Simple mastectomy + exploration and histological examination of parasternal and axillary lymph nodes.
   b) Modified radical mastectomy.
   c) Quadrantectomy + axillary dissection + radiotherapy can be considered in $T1_a$ NO-1 cases
3. Post-operative therapy:
   a) Axillary nodes negative: no further therapy, regular follow-up examinations.
   b) Axillary nodes positive: in all premenopausal women surgical adjuvant chemotherapy has to be considered, in high-risk patients it is obligatory. For postmenopausal women with ER^+ tamoxifen with ER^- chemotherapy may be considered but cannot be recommended as standard practice.
   c) Post-operative radiotherapy is accepted to reduce local recurrence but has no other role.

17.8.2 Inoperable (Stage III; T3b-4; N2; N3; MO) Without Distant Metastases

1. Needle biopsy.
2. Curative radiotherapy,
3. Palliative mastectomy prior to radiation may be considered in selected cases.
4. Chemotherapy; in ER^+ cases, combined hormonal and chemotherapy.

17.9 Single Agents Effective in Advanced Breast Cancer (Pooled Data)

Drugs	Number of evaluated cases	Number of remissions	Remission rate (%)
Mechlorethamine	92	32	35
Cyclophosphamide	529	182	34
Melphalan	177	38	22
Chlorambucil	54	11	20
Thiotepa	162	48	30
Mitolactol	53	22	41
Dacarbazine	37	3	8
Carnustine (BCNU)	82	19	23
Lomustine (CCNU)	206	24	11
Methyl-CCNU	110	4	4
Streptozotocin	19	2	10.5
Procarbazine	21	1	5
Methotrexate	356	120	34
Mercaptopurine	44	6	14
5-Fluorouracil	1263	324	26
Ftorafur	54	23	43
Cytarabine	64	6	9
Hydroxycarbamide	21	4	19
Hexamethylmelamine	54	11	20
Bleomycin	18	3	16
Dactinomycin	44	5	11
Daunorubicin	40	15	38
Doxorubicin	193	67	35
4-Epidoxorubicin	30	11	37
Bisantrene	56	7	13
Mitoxantrone	59	19	32
Amsacrine (m-AMSA)	77	3	4
Mitomycin	106	23	22
Spreptonigrin	13	3	23
Vincristine	226	47	21
Vinblastine	95	19	20
Vinblastine (continous infusion)	77	25	36
Etoposide	66	9	14
Maytansine	15	2	13

17.10 Hormones Effective in Advanced Breast Cancer

Drugs	Menopausal status	Number of evaluated cases	Remission rate (%)
Diethylstilboestrol (DES)	Premenopausal	63	9
	Postmenopausal	344	35
Turisteron (long-acting oestrogen)	Postmenopausal	40	30
Testosterone	Premenopausal	212	10
	Postmenopausal	222	24
Medroxyprogesterone acetate	Paramenopausal	28	29
	Postmenopausal	35	34
Aminoglutehimide	Postmenopausal	34	47
	All	57	30
Tamoxifen	Premenopausal	120	30
	Postmenopausal	83	25

17.11 Drug Combinations Effective in Breast Cancer

17.11.1 Results with the "Cooper Regimen" (CMFVP) and Its Variations

Combination	No. of studies or name of institution	No. of patients	No. (and percentage) of response
CMFVP	9	503	253 (51)
CMFV	3	118	63 (53)
CMFP	Eastern cooperative Oncology Group (ECOG)	88	52 (59)
CMF	3	366	183 (50)
FVP	Cancer and Acute Leukaemia Group B	82	30 (36)
CFV	Michigan University	46	20 (43)
CMV	Swiss Group	46	15 (32)
CMP	Swiss Group	67	29 (44)
CMFt	Berlin-Buch	33	14 (42)

C, cyclophosphamide; F, fluorouracil; P, prednisone; M, methotrexate; V, vincristine; Ft, ftorafur

Conclusions:

1. CMF, CMFt and CMFP give results similar to those of CMFVP.
2. The addition of prednisone increases the drug tolerance and maybe the remission rate by 10%–12%, possibly due to inhibition of adrenal function (results from three separate studies).

3. Remission duration varies between 6 and 13 months with the best combinations (CMF, CMFP, CMFVP), and seems to depend more on patient characteristics than on the drug regimen used.
4. Responders have a significantly longer median survival than non-responders; quality of response [complete remission (CR), good partial remission (PR)] influences survival more than the drug regimen employed.

17.11.2 Adriamycin and Its Combinations (Pooled Data)

Combination	No. of patients	No. and % response
CTX + ADM + 5-FU + MTX	61	36 (59)
CTX + ADM + 5-FU + VCR	46	7 (15)
CTX + ADM + VCR	65	42 (65)
CTX + ADM	156	84 (54)
CTX + ADM + 5-FU	183	87 (48)
CTX + ADM + 5-FU + MTX	105	51 (49)
CTX + ADM + 5-FU + VCR + PRD	77	44 (57)
ADM + VP-16-213	74	25 (34)

ADM, Adriamycin; CTX, cyclophosphamide; 5-FU, fluorouracil; PRD, prednisone; MTX, methotrexate; VCR, vincristine; VP-16-213, etoposide

17.11.3 Randomized Clinical Trials Comparing CMF-Type and Adriamycin (A)-Type Combinations

Drugs[a]	Study	No. of patients	Remission rate %	Mean duration of remission (months)
VCMF		57	44	11.8
vs	Bezwoda			
CAMF		51	55	12.9
VBL CMF		19	22	13
vs	Klefström			
VAC		21	47	12.5
CMF (low dose)		39	49	12
vs	Creech			
CAMF		39	62	12
CMF		53	47	8
vs	Brambilla			
AV		52	52	8.5

Drugs[a]	Study	No. of patients	Remission rate %	Mean duration of remission (months)
CMF		40	62	8.0
vs	Bull			
FAC		38	82	9.6
A		20	50	–
vs				
CFP	Ahman	16	50	–
vs				
VCFP		12	42	–
CMFVP		72	57	13
vs	Muss			
CAFVP		76	58	15
CMF		40	62	10
vs	Bull			
CAF		38	82	no significant difference
CMFVP		54	37	5,5
vs	Smalley			
CAF		59	64	8.0
CMF		79	57	8.4
vs				
CMFP	Tormey	86	63	4.5
vs				
AV		166	56	7.7
CMF		44	16	6
vs	Muss			
VAC		45	47	9
CMF		53	53	10,5
vs	Valagussa			
AV		52	51	10,5
AC		140	41	7.5
vs	Traunum			
FAC		160	48	13
vs				
A+CMFP		148	46	9

VBL, vinblastine; A, Adriamycin
[a] For drug combination acronyms, see Sect. 17.11.1.

Conclusions:

1. The response rates, the mean duration of remission and the survival time of CMF-type and A-type combinations are in the same range. A-type combinations show a tendency to give slightly higher remission rates.
2. Adriamycin is less effective after prior cytotoxic therapy.
3. Adriamycin combinations may produce more side effects than CMFVP, mainly in terms of the risk of cardiac toxicity.
4. Alternating CMFVP and Adriamycin combinations does not improve overall results.

17.12 Trials Combining Cytotoxic and Endocrine Therapy (Postmenopausal Patients)

Drug	No. of patients	Remission rate (%)	Mean duration of remission (months)
CMF	73	45	–
vs			
CMF + Tam	77	70	–
CT + Tam	118	44	–
vs			
CT→Tam	113	40	–
DES	38	37	10
vs			
DES + CTX	48	67	> 10
CMF	71	51	11.7
vs			
CMF + Tam	62	74	12.7
VAC	89	47	15
vs			
VAC + Tam	88	49	> 15
CFP	64	66	12
vs			
CFP + Tam	58	60	6
H→C	86	–	28.2
vs			
H + C	83	–	31.3 (mean survival)

C and CT; chemotherapeutic regimen; H, hormonal regimen; Tam, tamoxifen

Conclusions:
Although concomitant hormones + chemotherapy may produce higher remission rates than chemotherapy alone, survival is not generally affected. In postmenopausal ER^+ or unknown ER patients the optimal treatment is hormone therapy followed by chemotherapy.

17.13 Recommended Therapy for Metastatic Breast Cancer

17.13.1 Relatively Indolent Diesease, with Good-Prognostic Factors (if Three or More of the Criteria Below Are Met)

a) Disease-free interval of more than 5 years
b) Only one organ system involved, with limited tumour mass (loco-regional or osseous or nodular pulmonary disease)
c) Evolution of the disease estimated to be low
d) Normal performance status, no weight loss, no anaemia, no liver function abnormalities
e) ER^+ or unknown

1. Premenopausal patients:
   Oophorectomy alone: observe for 6–8 weeks
   - If response is seen: Observe until relapse, then use other hormonal treatment (tamoxifen, adrenalectomy, aminoglutethimide) until resistance to further hormonal manipulation is established: then combination chemotherapy.
2. Postmenopausal patients:
   Tamoxifen 20–30 mg daily: observe for 6–8 weeks
   - Response: Observe until relapse; after relapse, observe withdrawal effect (may produce another remission), then start other endocrine treatment. If unsuccessful, start chemotherapy.
   - Progressive disease: Start multidrug chemotherapy.

17.13.2 Intermediate Aggressive Disease (if Three or More of the Criteria Below Are Met)

a) Disease-free interval of 1–5 years
b) One organ system extensively involved or combined loco-regional and osseous metastases without visceral metastases
c) Moderate evolution of metastatic disease
d) Performance status 0–1, no weight loss, no anaemia, no liver function abnormalities

ER Content High, Intermediate or Unknown:
The same guidelines as in Sect. 17.13.1 apply, but chemotherapy should be started not only where there is progressive disease after 6–8 weeks' observation, but also where there is no objective tumour regression and clinical symptoms persist.

ER Content Either Low or Negative:
1. Premenopausal patients:
   Combination chemotherapy ± oophorectomy
2. Postmenopausal patients:
   Combination chemotherapy + tamoxifen

17.13.3 Aggressive Disease (if Three or More of the Criteria Below Are Met)

a) Disease-free interval below 1 year
b) Two or three organ systems involved, including visceral organs; or locally inoperable disease (especially with lymphangitic skin involvement) with or without distant metastases
c) Evolution of the disease judged to be rapid
d) Performance status 1 or more; weight loss, anaemia, liver function abnormalities

ER^+ (Low or High) or Unknown:
1. Premenopausal patients:
   Oophorectomy, combination chemotherapy
2. Postmenopausal patients:
   Tamoxifen followed by combination chemotherapy

ER^-:
1. Premenopausal patients:
   Multidrug chemotherapy initially (additional hormonal therapy may be considered later in addition to chemotherapy)
2. Postmenopausal patients:
   Chemotherapy with or without tamoxifen

17.14 Standard Schedules for Combination Chemotherapy

1. CMF	- CTX 100 mg/m^2/day p.o., days 1-14 - MTX 40 mg/m^2, days 1+8 i.v. - 5-FU 600 mg/m^2, days 1+8 i.v.	repeat every 4 weeks
2. FAC	- ADM 50 mg/m^2 day 1 or 30 mg/m^2 days 1+8 i.v. - 5-FU 500 mg/m^2 days 1+8 i.v. - CTX 500 mg/m^2 i.v. on day 1 or 100 mg/m^2 daily, days 1-14 p.o.	repeat every 4 weeks
3. CMF + prednisone, FAC + prednisone		
4. CMFt	- CTX 15 mg/kg/day i.v., days 1,8,15 - MTX 0.5 mg/kg/day i.v., days 1, 8, 15 - Ftorafur 25 mg/kg/day i.v., days 1, 8, 15	repeat every 4 weeks

17.15 Second- and Third-Line Chemotherapy

1. In patients resistant after oophorectomy or tamoxifen surgical or medical adrenalectomy or high-dose progesterone therapy may rarely induce a remission.
   Aminoglutethimide 4 × 250 mg/day
   Hydrocortisone 40-50 mg/day
   or
   Medroxyprogesteroneacetate (Depo-Provera) 1000 mg/day i.m. for 3-4 weeks; if remission is seen, maintenance therapy with 500 mg weekly.
2. The therapy of choice for patients who have previously received CMF-type chemotherapy is ADM alone or in combination as:
   ADM 60-75 mg/m^2/day 1 i.v.
   VCR 1.4 mg/m^2/day 1+8 i.v.
   every 28 days
   or
   ADM 40 mg/m^2/day 1 i.v.
   Dibromodulcitol 70 mg/m^2/day 2-6 p.o.
   Mitomycin C (MIT-C) 10 mg/m^2/day 1
   In patients who no longer respond to ADM-containing regimens, the choice of treatment is limited to one or more of the remaining drugs, i.e. the *Vinca* alkaloids and MIT-C either alone or in combinations.
   Second-line and particularly third-line treatment rarely result in CR and the potential for long-term control of disease is negligible.

17.15.1 Approaches for Third-Line Chemotherapy in Breast Cancer

Drugs[a]	No. of patients response/all	Remission rate (%)	Mean duration response (weeks)
CTX + VP-16-213	11/27	45.8	31.4
5-FU + MIT-C	18/35	51	-
High-dose MTX (HDMTX) + VBL	17/75	23	8
Hexamethylmelamine (HHM) + MIT-C	5/27	19	20
Mitolactol (DBD) + HMM	0/15	0	-
DDP + HMM + MIT-C	3/11	27	20
MIT-C + VBL	1/14	7	4
5-FU + MIT-C	14/35	41	31
BCNU + MIT-C + VCR + prednisone	2/20	10	-
MTX + L-asparaginase	10/33	30	36

17.16 Adjuvant Chemotherapy in Operable Breast Cancer (T1-3a; N1-2; MO)

17.16.1 Summary of Results with Adjuvant Treatments in Various Centres

Research group	Adjuvant therapy after radical mastectomy	Important findings
Istituto Tumori, Milan	Control vs CMF	Significant improvement of 5-year RFS and total survival in premenopausal women
	CMF 6 + 12 cycles	No difference: 6 vs 12 in premenopausal women
	CMF + Tam	No influence of ER status, no increased incidence of second neoplasms
National Surgical Adjuvant Breast Project	Melphalan (PAM) for 2 years PAM + 5-FU PAM + 5-FU + MTX PAM + 5-FU + Tam	Significant improvement of 5-year RFS and total survival in premenopausal with 1-3 nodes given PAM compared to controls. Significant improvement in postmenopausal women with < 3 nodes given PAM + 5-FU compared to PAM alone

Research group	Adjuvant therapy after radical mastectomy	Important findings
Mayo Clinic, Rochester	PAM vs CFP ± RT	Increased RFS in premenopausal women after CFP ± RT compared to PAM. Improved results over historical controls. No influence of postoperative RT
University of Arizona	AC ± RT	Improved results over historical controls, preliminary evidence of a dose-response effect
MD Anderson, Houston	FAC + BCG + RT	Increased RFS and total survival over historical controls. Best available RFS in women with > 3 nodes. No influence of postoperative RT. Role of BCG unsettled. No increased risk of second neoplasms
ECOG	PAM ± RT vs LMFP ± RT	Increased RFS after LMFP in patients with 1-3 nodes
East Swiss group (OSAKO)	CTR vs LMF + BCG	No increased RFS after LMF + BCG over CTR especially in premenopausal women
Southwest Oncology Group (SWOG)	CMFVP vs PAM	Continuous CMFVP is superior to intermittent PAM in increasing RFS and total survival in both pre- and postmenopausal women
Sidney Farber, Boston	AC 15 vs 30 weeks	No significant differences in the time to relapse
Sloan Kettering, New York	CMF vs CMF + levamisol	Levamisol has not extended RFS or total survival
Guy's Hospital, London	PAM	No significant differences in the time to relapse
Nissen-Meyer	Short-term CTX	Increased total survival
Berlin-Buch	In vitro predicted hormone - chemotherapy	Significant improvement of 5-year RFS and total survival in ER^+ and drug-sensitive patients
Inter-France	CMF vs AVCF	The ADM-containing regimen reduces significantly the rate of short-term relapses when compared to CMF in case of N^+

LMF, chlorambucil + methotrexate + fluorouracil; P, prednisone; CTR, concomitant control; RFS, relapse-free survival; RT, radiotherapy; BCG, Calmette-Guerin bacillus
N. B. In all series the RFS was analysed at more than 3 years.

Conclusions as to adjuvant chemotherapy in operable breast cancer:

1. Adjuvant chemotherapy is effective in significantly prolonging relapse-free survival and total survival in node-positive operable breast cancers in premenopausal women, and has to be considered in this defined subset of patients. In high-risk cases, surgical adjuvant chemotherapy is obligatory. There is not yet conclusive evidence to support the routine use of adjuvant chemotherapy in patients with negative axillary nodes.
2. Combination chemotherapy such as CMF produces better results than adjuvant single-agent chemotherapy, such as melphalan. Drugs should be given at full dosage and for prescribed durations, since lesser amounts of chemotherapy or changes in schedule have shown inferior results.
3. For postmenopausal women with positive nodes and ER^+, surgical adjuvant tamoxifen is the treatment of choice; in case of ER^- adjuvant chemotherapy may be considered, but cannot be recommended as standard practice.
4. For postmenopausal women with negative nodes, regardless of hormone receptor levels, there is no indication for routine adjuvant treatment.

17.17 Problems Under Study and Future Prospects

Some new drugs, such as spirogermanium or mitoxantrone, are under investigation at present, but nevertheless the development of new, more selective drugs remains the most fundamental problem of chemotherapy also in breast cancer. Considering the given drugs, problems as to the optimal drug combinations should be elaborated. An unsolved problem is still the optimal duration of drug application, particularly in surgical adjuvant chemotherapy. Hormonal treatment of breast cancer had a very dynamic development during the last decade. Further success can be expected. In general, cytostatic and hormonal treatment should also be more individualized in breast cancer, tailored to the patient. With the exception of hormone receptor assays, no methods to predict the optimal drug treatment are available, but they should be investigated.

18 Gastrointestinal Tumours

I. Oesophagus[1]

18.1 Suggested Chemotherapy for Oesophageal Cancer

There is no valuable chemotherapy for oesophageal cancer. Treatments that have been used and occasionally produce short-term responses are:

1. Methotrexate 40 mg/m^2 weekly i. v.
2. Bleomycin 10 mg/m^2 bi-weekly i. v.
3. *Cis*-platinum:
   a) 20 mg/m^2 daily × 5 – repeat every 3 weeks, or
   b) 100 mg/m^2 every 3 weeks

   N. B. Platinum therapy must be accompanied by vigorous hydration and diuresis with furosemide + mannitol when 100 mg/m^2 is given as a single dose.

II. Stomach

18.2 Extent of the Gastric Cancer Problem

Most common cancer in incidence in Japan (72/100000) and Chile (70/100000).

Sixth most common cause of cancer deaths in the United States (14000 deaths per year), although overall incidence (8/100000) is low.

18.3 Aetiological and Risk Factors in Gastric Cancer

1. Definitely of environmental origin. Most common in individuals with:
   a) High nitrate intake
   b) High smoked food consumption

---

[1] See also Chap. 38, Oesophageal Carcinoma.

c) High salted fish intake
d) Asbestos exposure
2. Other risk factors:
a) Pernicious anaemia
b) Adenomatous (villous) polyps
c) Gastric intestinal metaplasia
d) Familial (rare)
3. *Not* causally related to:
a) Blood group A
b) Atrophic gastritis

18.4 Prognostic Factors in Gastric Cancer

18.4.1 Pathological Staging (Higgins et al.)

Factor	5-Year survival with: Factor present (%)	Factor absent (%)
Linitis plastica	2	28
Lesion in cardias	13	28
Lesion >3 cm	23	40
Lymph nodes positive for tumour	17	38
Lymphatic invasion	18	37
Blood vessel invasion	12	29
Serosal penetration	18	36

18.4.2 Other Unfavourable Prognostic Factors

1. Poor performance status
2. Undifferentiated tumour (Broder's grade 3 or 4)

18.5 Pathology and Metastatic Sites in Gastric Cancer

1. Gross pathology:
a) Polypoid
b) Ulcerative
c) Scirrhous
2. Metastatic sites:
a) Regional nodes

b) Distant nodes
   - Left supraclavicular (Virchow's)
   - Left axillary (Irish's)
c) Direct extension:
   - Colon, pancreas, liver, bile ducts, oesophagus
d) Haematogenous dissemination
e) Peritoneal implantation:
   - Blumer's rectal shelf
   - Krukenberg's ovarian tumour
   - Umbilical nodule

18.6 Treatment

18.6.1 Surgery:

Disease-free 5-year survival in resected cases 30%–50%.

18.6.2 Radiation therapy (Moertel 1973):

1. No improved survival in unresectable or locally recurrent cases.
2. Radiation + 5-fluorouracil (5-FU) in unresectable cases may improve survival over radiation alone.

Treatment	Mean survival
4000 rads	6 months
4000 rads + 5-FU	14 months

3. Radiation + combination chemotherapy [5-FU-semustine (Me-CCNU)] may improve long-term survival in locally unresectable patients. 20% survival in treated patients is maintained at 2–3 years (Schein et al.)

18.6.3 Chemotherapy (MacDonald)

1. Single-agent chemotherapy:

Drug	Response (%)
Adriamycin	22-30
5-FU	21
Mitomycin C	20
Hydroxyurea	19
Carmustine (BCNU)	18
Chlorambucil	17
Methyl-CCNU	8

2. Combination chemotherapy:

Drug regimen	Response (%)
5-FU + Adriamycin + mitomycin C	40-55
5-FU + BCNU	41
5-FU + Methyl-CCNU	21-40
5-FU + mitomycin C	32
5-FU + cytosine arabinoside + mitomycin C	17-55

3. Suggested chemotherapy for advanced gastric cancer:

	Week								
	1	2	3	4	5	6	7	8	9
5-FU 600 mg/m^2	x	x			x	x			x
Adriamycin 30 mg/m^2	x				x				x
Mitomycin C 10 mg/m^2	x								x

This FAM regimen is well-tolerated and produces response in 40%-55% of patients, with duration of response being 7-12 months.

18.7 Suggested Strategy for Gastric Cancer Treatment

1. Localized disease:
   Total surgical resection is therapy of choice. Single-agent adjuvant chemotherapy is not of value. Results of randomized adjuvant combination chemotherapy trials are conflicting.
2. Locally Unresectable or Locally Recurrent Disease:
   The combination of radiation + 5-FU followed by combination chemotherapy (see above) can be used in these patients.
3. Metastatic Gastric Cancer:
   Combination chemotherapy with FAM or equivalent regimen can be utilized (see above).

III. Colon and Rectum

18.8 Extent of Colorectal Cancer Problem

100000 new cases in the United States each year with 50000 deaths per year. Results of surgical treatment have not improved within the last 30 years.

18.9 Aetiology and Risk Factors

1. Aetiology:
   Most common in Western industrial societies. Has been associated with low-fibre, high-fat diets
2. Risk factors:
   a) Adenomatous and villous polyps
   b) Familial polyposis
   c) Chronic ulcerative colitis
   d) Crohn's disease of colon

18.10 Prognostic Factors in Colon Cancer

18.10.1 Pathological Staging

1. Duke's staging of colorectal cancer:
   A Tumour confined to mucosa. No lymph node involvement

B.1 Tumour penetrating bowel wall muscle. Serosal surface not involved. No lymph node involvement
B.2 Tumour penetrating to serosa or beyond. No lymph node involvement
C.1 Proximal mesenteric nodes involved
C.2 Distal mesenteric nodes involved

Survival by stage in colorectal cancer following treatment by resection:

Duke's stage	5-year survival (%)
A	61-81
B	25-64
C	10-50

2. Tumour differentiation - Broder's classification:
   1, Well-differentiated
   2, Moderate differentiation
   3, Anaplastic
3. Site of tumour:
   Rectal cancer has poorer prognosis than other sites in colon.
4. Symptoms:
   Patients presenting with obstruction have poorer prognosis than those presenting with no obstruction.

18.11 Single-Agent Drug Activity in Large-Bowel Cancers (MacDonald et al.)

Drug	No. of responses	No. of patients	Response rate (%)
5-FUDR (5-fluoro-2-deoxyuridine)	144	617	23
5-FU	454	2107	21
Me-CCNU	7	40	18
Chlorozotocin	4	24	17
Mitomycin C	35	218	16

18.12 Drug Combinations in Large-Bowel Cancers (MacDonald et al. 1981)

Combination	No. of patients	No. of responses	Response rate %
5-FU + Me-CCNU	489	98	20
5-FU + Me-CCNU + vincristine	358	82	23
5-FU + Me-CNNU + DTIC	83	14	14
5-FU + Me-CCNU + vincristine + DTIC	71	11	15
5-FU + Me-CCNU + vincristine + streptozotocin	54	15	27
5-FU + BCNU	20	1	5

N.B. There is no convincing evidence that a combination of 5-FU with Me-CCNU is better than 5-FU alone.

18.13 Suggested Chemotherapy for Advanced Colorectal Cancer

1. 5-FU 15–20 mg/kg/once weekly i.v. or 10–12 mg/kg/day i.v. 4 times, repeated every 3 weeks or
2. Experimental protocol study evaluating new chemotherapy treatment

18.14 Combined-Modality Treatment for Duke's Stage C (< 50% 5-Year Survival)

Combined-modality treatment	Treatment results
1. Pre-operative/postoperative radiotherapy	Small non-significant improvements in disease-free survival. Current studies are evaluating radiation with chemotherapy
2. Single-agent adjuvant chemotherapy (5-FU)	
- Short-term therapy	No significant improvement in survival.
- Long-term therapy	All studies show improvement, but none demonstrates statistical significance
3. Combination adjuvant chemotherapy	
- Several adjuvant trials using combinations (5-FU + Me-CCNU)	No significant improvement in survival
4. Immunotherapy	No consistent improvement demonstrated

18.15 Recommended Strategy for Treatment of Colorectal Cancer

18.15.1 Localized Cancer

The only curative procedure is surgical removal of bowel and draining of mesenteric nodes. Pre-operative radiotherapy may have a favourable effect on rectal lesions, but definitive studies are still in progress.

Adjuvant Chemotherapy. Several studies on single-agent adjuvant therapy following surgery have been carried out. There is no definite evidence of improved survival, although some studies have shown a slight difference in favour of adjuvant chemotherapy. Definitive studies using combined chemotherapy (e.g. 5-FU + Me-CCNU) and/or immunotherapy are in progress.

18.15.2 Advanced Cancer

Palliative surgery or radiotherapy is of value in selected cases. There is no convincing evidence that multidrug chemotherapy is superior to 5-FU.

IV. Pancreas

18.16 Extent of Pancreatic Cancer Problem

Pancreatic cancer has an incidence rate of 11/100000 in the United States, with 22000 new cases each year. This disease is of importance because of its very poor prognosis, the fact that it is increasing in incidence, and is environmentally caused.

18.17 Aetiology and Risk Factors

1. Increased incidence of pancreatic cancer in patients who are cigarette smokers or have been exposed to chemicals (chemical industry workers)
2. Not causally related to:
   - Pancreatitis
   - Diabetes mellitus

18.18 Prognosis

Almost uniformly fatal – overall 5-year survival 1%–4%

18.19 Treatment

18.19.1 Surgery

1. Whipple's procedure (pancreaticoduodenal resection with preservation of the pancreatic tail).
2. Radical total pancreaticoduodectomy. Only 10%–20% of all patients are considered for surgical resection and the 3-year disease-free survival is 15%. Operative mortality is 10%–30%.

18.19.2 Radiation Therapy

In patients with locally unresectable pancreatic cancer, either 4000 or 6000 rads of split-course irradiation with concomitant 5-FU therapy produce improvement in survival compared to 6000 rads of radiation alone (Lockich et al.). The median survival for the 5-FU + radiation regimens is 12 months as opposed to 6 months for radiation therapy alone.

18.19.3 Chemotherapy

1. Single-agent chemotherapy (MacDonald et al. 1981):

Drug	No. of patients	No. of responses	Response rate (%)
5-FU	212	60	28
Mitomycin C	44	12	27
Streptozotocin	22	8	36
Adriamycin	15	2	13
Me-CCNU	34	3	9
Actinomycin D	28	1	
Methotrexate	25	1	
Razoxane (ICRF 159)	18	1	
Galactitol	20	1	
β-2-deoxythioguanosine (TgdR)	26	1	
BCNU	31	0	

2. Multi-drug chemotherapy:

Drug combinations	No. of patients	No. of responses	Response rate (%)
Streptozotocin + mitomycin + 5-FU	23	10	43
5-FU + Adriamycin + mitomycin C	25	10	40
5-FU + BCNU	45	14	31
5-FU + Me-CCNU	-	-	7
5-FU + mitomycin C	-	-	30

18.20 Recommended Treatment Strategy for Pancreatic Cancer

18.20.1 Localized Disease

Treatment of choice is surgical resection.

18.20.2 Locally Unresectable Disease

Radiation therapy + 5-FU to be followed with multidrug chemotherapy (if tolerated) is the treatment of choice.

18.20.3 Metastatic Pancreatic Cancer

Multidrug chemotherapy with either streptozotocin, mitomycin C, 5-FU (SMF) or FAM (Smith et al.)

N. B. For the therapy of insuloma, see Chap. 26, Endocrine Organ Tumours.

V. Liver[1]

18.21 Suggested Chemotherapy for Hepatic Carcinoma

First choice:
Adriamycin 60–75 mg/m² i.v. every 3 weeks
Maximum tolerable dose: 500–550 mg/m²
Second choice:
5-FU 15–20 mg/kg/once weekly i.v. or 10–12 mg/kg/day i.v. × 4 repeated every 3 weeks

Further Reading

Kemeny N, Yagoda A, Golbey R (1980) A prospective randomized study of methyl CCNU, 5-fluorouracil and vincristine (MOF) vs. MOF plus streptozotocin (MOF-STREP) in patients with metastatic colorectal carcinoma. Proc ASCO and AACR 21: 417
MacDonald JS, Schein PS, Woolley PV, Smythe T, Ueno W, Hoth D, Smith F, Boiron M, Gisselbrecht C, Brunet, R, Lagarde C (1980) 5-Fluorouracil, Doxorubicin and Mitomycin (FAM): Combination chemotherapy for advanced gastric cancer. Ann Intern Med 93: 533–536
MacDonald J, Gunderson L, Dohn I (1980) Stomach cancer. In: Principles and Practice of Oncology, DeVita VT, Hellman S, Rosenberg S (eds) Lippincott, Philadelphia
MacDonald JS, Gunderson L, Dohn I (1980) Pancreatic cancer. In: Principles and Practice of Oncology, DeVita VT, Hellman S, Rosenberg S (eds) Lippincott, Philadelphia
Moertel C (1973) Stomach cancer. In: Cancer Medicine, Frei E and Holland J (eds) Lead & Febiger, Philadelphia
Moertel C (1973) Pancreatic cancer. In: Cancer Medicine. Frei E and Holland J (eds) Lea & Febiger, Philadelphia
Moertel C (1973) Colon cancer. In: Cancer Medicine. Frei E, Holland J (eds) Lea & Febiger, Philadelphia
Nöthiger F, Oesch I (1978) Tumeurs Colo-rectales. Schweizerische Krebsliga, Bern
Piper DW (1978) Stomach Cancer, UICC Technical Report Series, Vol 34. UICC, Geneva
Sugarbaker P (1980) Colon cancer. In: Principles and Practice of Oncology, DeVita VT, Hellman S, Rosenberg S (eds) Lippincott, Philadelphia

[1] See also Chap. 39, Hepatocellular Carcinoma in the Tropics.

19 Lung Tumours

19.1 Incidence and Epidemiology

Most common cause of cancer deaths in the United States and an increasingly important cause of cancer deaths in all societies in which cigarette smoking is common - 117000 new cases per year in United States (59/100000). First cause of cancer deaths in males and second to breast cancer as a cause of cancer-related mortality in women.

19.2 Aetiology and Risk Factors

90% of all lung cancers are directly attributable to cigarette smoking.

Other aetiologies include: radiation exposure (uranium miners, atomic bomb survivors), chemical industry workers (methyl ethers, etc.).

19.3 Pathological Classification

1. Squamous cell carcinoma (epidermoid carcinoma)
   Variant
   a) spindle cell (squamous) carcinoma
2. Small-cell carcinoma
   a) Oat-cell carcinoma
   b) Intermediate cell type
   c) Combined
3. Adenocarcinoma
   a) Acinar adenocarcinoma
   b) Papillary adenocarcinoma
   c) Bronchiolo-alveolar carcinoma
   d) Solid carcinoma with mucus formation
4. Large-cell carcinoma
   Variants
   a) Giant-cell carcinoma
   b) Clear-cell carcinoma

Cell type	Incidence (%)
Epidermoid	40
Adenocarcinoma	22
Large-cell	15
Small-cell anaplastic	19
Other	3

19.4 Main Clinical Features

Haemoptysis
Cough
Dyspnoea
Pneumonitis
Pain
Wheeze
Weight loss

19.5 Diagnostic Procedures (Where Applicable)

1. Clinical examination
2. Sputum cytology
3. Bronchoscopy - Brush biopsy
   - Transbronchial biopsy
4. Open biopsy
5. Lymph node biopsy
6. Staging investigations may also include:
   a) Bone marrow aspirate (small-cell only)
   b) Bone scan
   c) Liver ultrasound

19.6 Staging of Lung Cancer

T1: Tumour size below 3 cm, within one lobe and surrounded by normal lung tissue
T2: Tumour size more than 3 cm, surrounded with atelectasis and/or pneumonic infiltration or extension into the hilar region. Tumour at least 2 cm distant from the carina
T3: Tumour of any size with extension into the neighbouring structure (chest wall, mediastinum, diaphragm) or less than 2 cm from carina
N0: No lymph nodes involved
N1: Ipsilateral hilar lymph nodes involved
N2: Mediastinal lymph nodes involved
Operable Stages (WHO Classification)
Stage I: T1, N0-N1 and T2, N0, M0
Stage II: T2, N1, M0
Stage III: Remainder

19.6.1 Small-Cell Lung Cancer

Limited disease: Limited to one hemithorax, mediastinum and ipsilateral supraclavicular area
Extensive disease: All other extensions and metastases

19.7 Prognosis and Treatment

19.7.1 Prognosis of Patients in Relation to Operability (see page 220)

19.7.2 Prognostic Factors in Patients with Inoperable Lung Cancer

1. Histological type: Best prognosis - squamous cell carcinoma
   Worst prognosis - small-cell carcinoma (if untreated)
   Intermediate - adenocarcinoma, large-cell carcinoma
2. Extent of disease: Limited disease has better survival and better response to therapy than extensive disease
3. Performance status: [Eastern Cooperative Oncology Group (ECOG) scale] 0 and 1 (fully ambulatory patients) have better survival and better response to therapy than 2, 3 or 4 (not fully ambulatory patients)
4. Weight loss: Worsens prognosis
5. Other systemic disease symptoms and/or abnormalities in haematological parameters or serum chemistry

19.7.3 Non-Surgical Treatment

19.7.3.1 Radiation Therapy

Non-Small-Cell Lung Cancer. At present there is no convincing evidence (with one possible exception) that irradiation of unresectable non-small-cell lung cancer improves patient survival (Muggia et al.). Although improved survival may not be achievable with irradiation, it may be possible to significantly palliate symptoms of pain or obstruction with radiation therapy. Radiation therapy combined with aggressive surgery may result in cure of up to 30% of patients with superior sulcus (Pancoast) tumours (Muggia et al.).

Survival of Patients with Undifferentiated Small-Cell Carcinoma of Lung by Clinical Diagnostic Stage

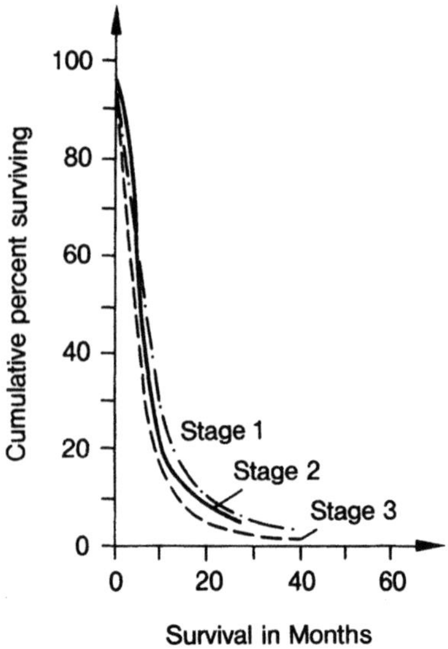

Survival of Patients with Squamous Cell Carcinoma of Lung by Clinical Diagnostic Stage

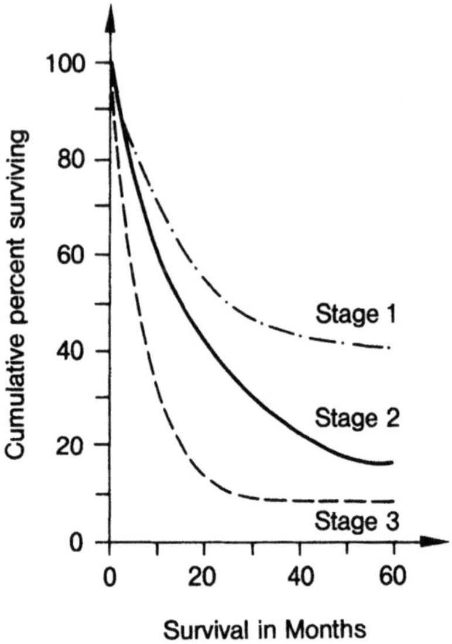

Survival of Patients with Adenocarcinoma and Undifferentiated Large-Cell Carcinoma of Lung by Clinical Diagnostic Stage

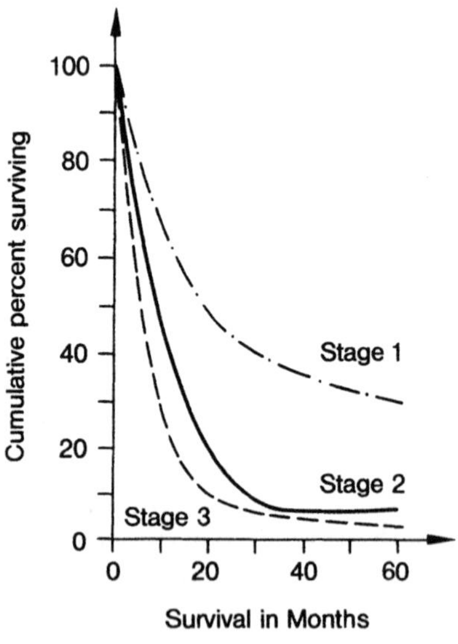

Small-Cell Lung Cancer. Irradiation of small-cell lung cancer results in objective regression of tumour in 70%-80% of cases. However, this does not significantly improve survival, since small-cell cancer is almost always disseminated at the time of diagnosis and requires systemic therapy in addition to local therapy.

19.7.3.2 Chemotherapy

1. Single drugs effective in lung cancer

Drug	Objective response (mostly small series) (%)			
	Epidermoid	Small-cell	Large-cell	Adenocarcinoma
Cyclophosphamide (CTX)				
- i.v. intermittent high dose (40 mg/kg)	19	85	30	?
- daily dose	17	56	27	?
Nitrogen mustard	20-25	40	30	?
Methotrexate (MTX)	15	30-40	12-25	30-35
Procarbazine (PCB)	All histologies together: 9			
Vincristine (VCR)	Below 10	33 (?)	Below 20	Below 20
Lomustine (CCNU)	10-41	13-33 (?)	?	?
Adriamycin (ADM)	15-20	35-45	20-30	Below 20
Mitomycin C (MIT-C)	15-20	25-35	?	?
Etoposide (VP-16-213)	Below 20	50	35	Below 20
Hexamethylmelamine	20	25-30	?	?
Cis-platinum (DDP)	Below 20	25-35	?	?
Vindesine	22 in non-small-cell carcinoma (10/46)			

2. Drug combinations in lung cancer (see p. 222)

Drugs	Institute or author	No. of patients	Objective responses (%)			
			Small-cell	Squamous-cell	Large-cell	Adenocarcinoma
CTX + CCNU	Eastern Cooperative Oncology Group (ECOG) 1977	83	45 (CR 12)	–	–	–
CTX + CCNU + MTX	NCI/VA 1977					
- standard dose		9	45	–	–	–
- high dose		23	96 (CR 30)	–	–	–
CTX + CCNU + MTX 6 weeks then ADM + VCR + PCB	NCI/VA 1977	50	89 (CR 56)	–	–	–
CTX + ADM + VP-16-213 (CTX high dose)	J. Hopkins, Baltimore, 1979	21	86 (CR 29)	–	–	–
CTX-MTX + VCR + PCB	Swiss Group 1973	114	62	24	–	–
CTX + MTX + VCR + PCB	Bern/St. Gall 1979	45	64	–	–	–
ADM + CTX + VCR (+ brain irradiation) (limited disease)	Einhorn	32	87 (CR 60)	–	–	–
3000 rads, then CTX + ADM + MTX + PCB (CAMP) Stage III-M_0	Bitran et al.	39	–	57	43	45
CTX + ADM + DDP (CAP I)	Mayo Clinic, Rochester, 1977	41		44 (8/18)	22 (2/9)	43 6/14)
CTX + ADM + DDP (CAP II)	Mayo Clinic 1979	42	–	–	48 (20/42)	48 (20/42)
5-Flourouracil (5-FU) + ADM + MIT-C	Georgetown University, Washington D.C., 1979	25	–	–	–	36 (9/25)
DDP + vindesine	Sloan Kettering, New York, 1979	59	–	47 (8/17)	50 (1/2)	42 (17/40)

19.8 Problems Under Study and Future Prospects: Conclusions as to the Therapy of Inoperable Lung Cancer

19.8.1 Small-Cell Carcinoma

1. Small-cell cancer of the lung represents approximately 20% of lung cancers in Western Europe and the United States.
2. Its incidence is closely related to smoking.
3. The presence of widespread metastases in the majority (80%) of patients at presentation means that the TNM staging system has little relevance to management.
4. Although marker substances may be produced, the low levels and lack of specificity make these of little value in diagnosis or management.
5. Surgery may be of value in the rare instance of localized peripheral tumour. The importance of reducing tumour volume has yet to be assessed.
6. Radiotherapy alone is less effective than chemotherapy for both limited and extensive disease. However, the studies contributing to this conclusion used suboptimal doses of radiotherapy.
7. Small-cell lung cancer is highly chemosensitive. The complete response rate may be improved by combining three to four drugs.
8. Radiotherapy to sites of bulk disease following chemotherapy may further increase the response rate, but an equivalent improvement in survival is only seen in patients with localized disease.
9. Assessment of response remains largely subjective.

19.8.2 Non-Small-Cell Carcinoma

1. Therapeutic results with chemotherapy and radiotherapy or any combination of both are generally still unsatisfactory, with limited benefit to most patients. Median survival does not seem to be affected significantly.
2. Response rates of over 40% with certain chemotherapeutic regimens have so far been reported only in small series. They have not yet been confirmed by additional studies and other investigators.
3. The first choice of treatment for symptomatic, limited disease of the squamous and large-cell type may still be local radiotherapy.

19.9 Suggested Treatment Regimens for Inoperable Lung Cancer

19.9.1 Small-Cell Carcinoma[1]

1. CCNU	70 mg/m² every 6 weeks p.o.
CTX	1500 mg/m² every 3 weeks i.v.
MTX	10 mg/m² twice weekly for 4–6 weeks p.o.
2. CTX	1500 mg/m² i.v. day 1
ADM	60 mg/m² i.v. day 1
VP-16-213	125 mg/m² i.v. slowly, or short infusion days 1–3
Repeated every 4 weeks	
3. ADM	50 mg/m² i.v.
CTX	750 mg/m² i.v.
VCR	1.5 mg/m² i.v.
Repeated every 3 weeks	
4. CTX	220 mg/m² i.v. or p.o. day 1–3
VP-16-213	125 mg/m² slowly i.v. (5') day 1–3
VCR	1.5 mg/m² i.v. day 1
MTX	40 mg/m² i.v. day 1

19.9.2 Non-Small-Cell Carcinoma

1. CTX	300 mg/m² days 1+8
ADM	20 mg/m² days 1+9
MTX	15 mg/m² days 1+8
PCB	100 mg/m² days 1–10
Repeated every 4 weeks	

		day 1	8	29	36	56
2. FAM						
5-FU	600 mg/m²	×	×	×	×	×
ADM	30 mg/m²	×		×		×
MIT-C	10 mg/m²	×				×

3. CAP I	
CTX	400 mg/m² day 1
ADM	40 mg/m² day 1
DDP	40 mg/m² day 1
Repeated every 3–4 weeks	
4. CAP II	
CTX	400 mg/m² day 1

---

[1] Surgery rarely indicated in small-cell carcinoma.

ADM	40 mg/m^2 day 1
DDP	60 mg/m^2 day 1
Repeated every 3-4 weeks	
5. DDP	120 mg/m^2 1 hour infusion with hydration, days 1, 29, 71, 113, 155
Vindesine	3 mg/m^2 i.v. weekly for 7 weeks, then every 2 weeks

Comments on Recommended Therapy Schedules:

1. Regimens 1 and 2 for small-cell carcinoma are high-dose, intensive treatments which may need hospitalization and supportive care.
2. Chemotherapy in small-cell carcinoma may be combined with prophylactic brain irradiation.
3. The "CAMP" regimen for non-small-cell lung cancer has been used after 3000 rads to the primary tumour with minimal toxicity.

Further Reading

Bitran J et al. (1976) CAMP chemotherapy. Cancer Treat Rep 60: 1225

Bunn P et al. (1977) Therapy of small cell anaplastic carcinoma of the lung. Cancer Treat Rep 61: 333

Butler TP et al. (1979) FAM chemotherapy in adenocarcinoma of the lung. Cancer 43: 1183

Cohen MD (1975) Lung cancer: A status report. J Natl Cancer Inst 55: 505

Gray N, Daube M (1980) Guidelines for Smoking Control. UICC Technical Report Series, Vol 52. UICC, Geneva

Hansen HH, Rork M (1981) In: Pinedo HM (ed) Cancer Chemotherapy. Excerpta Medica, Amsterdam

Lung Cancer (1980) II World Conference, Copenhagen

McKneally MF (1976) BCG immunotherapy. J Thoracic Cardiovasc Surg 72: 333

Mountain CF (1974) Surgical therapy. Semin Oncol I (3): 235

Roswit B et al. (1968) Radiation therapy as adjuvant. Radiology 90: 688

Small-cell lung Cancer (1981) Greco A, Oldham RK, Burn PA (eds) Grune & Stratton

Wynder EL, Hecht S (1976) Lung Cancer. UICC Technical Report Series, Vol 25. UICC, Geneva

Wynder, Hoffman (1976) Tobacco and etiology of lung cancer. Semin Oncol III (1): 5

20 Urogenital Tumours I: Kidney, Renal Pelvis, Ureter, Bladder

I. Kidney, Renal, Pelvis, Ureter

20.1 Incidence and Epidemiology

Male incidence rates are around 6/100000 per year, female rates are 50%-65% of those in males. The parenchyma/pelvis ratio is fairly constant around 5. Higher incidence in Sweden and Iceland, lower in United Kingdom, Eastern Europe, Africa, Asia.

20.2 Aetiology and Risk Factors

Aetiology of the majority of cancers of the kidney, renal pelvis and ureter is unknown.

20.3 Pathological Classification

1. Renal cell adenocarcinoma:
   a) Clear-cell carcinoma
   b) Granular-cell carcinoma
   c) Sarcomatoid
2. Carcinoma of the renal pelvis:
   a) Papillary transitional-cell carcinoma (90%)
   b) Squamous cell carcinoma
3. Carcinoma of the ureter:
   a) Transitional-cell carcinoma (>70%)
   b) Squamous cell carcinoma

20.4 Presenting Symptoms, Laboratory Abnormality, or Abnormality on Physical Examination and its Relation to Survival Rate in 309 Consecutive Patients Undergoing Nephrectomy for Renal Cell Carcinoma (Modified from Skinner et al.)

Presenting symptom, abnormal laboratory finding or abnormality on physical examination	Number of patients (and percentages of total)
Classic triad (gross haematuria, abnormal mass, pain)	29 (9%)
Haematuria	183 (59%)
Pain	127 (41%)
Abdominal mass	139 (45%)
Fever	21 (7%)
Weight loss	85 (28%)
Anaemia	64 (21%)
Erythrocytosis	10 (3%)
Hypercalcaemia	11 (3%)
Acute varicocele	7 (2%)
Tumour calcification on x-ray film	39 (13%)
Symptoms for metastases	31 (10%)
Cancer, an incidental finding (silent)	20 (7%)

20.5 Diagnostic Procedures for Mass Lesions of the Kidney (Lang)

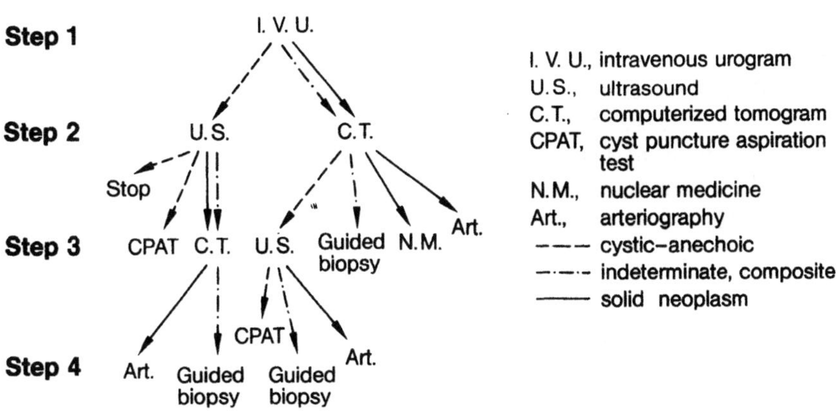

20.6 TNM Classification of Renal Cell carcinoma

T - Primary Tumour

In the absence of arteriography the symbol TX must be used

T0 No evidence of primary tumour.

T1 Evidence of a small tumour without enlargement of the kidney. There is a limited calyceal distortion or deformity and circumscribed vascular deformities, surrounded by renal parenchyma.

T2 Evidence of a large tumour with deformity *and/or* enlargement of the kidney *or* calyceal *or* pelvic involvement. The continuity of the cortex is preserved on artiography.

T3 Evidence of spread into perinephric fat, peri-pelvic fat or hilar renal vessels.

T4 Evidence of extension into neighbouring organs or abdominal wall.

TX The minimum requirements to assess the primary tumour cannot be met.

N - Regional and Juxta-Regional Lymph Nodes

N0 No evidence of regional lymph node involvement.

N1 Evidence of involvement of a single homolateral regional lymph node.

N2 Evidence of contralateral *or* bilateral *or* multiple regional lymph nodes.

N3 Evidence of involvement of fixed regional lymph nodes (assessable only at surgical evaluation).

N4 Evidence of involvement of juxta-regional lymph nodes.

NX The minimum requirements to assess the regional *and/or* juxta-regional lymph nodes cannot be met.

M - Distant metastases

M0 No evidence of distant metastases.

M1 Evidence of distant metastases.

MX The minimum requirements to assess the presence of distant metastases cannot be met.

20.7 Staging of Renal Cell Carcinoma (Robson 1963)

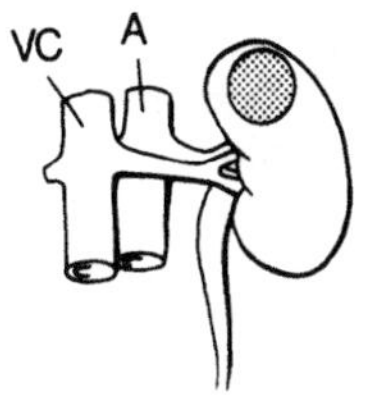

Stage I Tumour within capsule

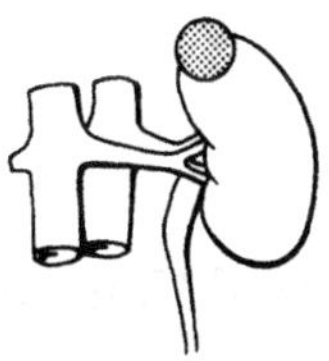

Stage II Tumour invasion of the perinephric fat

VC, Vena Cava
A, Aorta

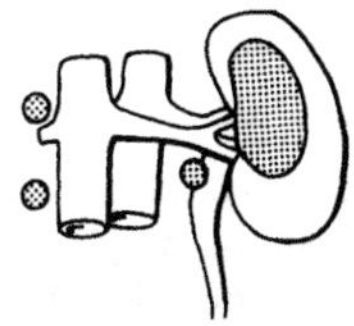

Stage III Tumour invasion of the pedicle and/or regional nodes

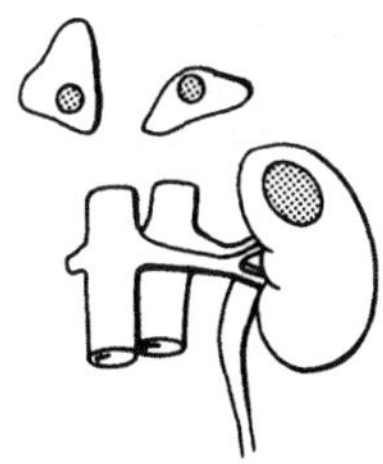

Stage IV distant metastases

20.8 Single Drugs Effective in Renal Cell Carcinoma

Systemic therapy for advanced renal cell carcinoma is extremely unsatisfactory. In 496 patients treated with 11 cytotoxic agents, the percentage of responders varied between 0 and 25% (mean value: 5.3%). Medroxyprogesterone (Provera) has been reported of value, and in the period 1967-1971, the response rate in a group of 228 patients reached 17%. Nevertheless, more recent data compiled on 415 patients from the period of 1971-1976 showed only 2% responders.

20.8.1 Response of Advanced Renal Cancer to Cytotoxic Agents and Hormones

Drug	No. of patients	Response rate (%)
Progesterone (1967-1971)	228	17
Progesterone (1971-1976)	415	2
Vinblastine (VBL)	135	25
Mitomycin C	26	11
Methyl-CCNU (Me-CCNU)	79	7
5-Fluorouracil	51	5
Hydroxyurea	45	5
Nitrogen mustard	35	4
6-Mercaptopurine (6-MP)	26	2

20.9 Drug Combinations Effective in Renal Cell Carcinoma

Combination chemotherapy produced a slightly improved response rate in patients with advanced renal carcinoma; however, the number of patients treated so far is low.

20.9.1 Response of Advanced Renal Cancer to Combination Chemotherapy

Drug combinations	No. of patients	Response rate %
Vincristine (VCR) + Adriamycin (ADM) + MedProg Ac + BCG	31	33
Lomustine (CCNU) + VBL	29	24
Me-CCNU + MedProg Ac	38	11
VBL + MedProg Ac	38	8
Me-CCNU + VBL	15	7

MedProg Ac, medroxyprogesterone acetate; BCG, Calmette-Guerin bacillus

20.10 Therapeutic Strategy

1. For tumours of the kidney and pelvis, radical surgery alone offers a chance for long-term survival or palliation. Advanced distant metastases, advanced lymph node involvement and infiltration of adjacent vital structures contraindicate surgery.
2. Solitary brain and lung metastases may be treated by surgical excision which occasionally leads to reasonable survival.
3. Pre- and post-operative irradiation has been used, but its value is questionable. Irradiation may be effective in long-term control of skeletal metastases.
4. Chemotherapy has a limited value, but may help in palliation.

20.11 Recommended Chemotherapy

No effective chemotherapy is known. Occasional responses have been reported with Depo-Provera.

20.12 Survival of Patients with Renal Adenocarcinoma in Relation to Stage (Robson et al.)

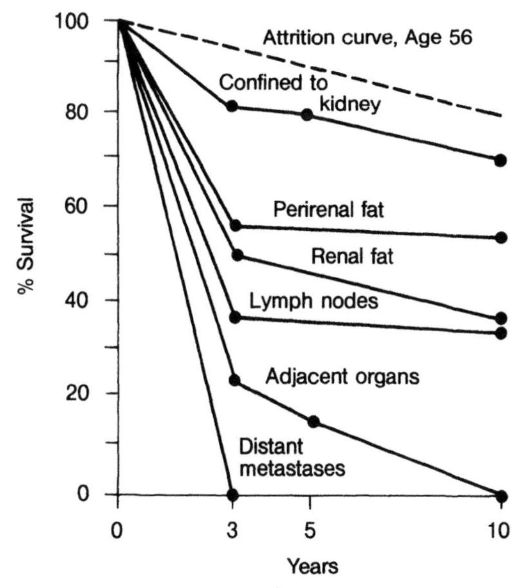

II. Bladder

20.13 Incidence, Epidemiology, Aetiology and Risk Factors

Bladder cancers (see also Chap. 40) account for about 3% of all malignant tumours. The incidence is higher in countries where schistosomiasis is endemic such as Egypt (20%) and Iraq. The peak incidence is in the 6th and 7th decades. The male: female ratio is 3:1.

Persons working with aniline dyes, synthetic rubber and various other chemicals have developed bladder cancer which could be attributed to the action of aromatic amines, benzidine, 2-naphthylamine, etc. Tumours may develop many years after exposure, as papillary transitional-cell carcinomas which are often multiple.

Urinary schistosomiasis (bilharziasis) which persists over 20-40 years induces squamous cell metaplasia, dysplasia, carcinoma in situ and ultimately invasive cancer which is mostly a well-differentiated squamous cell carcinoma.

N.B. A detailed description of the diagnostic procedures, staging and therapeutic strategy for bladder cancer can be found in Chap. 40.

21 Urogenital Tumours II: Prostate, Testis

I. Prostate

21.1 Incidence and Epidemiology

Death rates ranging from 10 to 20 per 100000 population, higher incidence in blacks. The incidence of prostatic cancer is increasing in the industrialized countries. More than 10% found at autopsy.

21.2 Risk Factors

Very rare under the age of 40, peak of incidence 7th and 8th decade.

21.3 Pathology

Adenocarcinoma accounts for 95% of prostatic cancer.
Histopathological grading:
G1 High degree of differentiation
G2 Medium degree of differentiation
G3 Low degree of differentiation or undifferentiated
GX Grade cannot be assessed

21.4 Main Clinical Features

1. Symptoms due to bony metastases
2. Symptoms of urethral obstruction
3. Occasional severe irritative bladder symptoms
4. Rare isolated haematuria

21.5 Diagnostic Procedures and TNM Classification

1. Rectal examination, transrectal (or transperineal) needle biopsy
2. Transrectal prostate ultrasound
3. Routine chest and pelvic roentgenograms, radioisotopic bone scanning
4. Lymphangiography
5. Prostatic acid phosphatase

Prostate	
T0	Incidental carcinoma
T1	Intracapsular/normal gland
T2	Intracapsular/deformed gland
T3	Extension beyond capsule
T4	Extension fixed to neighbouring organs
N1	Single homolateral regional
N2	Contra - or bi-lateral/multiple regional
N3	Fixed regional
N4	Juxta-regional

21.6 Relationship Between Staging Classifications for Prostatic Carcinoma. Preliminary Stage Classification (Paulson et al. 1982[a])

Stage	Stage	TNM Classification	Local lesion	Prostatic acid phosphatase	Bone metastases by bone roentgeno-gram
A. Focal	IA	$T_0N_0M_0$	Not palpable, focal	Not elevated	No
A. Diffuse	IB	$T_0N_0M_0$	Not palpable, diffuse	Not elevated	No
B	II	$T_1T_2N_0M_0$	Confined to prostate	Not elevated	No
C	III	$T_3N_0M_0$	Local extension	Not elevated	No
D	IVA	$T_4N_0M_0$	Any	Elevated	No
D	IVB	$T_{0\text{-}4}N_{1\text{-}4}M_0$[a]	Any	Any	No
D	IVC	$T_{0\text{-}4}N_{0\text{-}4}M_1$	Any	Any	Yes

[a] IVB patients cannot be assigned a stage classification until after node dissection as this category is reserved for patients with lymph node extension

21.7 Endocrine Therapy in Advanced Prostatic Carcinoma

There is good evidence that orchidectomy or oestrogen therapy is attended by useful palliation in stages III (extension to extracapsular structures) and IV (bone or any extrapelvic involvement).

Recent controlled studies have not shown any difference in survival between treated patients and controls; however, the controls also received endocrine therapy at a later date. Consequently, although the evidence is inadequate, endocrine treatment may prolong survival to some degree. It has been shown that survival is not impaired by withholding endocrine therapy until the patient is symptomatic; and, in view of the side effects and risks of endocrine therapy, most authorities recommend this approach.

Effect of endocrine therapy in different case series

Therapy	Stage	Survival at 5 years (%)	Survival at 9 years (%)	Survival at 10 years (%)
No hormone therapy	III	10		
No hormone therapy	IV	6		
Orchidectomy ± oestrogen therapy	III	44		
Orchidectomy 324	III	31		
Oestrogen therapy patients	III	29		
Orchidectomy + oestrogen therapy	IV	20		
Orchidectomy 263	IV	22		
Oestrogen therapy patients	IV	10		
Early orchidectomy ± oestrogen therapy	III	57		26.5
Oestrogen therapy	III	35		11.5
No hormone therapy	III	15		5.0
Orchidectomy + oestrogen therapy	IV	13.5		
Oestrogen therapy	IV	21		
Placebo	III	53	20–30	
Orchidectomy + placebo	III	54	20–30	
Diethylstilboestrol 5 mg/day	III	50	20–30	
Orchidectomy + diethylstilboestrol 5 mg/day	III	46	20–30	
Placebo	IV	25	5–15	
Orchidectomy + placebo	IV	25	5–15	
Diethylstilboestrol 5 mg/day	IV	26	5–15	
Orchidectomy + diethylstilboestrol 5 mg/day	IV	24	5–15	

21.8 Chemotherapy of Advanced Prostatic Carcinoma

Single-agent or multi-drug chemotherapy is indicated for patients refractory to hormonal therapy. The following response rates were achieved: *cis*-platinum (DDP): 43%; mechlorethamine (HN2): 39%; 5-fluorouracil (5-FU): 29%; Adriamycin (ADM): 26%; CTX: 14%.

Among combined regimens, estramustine (15 mg/kg/day/p.o.) and 5-FU (600 mg/m^2/week/i.v.) produced 32% response rate with 12 weeks duration, while ADM (30 mg/m^2/i.v./day 1) and CTX (100 mg/m^2/day/p.o. day 1-14) achieved 33% partial remission (PR) with median duration over 11 months. More recently, response rates of close to 50% have been reported with ADM and DDP. Nevertheless, there are randomized trials which do not show any differences among the results obtained by either single-agent or multi-drug chemotherapy.

21.9 Remission Following Hormonal Therapy (Prout)

Subjective evidence	Objective evidence
Relief of pain	Return of serum acid phosphatase to normal
Return of sense of well-being	Decrease in size and induration of primary tumour
Relief or anorexia	Decrease in size and number of metastases
	Correction of anaemia
	Weight gain

21.10 Therapeutic Strategy

1. T_1, T_2, T_3 lesions (tumours localized to the prostate) can be treated by radical prostatectomy or radical irradiation.
2. T_4 and M_1 lesions can be treated by endocrine therapy (ablative or additive). Urinary obstruction, if present, can be relieved by a limited transurethral resection.
3. Disease unresponsive to endocrine therapy can be treated with chemotherapy.

21.11 Prognostic Factors

1. Survival is directly related to stage:
   Stages I and II ~ 70% at 5 years
   Stage III ~50% at 5 years
   Stage IV ~25% at 5 years
2. Degree of differentiation is an important factor in prognosis: differentiated carcinomas have better prognosis.

II. Testis

21.12 Incidence and Epidemiology

Testicular cancer accounts for 1%-2% of all malignant diseases in males. The annual incidence is 1-2 per 100000 of the male population. It is the most common type of cancer in males between 20 and 34 years of age. The disease appears to be more frequent in the white population than in other races.

21.13 Aetiology and Risk Factors

The aetiology of testicular cancer is unknown. Patients with cryptorchidism have a greatly increased risk of developing cancer not only in the maldescended but also in the normally descended testis. Orchiopexy, even before the age of 6 years, does not diminish this risk appreciably.

21.14 Histological Classifications of Testicular Tumours

A. British Testicular Tumours Panel (1975)	B. US Armed Forces Institute of Pathology	C. WHO Classification
Teratoma - differentiated Malignant teratoma - intermediate (formerly MTIA) Malignant teratoma - undifferentiated (formerly MTIB)	*Germinal origin:* 1. Seminoma a) Typical (classical) b) Anaplastic c) Spermatocytic (atypical) 2. Embryonal carcinoma 3. Teratoma	Tumours of one histological type: Typical seminoma Anaplastic seminoma Spermatocytic seminoma Embryonal carcinoma Yolk sack tumour (infantile embryonal carcinoma)

Malignant teratoma - trophoblastic WHO classification (1975) Teratoma - mature - immature Embryonal carcinoma Choriocarcinoma with or without embryonal carcinoma	4. Teratoma with malignant areas (teratocarcinoma) 5. Choriocarcinoma 6. Compound tumour *Non-germinal origin:* 1. Interstitial cell tumour 2. Gonadal-stromal tumours Miscellaneous	Teratoma Mature teratoma Immature teratoma Teratoma with malignant transformation Choriocarcinoma pure Tumours of more than one histological type: Relative amounts of each component to be specified

21.15 Main clinical features

1. Painless hard testicular swelling which does not transilluminate.
2. Many patients seek medical advice not because of the testicular tumour but because of severe back pain or an abdominal mass due to extensive involvement of the retroperitoneal lymph nodes, or gynaecomastia due to the production of chorionic gonadotropin by the tumour.

21.16 Necessary Procedures for Staging of Testicular Tumours

Tumour markers: Beta-human chorionic gonadotropin (β-HCG), alpha-foetoprotein (α-FP), lactic dehydrogenase (LDH)
Primary tumour: Inguinal orchidectomy and pathological examination
Retroperitoneal nodes:
- Clinical examination
- Lymphangiogram, intravenous pyelogram and phlebography in selected cases
- Computed tomography (CT) scan, where available

Supraclavicular nodes: Clinical examination
Mediastinum and lungs:
- Chest x-rays
- Full-lung tomograms in patients with extended retroperitoneal involvement and negative chest x-rays

Other sites:
- Complete clinical examination (including neurological)
- Liver function tests

21.17 Tumour Markers in Germ Cell Tumours (Jovadpour)

	alpha-FP	β-HCG	SP_1[a]
Results in 97 men with testicular tumour			
Seminoma	–	–	–
Embryonal carcinoma	+	+	–
Embryonal carcinoma or terato carcinoma with synctiotrophoblastic giant cells	+	+	+
Choriocarcinoma	–	+	+

[a] New placental protein (pregnancy-specific beta 1 glycoprotein)

21.18 Value of Tumour Markers (TM) in Non-Seminomatous Germ Cell Tumours

α-FP in 70%-90%
β-HCG in 40%-60%

Elevated prelymphadenectomy tumour markers indicate a far worse prognosis than in patients with normal tumour markers.

Tumour marker determination may reduce the clinical staging error to the 10%-15% range.

Elevated tumour markers after orchidectomy and/or lymphadenectomy presence of residual tumour: need for further treatment.

Serial measurement of tumour markers is a sensitive indicator or response to chemotherapy.

21.19 Proposal for Staging Testicular Cancer (Cavalli et al. 1980)

Stage I:	No evidence of metastatic spread
I A:	Tumour confined to the testis and its appendages (category T1, T2 and T3 of the TNM classification)
I B:	Tumour infiltrating the spermatic cord (category T4 a) or a tumour arising in an undescended testis
I C:	Tumour infiltrating the scrotum (T4 b) or arising after inguinal or scrotal surgery, or managed by transcrotal biopsy or orchidectomy
I X:	The extension of the primary tumour cannot be assessed.

Stage II:	Metastases to infradiaphragmatic nodes only
II A:	All metastatic nodes are ≤2 cm
II B:	At least one metastatic node is between 2 and 5 cm
II C:	Retroperitoneal metastasis larger than 5 cm
II D:	Palpable abdominal mass or fixed inguinal nodes (N_3)
Pathological staging	Specify number and location of metastatic nodes in operated patients Specify extracapsular growth and invasion of veins.
Stage III:	Mediastinal and supraclavicular node involvement, distant metastases
III A:	Mediastinal and/or supraclavicular node involvement without any distant metastasis (N_4)
III B:	Distant metastases only to the lung 'Minimal pulmonary disease': less than 5 nodules in each lung field no one >2 cm 'Advanced pulmonary disease': more than 5 nodules in each lung field or a nodule >2 cm or a pleural effusion
Pathological staging	Specify the extent of concomitant lymph node disease
III C:	Any haematogenous spread outside the lungs
III O:	Persistent positive biological markers after definite therapy and without any other evidence of disease.

Stage I and stages II A and B are considered "early stages"; stages II C and D as well as stage III represent 'advanced disease'.

21.20 Single Agents Effective in Testicular Carcinomas: Cumulative Data from Published Literature

Agent	No. evaluated	Reported response rate	
		CR (%)	CR + PR (%)
Actinomycin (Act-D)	61	18	33
CTX	14	28	86
Mithramycin	501	10	35
Vinblastine (VBL)	41	12	37
Bleomycin (BLM)	54	11	43
ADM	29	0	17
DDP	70	21	66
Etoposide (VP-16-213)	24	12	46

CR, complete remission PR, partial remission

21.21 Principal Drug Combinations (Not Including Cis-Platinum) Effective in Testicular Carcinomas

Combination	No. evaluated	Reported response rate	
		CR (%)	CR + PR (%)
Act-D, methotrexate, chlorambucil	28	36	50
CTX, vincristine, act-D ± mithramycin	58	12	39
CTX, vincristine, methotrexate, 5-FU (COMF)	17	29	41
ADM, BLM, vincristine	25	32	80
VBL, BLM infusion	57	49	81

21.22 Outline of PVB (Einhorn) and VAB VI (Memorial Sloan-Kettering Cancer Center) Combinations

Scheme	Drug and drug schedule during induction phase				
	VBL	Act-D	BLM	DDP	CTX
PVB	6 mg/m² Day 1 and 2	–	30 mg Day 2, 9 and 16	20 mg/m² Day 1-5	–
VAB VI	4 mg/m² Day 1	1 mg/m² Day 1	30 mg/m² Day 1 + 20 mg/m² from day 1 to 3 through continuous infusion	120 mg/m² Day 4	600 mg/m² Day 1

PVB, *cis*-platinum + vinblastine + bleomycin

N. B. These combinations are to be administered in centres experienced in treatment and prevention of agranulocytic sepsis, renal failure and lung fibrosis. To decrease the risk of irreversible bone marrow toxicity, the lower VBL dosage is suggested.

21.23 Results after PVB and VAB VI in United States

Author	No. of patients evaluated	CR %
Einhorn (PVB)	47	70
Stoter (PVB)	40	60
Samson (PVB)	143	59
MSKCC (VAB VI)	21	90[a]

[a] Also reductive surgery after induction.

21.24 Response to PVB Related to the Extent of Disease (Einhorn)

Disease	No. of patients	CR %
Minimal pulmonary	10	80
Advanced pulmonary	9	67
Minimal abdominal and pulmonary	9	88
Advanced abdominal	16	50
Elevated HCG alone	3	100

21.25 Average Results with PVB and VAB in Advanced Testicular Carcinomas

CR after 3-5 courses: 65%-80%
Total CR after surgery: 80%-95%
Most patients with mature teratoma and/or fibrous tissue remain with no evidence of disease
Total relapse rate in CR: 5%-15%
Further chemotherapy is required in patients with residual tumour after surgery

21.26 Conclusions from Results Achieved with PVB and VAB in Advanced Testicular Carcinomas

1. Induction is the most effective part of treatment
2. CR usually within first three cycles, relapse rate in CR: 5%-12%
3. Long maintenance programme is probably not necessary
4. Bulky metastases frequently have incomplete regression
5. Long-term CR can be achieved with complete resection or residual tumour and additional chemotherapy

21.27 Results of Combination Chemotherapy in Advanced Seminoma

Author	Combinations	No. of evaluable patients	Response		CR + PR (%)
			CR (%)	PR (%)	
Whitmore	CLB + Act-D	4	2 (50)	-	2 (50)
McKenzie	CLB + MTX + Act-D	4	-	2 (50)	2 (50)
Samuels	VBL + BLM	2	-	2 (100)	2 (100)
Yagoda	CTX + DDP	9	3 (33)	4 (45)	7 (78)
Einhorn	VBL + BLM + DDP	14	7 (50)	7 (50)	14 (100)
	VBL + BLM + DDP + ADM	5	5 (100)	-	5 (100)
Pinedo	VBL + BLM + DDP	3	3 (100)	-	3 (100)
Cortes-Funes	VBL + BLM + DDP	54	37 (69)	14 (25)	51 (94)

MTX, methotrexate; CLB, chlorambucil

21.28 Testicular Carcinomas: 5-Year Survival after Radical Retroperitoneal Lymph Node Dissection

1. Orchidectomy plus radical retroperitoneal lymph node dissection
   N – 75%-80%
   N + 50%-60%
2. Post-operative radiotherapy provides comparable results only in the presence of very small (<2 cm) or microscopic nodal metastases.

21.29 Adjuvant PVB × Two Cycles in Comparison with PVB at Relapse (Einhorn)

	PVB	No therapy	Act-D
No. of patients	13	30	30
Follow-up 18 months	13	30	30
Follow-up 36 months	6	16	30
No. relapsing	0	11 (37%)	14 (47%)
No. free of disease	13 (100%)	29 (97%)	29 (97%)
No. dead	0	1 (other causes)	1

21.30 Adjuvant Chemotherapy after Radical RPLND in Testicular Carcinoma

1. Adjuvant PVB and VAB after RPLND in patients with positive retroperitoneal nodes have been effective in minimizing relapse rate.
2. With close follow-up it is possible in the majority of patients relapsing after surgery (RPLND) alone to induce a CR by means of PVB and VAB.
3. Since 50% of patients with positive retroperitoneal nodes can be cured with surgery alone, adjuvant PVB and VAB should probably be administered in high-risk patients (N+ ≥5 and/or ≥2 cm).

21.31 Therapeutic Strategy in Testicular Seminoma after Orchidectomy

Stage IA	Prophylactic radiotherapy to regional lymph nodes after orchidectomy (2500-3000 rads in 3-4 weeks to the para-aortic regions and ipsilateral inguino-iliac area).
Stage IB	As above, but extending the radiation therapy field to the crural area.
Stage II	
- 1st step	Radical radiotherapy to the regional lymph nodes (3000-3500 rads in 4 weeks to the para-aortic regions and to ipsilateral inguino-iliac area). An extra dose of 500-1000 rads to the neoplastic mass may be given in stage IIB).
- 2nd step	Prophylactic radiotherapy to juxta-regional lymph nodes (2500-3000 rads in 3-4 weeks to the mediastinum and both supraclavicular fossae). In cases with extended retroperitoneal metastases (IIB) prophylactic radiotherapy should also be given to the contralateral inguino-iliac lymph nodes.

Stage IIIA	Radical radiotherapy to regional and juxtaregional lymph nodes (3000-3500 rads to para-aortic inguino-iliac, mediastinal and supraclavicular regions).
Stage IIIB	Combination chemotherapy as for carcinomas (PVB, VAB). Palliative radiotherapy to the most involved lymph node regions (3000-3500 rads in 3-4 weeks), in case of CR not achieved with chemotherapy.
Solitary metastasis	Radical radiotherapy (3000-4000 rads in 3-4 weeks).

21.32 Therapeutic Strategy for Stage I and IIA, IIB, IIC Testicular Carcinoma after Orchidectomy

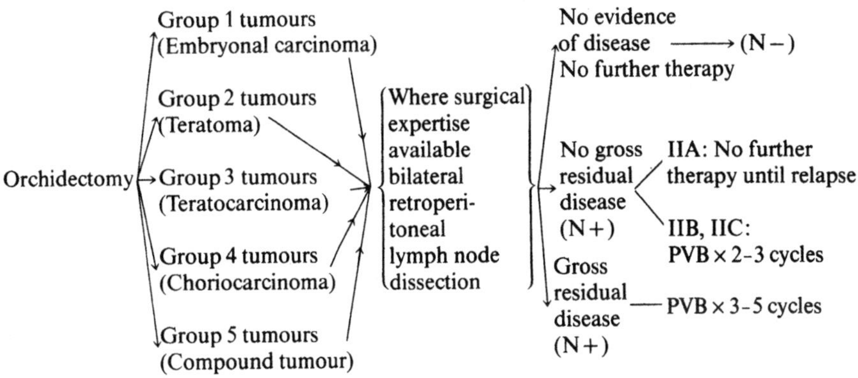

21.33 Therapeutic Strategy for Advanced Testicular Carcinomas (IID, IIIA, IIIB, IIIC, IIIO)

1st choice

PVB × 3-5 cycles

↓

No CR achieved

↓

Consider surgery to eliminate residual tumour

↓

Residual disease after surgery
Surgery not feasible

↓

DDP + VP-16-213 (± BLM) until CR

↓

No response or progression

↓

Act-D + CTX until CR

21.34 Recommended Chemotherapy

PVB and VAB combination, including DDP, can be considered of equivalent value; PVB is recommended, since its administration is easier.

21.35 Prognostic Factors

1. Carcinomas:
   a) Survival is related to stage, but to a lesser extent than in the past because of the progress of combination chemotherapy.
   b) Extended abdominal and/or pulmonary disease is an unfavourable prognostic factor.
2. Seminomas:
   a) Survival is directly related to stage and adequacy of treatment.
   b) Anaplastic seminoma has a slightly lesser survival in any stage compared to typical seminoma.

21.36 Survival in 65 Patients with Testicular Carcinoma According to Stage before the Era of Modern Intensive Combination Chemotherapy (INT Milan, Case Series, 1968–1978)

Actuarial survival according to stage in 65 patients with testicular carcinoma treated before the era of modern aggressive combination chemotherapy at the Istituto Nazionale per lo Studio e la Cura dei Tumori, Milan.

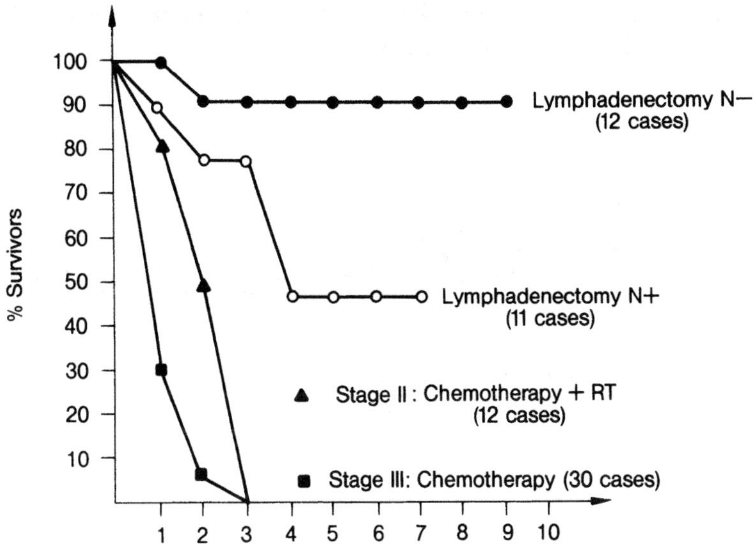

21.37 Sites of Relapse or Progression after Radiotherapy in 166 Patients with Seminoma (INT Milan, Case Series, 1968–1978)

Stage	Nodal relapse		Distant Metastases	Total
	Irradiated site	Non-irradiated site		
I	–	2	–	2/85
NX	–	1	–	1/8
II A–C	3	1	5	9/51
II D	1	–	1	2/15
III A	1	–	3	4/7
Total	5	4	9	18/166

21.38 Survival in 166 Patients with Seminoma after Radiotherapy (INT Milan, Case Series, 1968–1978)

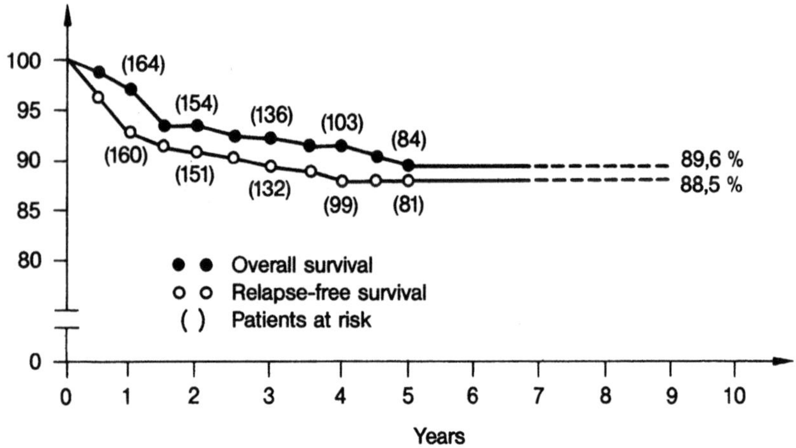

21.39 Problems Under Study

1. Therapy of advanced cases:
   a) Reduction of toxicity (bone marrow, lungs, kidney)
   b) Integration with surgery
   c) Development of alternative drug combinations
2. Adjuvant chemotherapy after RPLND in patients with positive lymph nodes:
   a) Selection of high-risk patients
   b) Early vs chemotherapy on relapse
   c) Type and number of drugs
   d) Duration of adjuvant therapy

Further Reading

Bladder Cancer (1981) UICC Technical Report Series, vol 60. Edited by Skrabanek P and Walsh A

Cavalli F, Monfardini S, Pizzocaro G (1980) Report on the International Workshop on Staging and Treatment of Testicular Cancer. Europ J Cancer 16: 1367

Coffey DS, Isaacs JT (1979) Prostate Cancer. UICC Technical Report Series, vol 48. UICC, Geneva

Friedell KE, Greenfield KE, Hilgar AG (Guest Eds) Urinary bladder cancer. Semin Oncol, June 1979

Murphy GP (Guest Ed) Carcinoma of the prostate. Semin Oncol, June 1976

Paulson DF, Perez CA, Anderson T (1982) Genito-urinary malignancies, pp 732-778 in: De Vita VT, Hellman S, Rosenberg SA (ed) "Cancer Principles and practice of Oncology". J. B. Lippincott Company, Philadelphia-Toronto

Paulson DF, Einhorn LH, Peckam MJ, Williams JD (1982) Cancer of the Testis, pp 786-816 in: De Vita VT, Hellman S, Rosenberg SA (ed) "Cancer Principles and practice of Oncology. J. B. Lippincott Company, Philadelphia-Toronto

Sufrin G, Beckley SA (1980) Renal Adenocarcinoma. UICC Technical Report Series, vol 49. UICC, Geneva

Veronesi U, Lasio E, Emanuelli H, Pizzocaro G, De Leman (1982) I Tumori Urologici Casa editrice Ambrosiana, Milano

Yagoda A, Golbey RB (Guest Eds) Germ cell tumours. Semin Oncol, March 1979

22 Gynaecological Tumours

I. Cervix

22.1 Incidence and Epidemiology

Average incidence in Europe and United States 30–35/100000 female population per year

Accounts for 10%–15% of all malignancies in women
Second or third most common form of cancer in the female population
Incidence falling off

22.2 Aetiology and Risk Factors

1. Rare in virgins, incidence higher in married than in single women and in women who married young or began sexual intercourse early
2. Incidence rises with the number of pregnancies
3. Incidence higher in the low-income groups
4. Rare in communities that practise male circumcision
5. Herpes virus infection may be a risk factor

22.3 Pathological Classification

95%–97% epidermoid or squamous cell carcinomas, the remainder being adenocarcinomas, undifferentiated cancers and very rarely sarcomas

22.4 Main Clinical Features

1. In early stages symptomless or in the form of a superficial erosion
2. In advanced stages exophytic, endophytic or ulcerating

22.5 Diagnostic Procedures

1. Pap smear
2. Thorough gynaecological examination
3. Biopsy of the cervical lesion
4. Endocervical exploration and hysterography
5. Cystoscopy
6. Schiller's test
7. Cone biopsy
8. Colposcopy
9. Lymphography

22.6 Staging Classification

UICC		Cervix	FIGO	
Tis		Carcinoma in situ	0	
T1		Confined to cervix	1	
	T1a	Micro-invasive		1a
	T1b	Invasive		1b
T2		Extension to vagina (not lower third) Parametrium/not pelvic wall	II	
	T2a	Vagina (not lower third)		IIa
	T2b	Parametrium		IIb
T3		Extension to lower third vagina/ parametrium/pelvic wall	III	
	T3a	Vagina/lower third		IIIa
	T3b	Parametrium/pelvic wall		IIIb
T4		Extension to bladder/rectum/beyond true pelvis		IVa
M1		Distant organs		IVb

FIGO, International Federation of Gynaecologists and Obstetricians

22.7 Prognostic Factors

Average 5-year-survival: T1, 70%-85%; T2, 40%-60%; T3, about 30%; T4 < 10%

22.8 Single Agents Effective in Cervical Cancer

Drug	Number of evaluated cases	Overall regression (%)
Cyclophosphamide	229	20
Melphalan	20	25
Chlorambucil	62	24
Methyl-CCNU (Me-CCNU)	32	13
Hexamethylmelamine	44	27
Methotrexate	52	25
Methotrexate i. a.[a]	71	47
5-Fluorouracil	263	20
Bleomycin (BLM)	83	12
Adriamycin	114	23
Mitomycin	23	22
Cis-platinum (DDP)	47	32

[a] i. a. = intraarterial

Conclusion. There is drug response of cervical cancer but up to now there is evidence only of a limited sensitivity of this type of tumour. Maybe DDP is a promising approach. In general, chemotherapy has been tested only minimally in cervical cancer.

22.9 Drug Combinations Active in Cervical Cancer

Drug combination	No. of patients response/total	Response rate (%)	Mean survival (months)
Cyclophosphamide + vincristine	2/19	10	19 (responder)
Cyclophosphamide + methotrexate	10/23	43	
BLM + methotrexate	8/14	57	
BLM + Adriamycin	3/26	12	4.3 19 (responder)
Adriamycin + DDP	6/19	32	
Adriamycin + vincristine	9/54	17	5.5
Adriamycin + 5-fluorouracil + vincristine	3/31	10	7.5

22.10 Therapeutic Strategy in Cervical Cancer

Surgery is the treatment of choice. Radiotherapy may be given in all stages of invasive cervical cancer. Chemotherapy is used for management of advanced stages of disease, but the efficacy of single drugs and drug combinations is marginal. Surgical adjuvant chemotherapy in cervical cancer is still experimental (no confirmed data available).

22.11 Recommended Chemotherapy

1. BLM	10 mg/m^2 i.m. once weekly	normal renal function
Methotrexate	10 mg/m^2 p.o. twice weekly	
2. Adriamycin	20–50 mg/m^2 i.v.	
DDP	50 mg/m^2 i.v. with proper hydration	

Courses repeated every 3 weeks

II. Ovary

22.12 Incidence and Epidemiology

Average incidence in Europe and United States 15–20/100000 female population per year

Accounts for 5%–6% of all malignancies in women

22.13 Aetiology and Risk Factors

1. Often associated with breast cancer
2. Incidence higher in the high-income group

22.14 Pathological Classification

I. Common "epithelial" tumours
   A. Serous
   B. Mucinous
   C. Endometrioid

D. Clear-cell (mesonephroid)	a) Benign
E. Brenner	b) Of borderline malignancy
F. Mixed epithelial	c) Carcinomas
G. Undifferentiated carcinoma	
H. Unclassified	

II. Sex cord stromal tumours

A. Granulosa-theca cell	
B. Androblastoma (Sertoli-Leydig)	a) Benign
C. Gynandroblastoma	b) Malignant
D. Unclassified	

III. Lipid cell tumours

IV. Germ cell tumours
- A. Dysgerminoma
- B. Endodermal sinus tumour
- C. Embryonal carcinoma
- D. Polyembryoma
- E. Choriocarcinoma
- F. Teratomas: Immature
  Mature (solid or cystic)
  Monodermal (stroma ovarii and/or carcinoid, others)

22.15 Main Clinical Features

Spread to the para-aortic, mediastinal and supraclavicular lymph nodes and metastasize late to distant organs, chiefly the liver. Ascites is the most common intra-abdominal problem.

22.16 Diagnostic Procedures

1. Gynaecological examination, abdominal palpation.
2. Ultrasonography, computerized axial tomographic (CAT) scan, laparoscopy.
3. Explorative laparotomy is the most useful diagnostic procedure.

22.17 Staging Classification

UICC TNM Pre-treatment Clinical Classification and FIGO Staging System for Carcinoma of the Ovary

UICC		Ovary	Figo	
T1		Limited to ovaries	I	
	T1a	One ovary, no ascites		Ia
	T1b	Both ovaries, no ascites		Ib
	T1c	One or both ovaries, with ascites		Ic
T2		With pelvic extension	II	
	T2a	Uterus and/or tubes, no ascites		IIa
	T2b	Other pelvic tissues, no ascites		IIb
	T2c	Other pelvic tissues, with ascites		IIc
T3		Extension to small bowel/omentum in true pelvis or intraperitoneal metastases/retroperitoneal nodes	III	
M1		Distant organs	IV	

22.18 Prognostic Factors for Survival and Response to Chemotherapy in Inoperable or Non-Radically-Operated Ovarian Cancer

1. Maximum size of (residual) tumour masses:
   a) Lesions less than 1.5 cm: potentially curable by chemotherapy
   b) Lesions more than 1.5 cm: unfavourable prognosis
2. Degree of histological differentiation (grading):
   (Percentage of undifferentiated cells in the tumour, and the degree to which the tumour is forming papillary structures or gland vs solid tumour) Broder's grade I-IV.
3. Best responses to chemotherapy are found in tumours of Broder's grade II and III.
4. Previous radiotherapy and chemotherapy decreases responsiveness.

22.19 Single Agents Effective in Ovarian Carcinoma

Drug	Number of evaluated cases	Overall regression (%)
Cyclophosphamide (CTX)	335	43
Melphalan	541	47
Chlorambucil	422	52,5
Thiotepa	574	31
Lomustine (CCNU)	69	32
Carmustine (BCNU)	34	6
Methotrexate (MTX)	26	19
5-Fluorouracil (5-FU)	141	26,5
Hexamethylmelamine (HMM)	54	39
Adriamycin (ADM)	114	35
Vinblastine (VBL)	20	15
Vincristine (VCR)	17	0
DDP	49	27
Iphosphamide	16	56

Conclusion. Alkylating agents are the most active drugs in ovarian carcinoma. Doxorubicin, hexamethylmelamine and 5-fluorouracil are valuable alternatives. The recent results with DDP underline that this compound seems to be a very promising approach for ovarian carcinoma chemotherapy.

22.20 Drug Combinations in Ovarian Carcinoma

1. Results with polychemotherapy

Combination	Author or Institution	Number of evaluated cases	Overall regression (%)	CR (%)	Survival (months)
Melphalan/ADM	Trope	72	63	30	16.8
Melphalan/HMM	Omura	94	52	28	14.3
CTX/HMM/MTX/5-FU	Young	41	75	33	29.0
CTX/HMM/MTX/5-FU	Sturgeon	31		19	17.0
CTX/HMM/ADM/DDP	Vogl	127	50	30	19.0
CTX/ADM	Omura	72	49	32	13.7
CTX/ADM/DDP	Mangioni	40	63	32	-
CTX/ADM/DDP	Bernath	18	38	17	13.5
CTX/ADM/DDP	Einhorn	56	80	41	-
CTX/5-FU	Barlow	22	32	19	15.0
CTX/5-FU	Barlow	21	67	48	14.0
CTX/HMM/ADM	Mangioni	37	57	11	-
HMM/ADM/DDP	Bernath	21	33	19	7.5
CTX/MTX/5-FU	ECOG 1974	53	38		-

2. Controlled clinical studies comparing mono- and polychemotherapy

Combination	Author or Institution	Number of evaluated cases	Overall regression (%)	CR (%)	Survival (months)
Melphalan		39	54	16	17.0
vs	Young et al.				
Hexa-CAF		41	75	33	29.0
Melphalan		119	36	16	17.6
vs	Vogl et al.				
CHAP		127	50	30	19.0
Melphalan		70	40	10	10.7
vs	Trope				
ADM-melphalan		72	63	30	16.8
Melphalan		64	37	20	12.3
vs					
HMM-melphalan	Omura et al.	97	52	28	14.3
vs					
ADM-CTX		72	49	32	13.7
Melphalan		29	-	14	
vs					
Hexa-CAF	Sturgeon	31	-	19	17.0
vs					
CAP		28	-	54	

Hexa-CAF, hexamethylmelamine + cyclophosphamide + methotrexate + fluorouracil; CHAP, cyclophosphamide + hexamethylmelamine + Adriamycin + *cis*-platinum; CAP, cyclophosphamide + Adriamycin + *cis*-platinum

22.21 Therapeutic Strategy in Ovarian Carcinoma

Surgery is the treatment of choice. Surgical treatment is also important in patients with extensive disease even though all the tumour cannot be removed. The surgical "debulking" allows both chemotherapy and radiotherapy to be used more effectively. In early radically operated cases surgical adjuvant chemotherapy is acceptable only in controlled clinical studies.

22.22 Recommended Chemotherapy in Ovarian Carcinoma

22.22.1 Single-Agent Chemotherapy

1. Melphalan 0.2 mg/kg/day × 5 repeated at intervals of 4 weeks. Results of a study on 494 patients with 47% responders (20% complete)

Histological disease type	Response	Median duration (months)	Range (months)
Serous	49%	9	3-44
	(22% complete)	20	3-94+
Mucinous	44%	10	5-34
	(22% complete)	46,5	11-99+
Undifferentiated	42%	6	3-20
	(22% complete)	16,5	4-94+

2. CTX 30-40 mg/kg/day × 2 i.v. repeated at intervals of 4 weeks.

22.22.2 Combination Chemotherapy

1. CMF:
   CTX 150 mg/m^2 p.o. daily for 14 days
   5-FU 600 mg/m^2 i.v. day 1 and 8 (push)
   MTX 40 mg/m^2 i.v. day 1 and 8

Courses repeated every 4 weeks
Dose modifications on day 8 of each course and before starting a new course.

2. CHAD:
   CTX 600 mg/m^2 i.v. day 1
   ADM 25 mg/m^2 i.v. day 1
   DDP 50 mg/m^2 i.v. day 1 (with hydration)
   HMM 150 mg/m^2 p.o. day 8-21
3. HAD (for patients resistant to alkylating agents):
   ADM 30 mg/m^2 i.v. day 1
   DDP 50 mg/m^2 i.v. day 1
   HMM 150 mg/m^2 p.o. day 8-21

Course repeated every 3 weeks

4. AD:
   ADM 50 mg/m^2/day 1 i.v.
   DDP 50 mg/m^2/day 1 i.v.

Course repeated every 3-4 weeks

Conclusions

1. There exist considerable variations in the results reported using the same single agents and the same or similar multidrug chemotherapies. These variations probably reflect differences in patient populations

with regard to extent of disease (tumour mass, largest diameter of tumour lesions) and tumour differentiation (grading) as well as previous treatment. Poorly differentiated tumours are less sensitive. Previous radio- or chemotherapy decreases drug response. In addition, evaluation of response is often difficult.

2. Debulking surgery has a definitive place in the treatment plan of ovarian carcinoma. The size of residual disease significantly influences the response to chemotherapy, the survival and possible chemotherapeutic cure.
3. The best results with likelihood of long-term survival are provided by drug combinations which include CTX, hexamethylmelamine, ADM and DDP although these drugs may produce severe side effects.
4. Ongoing and future studies will have to answer the question as to what kind of subsets of patients have to be treated aggressively with the most potent drugs and which subsets of patients may fare as well with less aggressive therapy or even with single-agent treatment only. At present single-drug treatment is recommended for patients with insufficient drug tolerance but highly differentiated tumours.

III. Endometrium

22.23 Incidence and Epidemiology

Average incidence in Europe and United States 15-23/100000 female population per year

Accounts for 5%-7% of all malignancies in women
Incidence rising
75% after the age of 50, mean age 61 years

22.24 Aetiology and Risk Factors

1. Incidence higher among high-income group.
2. Incidence higher among nulliparous women.
3. Frequently associated with metabolic disorders such as obesity, hypertension and diabetes.
4. Oestrogens given in perimenopausal women increase risk.

22.25 Pathological Classification

Adenocarcinoma, usually well-differentiated. In some cases squamous metaplasia may be present (adenoacanthoma). Uterine sarcomas are very rare.

22.26 Main Clinical Features

Spread occurs in the later stages of the disease involving mainly the external iliac and hypogastric lymph nodes. Haematogenous metastases: lung, bone. Progression of the disease relatively slow.

22.27 Diagnostic Procedures

1. History (abnormal, i.e. postmenopausal bleeding)
2. Curettage
3. Endometrial aspiration

22.28 Staging Classification

T1 (Stage I)	Carcinoma confined to the corpus
T2 (Stage II)	Carcinoma involving the cervix but not extending outside the uterus
T3 (Stage III)	Carcinoma extending outside the uterus, including spread to the vagina, but remaining within the true pelvis
T4 (Stage IV)	Carcinoma involving the mucosa of the bladder or rectum and/or extending beyond the true pelvis

22.29 Prognostic Factors

Five-year survival in Tis and T1 cases may be as high as 90%. With myometrial involvement, it drops to 70%, and with involvement of the cervix to 50%.

22.30 Single Agents Effective in Endometrial Carcinoma

22.30.1 Single-Agent Chemotherapy

Drug	Number of evaluated cases	Overall regression (%)
CTX	52	13
Chlorambucil	16	0
Mercaptopurine	10	0
5-FU	60	27
Cytembena	30	33
ADM	39	28
DDP	50	38

Conclusion. Due to the good results of surgery and radiotherapy there are only few data about chemotherapy in this type of tumour. Nevertheless, endometrial carcinoma seemed to be a tumour localization with low drug sensitivity. Better results have been achieved with hormones. Regression rate 30%-40%.

22.30.2 Hormones (High Doses of Progestins)

1. Probably act by a direct effect on endometrial cancer cells: only differentiated adenocarcinomas are responsive.
2. Response rate 30%-40% with a mean duration of 25 months (4-68 months).
3. Response rates are better for patients below the age of 50 years, for late-recurring cancers and for pulmonary and osseous metastases than for pelvic disease (especially after pelvic radiotherapy).
4. Regression rate in progesterone-positive patients 70%-100%.

22.31 Drug Combinations

Up to now no better results than with single agents

22.32 Recommended Chemotherapy in Endometrial Carcinoma

Indications of chemotherapy for stages III and IV and for recurrences:

First choice: progestin for 2 months (medroxyprogesterone acetate – Provera 200–600 mg p.o. daily – Depo-Provera 1000 mg i.m. weekly) (Differentiated carcinomas are more responsive to progestin than are nondifferentiated carcinomas)
No response or progression

Second choice: CTX 100 mg/day p.o. × 14 days
5-FU 600 mg/m^2 i.v. day 1 and 8
MTX 40 mg/m^2 i.v. day 1 and 8

Third choice: ADM 60–75 mg/m^2 i.v. every 3 weeks

IV. Trophoblastic Disease (Choriocarcinoma)

22.33 Forms of Gestational Trophoblastic Diseases

22.33.1 Benign Form: Hydatiform Mole (Molar Disease)

This develops in 5%–7% of cases into invasive mole, and in 3%–5% of cases into choriocarcinoma. Beta-human chorionic gonadotrophin (β-HCG) falls to zero within 2 months after evacuation.

If HCG does not normalize within 2 months = *persistent molar disease:* this disease has a 50% risk of developing into choriocarcinoma.

22.33.2 Malignant Gestational Trophoblastic Neoplasms

50% occur after molar pregnancy, 25% after full-term delivery and 25% after spontaneous abortion.

Diagnostic signs and symptoms:

a) Vaginal or uterine bleeding
b) In some cases, symptoms from metastases: lung, bone, etc.
c) Persistent elevation of HCG (beta fraction)

1. Non-metastatic malignant trophoblastic neoplasm:
   No evidence of spread beyond uterus. Can be cured in more than 90% of cases without hysterectomy.
2. Metastatic malignant trophoblastic neoplasm:
   Low risk - Metastases in pelvis and/or lung only
   - HCG titer below 100000 IU in 24-h urine
   - Treatment started within 4 months of apparent onset of the disease

High risk - Metastases elsewhere than lung and/or pelvis (bone, liver, brain)
- HCG titer more than 100000 IU in 24-h urine
- Treatment started more than 4 months after apparent onset of disease

22.34 Treatment of Malignant Gestational Trophoblastic Neoplasms

22.34.1 Single Agents and Combinations Effective in Trophoblastic Malignant Neoplasms (from Clarysse et al. 1976)

Single drugs and drug combinations	No. evaluated	Response rate (%)
MTX	63	48
	144	65
6-Mercaptopurine	93	56
Alkylating agents	19	48
Actinomycin D	8	8
	32	90
MTX + 6-mercaptopurine	100	78
MTX + actinomycin D sequentially	75	74
MTX + actinomycin D sequentially	29	72
MTX + actinomycin D	85	88

22.34.2 Treatment According to Stage and Risk Group of Disease

Non-Metastatic Malignant Trophoblastic Choriocarcinoma:
More than 90% cure with single-agent chemotherapy using methotrexate.
Only 10% need hysterectomy in addition.
MTX 50 mg/day 1, 3, 5, 7
Calcium folinate 6 mg/30 h after MTX
repeated every 7-10 days

Duration of treatment: until complete remission [i.e. until HCG titer is normal in three successive weekly determinations - β-HCG titer, other HCG down to normal luteinizing hormone values].

HCG monitoring must be continued.

If HCG does not normalize but reaches a plateau: hysterectomy. If HCG starts to rise again after 3 weeks of normal values: change to multi-drug chemotherapy and/or hysterectomy.

Metastatic Malignant Trophoblastic Choriocarcinoma:

1. Low-risk group: near 100% cure by single-agent chemotherapy
   a) MTX 50 mg/day 1, 3, 5, 7
   Calcium folinate 6 mg/30 hours after MTX
   repeated every 7-10 days
   b) Actinomycin D 10 µg/kg i.v. daily for 5 days, repeated after full recovery from haematological and other toxicity

   Duration of treatment and guidelines for change of treatment are the same as for non-metastatic disease.
2. Medium-risk group: Sequential treatment with:

Course A	Hydroxyurea	2 × 500 mg/day 1 p.o.
	MTX	50 mg/day 2, 4, 6, 8 i.m.
	Calcium folinate	6 mg 30 hours after MTX
	Mercaptopurine	75 mg/day 3, 5, 7, 9, p.o.
Course B	Actinomycin D	0,5 mg/day × 5 i.v.
Course C	VCR	0,8 mg/m²/day 1, 3 i.v.
	CTX	400 mg/m²/day 1, 3 i.v.

Every 7-14 days one course in the sequence A B C

3. High-risk group: Only 36% achieve complete remission and cure with single-agent therapy. Therefore, multidrug chemotherapy has to be applied.
   a) Chamoca protocol:

Day 1	Hydroxyurea	2 × 500 mg p.o.	
Day 2	VCR	1.0 mg/m²	10 a.m.
	MTX	100 mg/m²	3 p.m.
	MTX	200 mg/m²	12 h infusion
Day 3	Calcium folinate	15 mg i.m./p.o.	3 p.m.
Day 4	Calcium folinate	15 mg i.m./p.o.	8 a.m.
	CTX	600 mg/m²	10 a.m.
	Dactinomycin	0,5 mg	
	Calcium folinate	15 mg i.m./p.o.	3 p.m.
Day 5	Calcium folinate	15 mg i.m./p.o.	8 a.m.
	Dactinomycin	0,5 mg	10 a.m.
Day 6	Dactinomycin	0,5 mg	
Day 7	and 8 free		
Day 9	ADM	30 mg/m² i.v.	
	CTX	400 mg/m²	

   Minimal break between cycles 7 days, but interval adapted to tolerance

   b) MAC protocol:
   MTX 0.3 mg/kg/day × 5 i.v.

Actinomycin D 0.008 mg/kg/day × 5 i.v.
CTX 3 mg/kg/day × 5 i.v.
repeated every 3 weeks
c) VBL 9 mg/m^2/day 1 i.v.
BLM 0.02 mg/m^2/week i.m.
DDP 20 mg/m^2/day 1-5 i.v.
repeat VBL and DDP every 3 weeks
Brain metastases: additional brain irradiation
Other drugs to be used in recurrent or resistant disease:
- Etoposide (VP-16-213)
- Iphosphamide
- Mitoxantrone

22.35 Prophylactic Chemotherapy After Evacuation of a Mole

Not generally indicated, if sensitive assay for HCC is available.
Indication: Persistence of elevated HCG titers 8 weeks after evacuation of a mole: then single-agent chemotherapy as outlined above.

Further Reading

Clarysse A, Kenis Y, Mathé G (1976) Cancer chemotherapy - its role in the treatment strategy of hematologic malignancies and solid tumors. Springer, Berlin-Heidelberg-New York
Griffiths CT, Fuller AF (Eds) (1983) Gynecologic Oncology. Martinus Nijhoff Publ
Morrow CR (Ed) (1983) Recent clinical developments in gynecologic oncology. Raven Press, New York
Murphy ED, Beamer WG (Eds) (1980) Biology of Ovarian Neoplasia, UICC Technical Report Series, Vol 50, UICC, Geneva
Tanneberger S (Ed) (1986) Experimentelle und Klinische Chemotherapie. Akademie-Verlag, Berlin
Van Osterom AT, Muggia FM, Cleton FJ (Eds) (1980) Therapeutic Progress in Ovarian Cancer, Testicular Cancer and the Sarcomas. Leiden University Press, Leiden
Williams CJ, Michael J, Whitehouse A Cancer of the Female Reproductive System. In: Cancer Investigation and Management. Whitehouse, JMA, Williams CJ, Canellos GP (Eds)
Young RC (1980) Gynecologic Malignancies. In: Cancer Chemotherapy 1980. Pinedo HM (ed), Excepta Medica, Amsterdam

23 Skin Tumours

23.1 Malignancies Affecting Skin

Basal-cell carcinoma
Squamous cell carcinoma
Kaposi's sarcoma
Malignant melanoma

23.2 Precancerous Lesions

Bowen's disease
Keratosis senilis
Cornu cutaneum
Paget's disease
Keratoacanthoma (molluscum sebaceum)
Erythroplasia Queyrat

23.3 Differential Diagnosis

Glomus tumour
Dermatofibrosarcoma protuberans
Neurofibromatosis
Mycosis fungoides
Xeroderma pigmentosum
Basal-cell naevoid syndrome
Malignant lymphoma
Turban tumour

I. Malignant Melanoma

23.4 Epidemiology, Aetiology, Course of the Disease

Rare disease, incidence below 1-2/100000 almost everywhere, except Australia, where it is 16 per 100000. It accounts for 1%-3% of all malignant tumours.

Possible aetiological factors include exposure to sun, repeated injury to naevi.

5-year cure rates 24%-42%: stage I - about 30%; stage II, with microscopic node invasion - 15%; with clinically positive nodes - 10%.

Course of the disease unpredictable: with the same prognostic factors (see Sect. 23.6), early haematogenous spread or late local recurrence or distant metastases (after several years) may develop. Prognosis for females better than for males.

Spontaneous regressions occur in about only 0.08% of cases.

23.5 Histological Grading of Melanoma (McGovern et al.)

1. Diagnosis according to histogenetic-pattern:
   a) Malignant melanoma, invasive, with adjacent intra-epidermal component of Hutchinson's melanotic freckle type.
   b) Malignant melanoma, invasive, with adjacent intra-epidermal component of superficial spreading type.
   c) Malignant melanoma, invasive, with adjacent intra-epidermal component, unclassified.
   d) Malignant melanoma, invasive, without adjacent intra-epidermal component.
2. Cross-sectional-profile of section on slide:
   a) Flat or uneven.
   b) Convex or plateau of measurable height.
   c) Polypoidal.
3. Levels of invasion:
   a) Intra-epidermal.
   b) Papillary-dermal.
   c) Papillary-reticular interface.
   d) Reticular-dermal.
   e) Subcutaneous fat.
4. Ulceration, more than 6 mm in extent.

5. Vascular invasion:
   a) Lymphatics,
   b) Blood vessels.
6. Mitotic activity, assessed on at least ten high-power (×300) fields (h.p.f.):
   a) Fewer than 1/5 h.p.f.
   b) Between 1/5 h.p.f. and 1/h.p.f.
   c) 1/h.p.f. and over.
7. Other parameters such as cytology, pigmentation, "lymphocytic" infiltrates, evidence of spontaneous regression, associated naevi and solar changes in the dermis are mainly of research interest at present, and their recording is left to the individual histologist's discretion.

23.6 Prognosis in Melanoma by Type of Primary, Depth of Invasion and Stage

1. Type of primary:	5-year survival (Clark)
Lentigo maligna melanoma (Hutchinson's melanotic freckle)	55.2%
Superficial spreading melanoma	46.5%
Nodular melanoma	27.3%
2. Depth of invasion of primary:	5-year survival (Mehnerd and Heard)
Dermis to superficial rete pegs	77.6%
Dermis to base of deepest sweat glands	38.6%
Subcutaneous invasion	8.0%
3. Stage and definition:	5-year survival
I No metastases	60%–80%
II Local skin metastases	30%–50%
III Regional metastases	10%–25%
IV Distant metastases	<5%

23.7 Prognostic Factors in Malignant Melanoma

1. Primary tumour
   - Site (e.g. trunk worse than limbs)
   - Size

   - Superficial, nodular, lentigo maligna
   - Depth of invasion
   - Histological grade
2. Stage
3. Site of any metastatic disease (metastases of bone and liver carry worse prognosis than those of nodes, and skin)
4. Sex (female patients have better prognosis)
5. Presence of urinary melanogens indicates worse prognosis
6. Host condition
   - Immune status
   - Physical status

   when impaired, prognosis is worse

23.8 Single Agents Effective in Melanoma

1. Agents with response rates of 20% or more:
   Dacarbazine (DTIC)
   Methyl-CCNU(Me-CCNU)
2. Agents with response rates of 10%–20%:
   Cyclophosphamide
   Procarbazine
   Vinblastine
   CCNU
   Actinomycin
   Vindesine
   Actinomycin D
   Hydroxyurea
3. Agents with response rates of less than 10%:
   Most alkylating agents (mustine, thiotepa, chlorambucil, melphalan; response rate higher when given by intra-arterial infusion)
   Antimetabolites (6-mercaptopurine, cytosine arabinoside, methotrexate, 5-fluorouracil)

23.8.1 General Remarks as to the Chemotherapy of Malignant Melanoma

1. Response rates higher for skin, nodal or soft-tissue disease than for visceral metastases.
2. Complete response rate not higher than 5%.
3. The only drugs which are potentially effective for brain metastases are the nitrosoureas (Me-CCNU).

4. There is no agent or combined therapy which has been clearly demonstrated to be more effective than DTIC alone in the treatment of disseminated melanoma.
5. It remains controversial as to whether the results of chemotherapy are improved by concurrent non-specific immunotherapy (BCG, MER) - except intralesional BCG treatment, which alone produces a high rate of regressions of melanoma nodules. (BCG, Calmette-Guerin bacillus; MER, methanol extracted residue of BCG).

23.9 Recommended Chemotherapy for Melanoma

1. DTIC: 200-300 mg/m^2 push i.v. for 5 days, repeated every 3-4 weeks
2. Me-CCNU: 200 mg/m^2 p.o. as single agent every 6 weeks

1. and 2. may be combined.

23.10 Adjuvant Chemotherapy in Malignant Melanoma After Wide Excision

Remains controversial, with conflicting results in clinical trials. A newer large clinical trial claims some improvement of 5-year cure rates with combined DTIC treatment and BCG immunotherapy, compared with controls, BCG alone or DTIC alone.

These findings have not been confirmed on a large scale. Intratumoral BCG treatment can be of some benefit.

II. Cancers Affecting Skin Other Than Melanoma

23.11 Epidemology and Aetiology

The most common cancers in man, but with the highest cure rate (>90%)
Great variation in incidence from country to country; accounts for between 3% and 5% of all cancers
Predisposing factors:
- Exposure to sunlight
- Exposure to ionizing radiation
- Exposure to arsenic, tar, pitch
- Scars of severe burns
- Racial differences

23.12 TNM Classification of Skin Tumours (Excluding Melanoma)

TIS	Pre-invasive carcinoma (carcinoma in situ)
TO	No evidence of primary tumour
T1	Tumour 2 cm or less in its largest dimension, strictly superficial or exophytic
T2	Tumour more than 2 cm but not more than 5 cm in its largest dimension or with minimal infiltration of the dermis, irrespective of size
T3	Tumour more than 5 cm in its largest dimension or with deep infiltration of the dermis, irrespective of size
T4	Tumour involving other structures such as cartilage, muscle or bone
N0	No palpable nodes
N1	Movable homolateral nodes
N2	Movable contralateral or bilateral nodes
N3	Fixed
M0	No evidence of distant metastases
M1	Distant metastases present including lymph nodes beyond the region in which the primary tumour is situated or satellite nodules more than 5 cm from the border of the primary tumour

23.13 Clinical Course and Therapy of Skin Cancers (Excluding Malignant Melanoma)

23.13.1 Basal-Cell Carcinoma

1. If untreated, slow spread to surrounding and deep structures
2. Rarely metastasizes to regional nodes or distant nodes

Therapy only after biopsy:

a) Wide excisional surgery
b) Radiation therapy
c) Electrosurgery, chemosurgery, cryosurgery
} cure rate 97%

d) Topical chemotherapy – indicated mainly in the case of multiple, recurrent, superficial carcinomas in elderly patients:
5-Fluorouracil cream: Efudix 5%
Local application with occlusive dressing changed daily for 4–6 weeks

e) Systemic chemotherapy – indicated only in systemic disease not accessible to surgery or radiation therapy, or as adjuvant therapy in marginally operable or irradiated cases:
Bleomycin: 15–30 mg i.v. twice weekly
7.5–15 mg i.v. daily × 5 in a 24-h infusion

23.13.2 Squamous Cell Carcinoma

1. May be more undifferentiated
2. Higher tendency of spread to regional nodes and distant metastases
   Therapy:
   a) In principle the same as in basal cell carcinoma.
   b) In undifferentiated types, more aggressive surgery and/or radiation therapy is required.
   c) Surgical dissection of lymph node metastases.

23.13.3 Kaposi's Sarcoma

1. Rare in Europe or United States, widespread in many parts of Africa
2. Predominantly cutaneous, but may involve many tissues in the body
3. Natural history varies from a relatively benign to a more aggressive course
4. It is being observed with increasing frequency in patients with acquired immunodeficiency syndrome (AIDS).

Clinical Types of Kaposi's Sarcoma:

A. Nodular pattern: relatively benign course, limited to skin
B. Florid type: exulcerating exophytic lesions; more frequent infiltration of neighbouring structures (nodes, bone)
C. Infiltrating type: extending to underlying structures
D. Lymphadenopathic type: skin and indolent malignant lymphadenopathy, more often with distant metastases (visceral organs, bone)

Therapy:

a) Local excision and/or radiotherapy (good radiosensitivity)
b) If extension beyond the range of curative surgery and radiotherapy is present or suspected, adjuvant chemotherapy

Types B + D	Actinomycin D	0.5 mg i.v. daily × 5	every 2–3 weeks	70% complete remission
	Vincristine	1.3 mg/m^2 day 1 + 8		
Types A + C	Cyclophosphamide	1.4 g/m^2 every 3 weeks		
	Vincristine	1.3 mg/m^2 every 2 weeks		

Other drugs effective:

In Kaposi's sarcoma:
- DTIC
- Carmustine
- Bleomycin

Further Reading

1. Cancer of the skin (1970) In: Cancer. Ackerman LV, del Regato JA, Mosby St. Louis
2. Clark WH, Mastrangelo M, Goldman LI (Eds) (1980) Human Malignant Melanoma. Grune & Stratton New York
3. Rumke P (1980) Malignant melanoma. In: Cancer Chemotherapy 1980. Pinedo HM (Ed). Excerpta Medica, Amsterdam

24 Head and Neck Tumours

24.1 Incidence and Epidemiology

Cancers of the head and neck region represent approximately 5% of the total new cases in the USA.

M:F ratio 3:1. Most tumours occur over the age of 40, but salivary gland and nasopharyngeal tumours may occur in younger age groups.

Higher incidences: nasal cavity and paranasal sinuses - Japan, Hawaii; larynx - Asian, United States black population

24.2 Aetiology and Risk Factors

Prolonged exposure to alcohol, tobacco, snuff, poor oral hygiene, chromium, nickel, leather dust, wood dust

Role of Epstein-Barr virus uncertain

24.3 Pathological Classification

The majority of tumours derive from the surface epithelium, giving rise to squamous cell carcinoma or variant (lymphoepithelioma, spindle-cell carcinoma, verrucous carcinoma, undifferentiated carcinoma). Adenocarcinoma and tumours of mesenchymal origin.

24.4 Main Clinical Features

Epidermoid tumours begin as surface lesions. Lesions from ducts of minor salivary glands arise below surface as nodule. Muscle invasion is common. Bone or cartilage invasion is late event. Lymph node extension is common with poorly differentiated tumours and is a common feature of presentations involving the nasopharynx, the base of tongue, pharyngeal walls and hypopharynx.

24.5 Diagnostic Procedures

Use direct or indirect endoscopy for nasopharygeal examination. Careful clinical examination of all lymph node groups of the neck. Incisional or when indicated excisional biopsy (small lesions only) for histological diagnosis.

It should be remembered that surgery and radiotherapy are the only curative treatments of carcinomas of the head and neck. Initial surgery must therefore be planned with care.

24.6 Staging Classification

Use UICC TNM system.
T relates to primary lesion site (see below).
N is common to all head and neck sites.

Lip	Larynx	Pharynx
T1 ≤2 cm } limited to lip	*Glottis*	*Oropharynx*
T2 >2-4 cm } limited to lip	T1 Limited/mobile	T1 ≤2 cm
T3 >4 cm } limited to lip	a. One cord	T2 >2-4 cm
T4 beyond lip	b. Both cords	T3 >4 cm
	T2 Extension to supra or sub-glottis/mobile,	T4 Extension to bone, muscle, etc.
Oral cavity	T3 Fixation of cord(s)	
T1 ≤2 cm	T4 Extension beyond larynx	*Nasopharynx*
T2 >2-4 cm		T1 One site + biopsy
T3 >4 cm		T2 Two sites
T4 Extension to bone, muscle, etc.	*Supra- and Sub-Glottis*	T3 Extension to nose, oropharynx
	T1 Limited/mobile	T4 Extension to skull Cranial nerve involvement
	T2 Extension to glottis/ mobile	
	T3 Fixation of cord(s)	
	T4 Extension beyond larynx	*Hypopharynx*
		T1 One site
		T2 Extension to adjacent site or region without larynx fixation
		T3 With larynx fixation
		T4 Extension to bone, neck etc.

The American Joint Committee cervical node classification system is useful and applicable for all head and neck sites.

NX Nodes cannot be assessed
NO No clinically positive node
N1 Single clinically positive homolateral node 3 cm or less in diameter
N2 Single clinically positive homolateral node more than 3 but not more than 6 cm in diameter, or multiple clinically positive homolateral nodes, none more than 6 cm in diameter
N2A Single clinically positive homolateral node more than 3 cm but not more than 6 cm in diameter
N2B Multiple clinically positive homolateral nodes, none more than 6 cm in diameter
N3 Massive homolateral node(s), bilateral nodes, or contralateral node(s)
N3A Clinically positive homolateral node(s), one more than 6 cm in diameter
N3B Bilateral clinically positive nodes (in this situation, each side of the neck should be staged separately; that is, N3B: right, N2A: left, N1)
N3C Contralateral clinically positive node(s) only

24.7 Prognostic Factors

1. Extensive disease at presentation
2. Poorly differentiated tumours
3. Malignant change within an area of pre-existing pathology

24.8 Therapeutic Strategy

Most early squamous cell tumours of the head and neck can be cured by surgery alone. Surgery is indicated as the primary treatment when tumour volume is relatively small and is discrete. Radiation therapy is then reserved for treatment failure. Radiotherapy alone may offer tissue anatomical conservation. Treatment of this anatomical region is complex and requires specialist experience. Some sites (nasopharynx) can be treated only with radiation therapy (RTX). Chemotherapy remains essentially experimental, having no curative role when used alone. Its role as an adjunct to surgery and radiotherapy is under investigation. Complex schedules devised on the basis of cell kinetic principles have not been shown to have any advantage over simpler regimes.

24.9 Single Agents Effective in Head and Neck Cancer

Drug	No. of cases	Response rate %
Methotrexate (weekly or twice a week)	100	50
Cis-platinum	108	33
Bleomycin	298	18
Hydroxyurea	18	39
Cyclophosphamide	77	36
Vinblastine	35	29
Doxorubicin hydrochloride (Adriamycin)	34	23
5-Fluorouracil	118	15

24.10 New-Agent Activity in Head and Neck Squamous Cancer

Drug	No. of cases	Response rate %
Vindesine	62	16
Etoposide (VP-16-213)	24	4
Maytansine	24	4
Pyrazofurin	22	5
Dianhydrogalactitol	19	–
Ftorafur	17	6

24.11 Drug Combinations in Head and Neck Cancer

Drugs	No. of Cases	Response Rate (%)
DDP/BLM	40	71
BLM/MTX/DDP	46	63
VCR/BLM/MTX/5-FU/ hydrocortisone ± ADM	117	67
BLM/CTX/MTX/5-FU	48	58
BLM/VCR/MTX	60	30–62
BLM/DDP/MTX ± VCR	58	18–58
BLM/DDP/MTX/MITC	33	61
BLM/DDP/VBL	22	45
CTX/ADM/DDP	25	64
MTX/5-FU	24	75

DDP, *cis*-platinum; BLM, bleomycin; MTX, methotrexate; VCR, vincristine; 5-FU, 5-fluorouracil; MIT-C, mitomycin C; VBL, vinblastine; ADM, doxorubicin hydrochloride/Adriamycin; CTX, cyclophosphamide

Response durations for patients with prior therapy are very short.

There is no persuasive evidence that any drug combination is more effective than MTX or DDP used alone.

Further Reading

Cachin Y, Richard J, Eschwege F, Micheau C (1979) Les Cancers du Larynx. Masson, Paris

Kramer S (Ed) (1977) Head and neck cancer. Semin Oncol, December

Management Guidelines for Head and Neck Cancer (1977) US Department of Health, Education and Welfare. Public Health Service. National Institute of Health, Bethesda

Million RR, Cassisi NJ, Wittes RE (1982) Cancer in the Head and Neck. In: Principles and Practice of Oncology, DeVita VT, Hellman S, Rosenberg SA, Lippincot, Philadelphia

Shedd DP (1973) Cancer of head and neck. In: Cancer Medicine. Holland JF, Frei E, Lea & Febiger, Philadelphia

Suen JY, Myers EN (1981) Cancer of the Head and Neck. Churchill Livingston, London

Taylor SG (1980) Head and neck cancer. In: Cancer Chemotherapy 1980. Pinedo HM (Ed). Excerpta Medica, Amsterdam

25 Soft-Tissue Sarcoma

25.1 General

Soft-tissue sarcomas are a rare group of tumours comprising approximately 1% of all malignant tumours. The annual age-adjusted incidence is 2 per 100000. Conventional management has relied heavily on surgery, but the inadequacy of this approach is reflected by local recurrence rates of 40%–80% in adult sarcomas and of as high as 90% in childhood sarcomas. Suit et al., treating 100 patients with localized soft-tissue sarcoma using limited surgery and high-dose radiation therapy, made the following observations:

1. Histological grade affected prognosis (disease-free survivals of 86% for grade I tumours compared with 17% for grade III).
2. Size of the primary tumour determined the subsequent local recurrence rate (18% for tumours <5 cm compared with 8% for those 5 cm).
3. Site of the primary tumour was important (local recurrence rate 33% for proximal site compared with 5% for a distal site).

25.2 Staging of Adult Soft-Tissue Sarcomas (Adapted from Russel et al.)

T	Primary tumour	T_1	≤ 5 cm
		T_2	>5 cm
		T_3	Any size invading bone, major vessel or nerve
N	Regional nodes	N_0	Not involved
		N_1	Histologically verified involved
M	Distant metastases	M_0	No distant metastases
		M_1	Distant metastases
G	Histological grading	G_1	Low
		G_2	Moderate
		G_3	High

Stage I: Grade I tumour with no nodal or distant metastases

Ia <5 cm

Ib >5 cm

Stage II: Grade 2 tumour with no nodal or distant metastases

IIa <5 cm

IIb >5 cm

Stage III: Grade 3 tumour with no nodal or distant metastases

IIIa <5 cm

IIIb >5 cm

but: IIIc tumour of any grade or size with regional lymph nodes involved but without distant metastases

Stage IV: IVa tumour of any grade grossly invading bone, major vessel or major nerve with or without nodal metastases but without distant metastases

IVb tumour with distant metastases

25.3 Histopathological Varieties of Soft-Tissue Sarcoma (Russell)

Histopathological variety	Proportion of total cases (%)[a]
Rhabdomyosarcoma	19.2
Fibrosarcoma	19.0
Liposarcoma	18.2
Malignant fibrohistiocytoma	10.5
Sarcoma of soft-tissue, type unspecified	10.0
Synovial sarcoma	6.9
Leiomyosarcoma	6.5
Malignant schwannoma	4.9
Angiosarcoma	2.7
Other types	1.9

[a] Prepared from data (Russell 1977) from a study of 1215 soft-tissue sarcomas.

25.4 Natural History and Prognostic Factors of Soft-Tissue Sarcomas

Overall 5-year survival is about 40%.

Cure rate, rate of local recurrence and distant metastases depend on the following *prognostic factors:*

1. Size of the primary tumour (more or less than 5 cm): influences probability and extent of local invasion and radicality of surgery.
2. Tumour grade (see Sect. 25.2) and stage (see Sect. 25.2).
3. Radicality of surgery.
4. Site of primary tumour: proximal sites (trunk) worse than distal sites (extremities), probably because site influences radicality of surgery.

The bad prognosis of soft-tissue sarcomas is due to:

1. Tendency for local invasion into surrounding tissues along anatomical planes such as nerve fibres, muscle bundles, fascial planes and blood vessels. This accounts for the high rate of local recurrences, especially after inadequate surgery. Even after wide local excision beyond the pseudocapsule, the local recurrence rate is about 50%. 80% of all local recurrences occur within 2 years. Local recurrence is a poor prognostic sign; 1/3 develop distant metastases.
2. Tendency for haematogenous spread, mostly lung metastases. Spread to lymph nodes is rare and occurs in synovial sarcoma and rhabdomyosarcoma.

25.5 Therapeutic Strategy in Soft-Tissue Sarcoma

25.5.1 Primary Treatment

1. Wide local excision beyond pseudocapsule; should include:
   a) All normal tissue in the tumour area
   b) All skin and subcutaneous tissue near the tumour
   c) All scars and areas of previous biopsy
2. Pre- or/and post-operative radiotherapy: at least 5000 rads over 4–5 weeks; improves local control
3. Experimental: Adjuvant chemotherapy
   Usually Adriamycin (ADM) or ADM combinations

25.5.2 Treatment of Local Recurrence

1. After local recurrence at an extremity, amputation should be considered.
2. Other local recurrences: surgery and radiotherapy if possible, followed by adjuvant chemotherapy.

25.5.3 Metastatic (Systemic) Disease

Chemotherapy

25.6 Chemotherapy of Soft-Tissue Sarcoma

25.6.1 Single Agents

	No. patients	No. Response (%)
Activity > 10%		
ADM 45–90 mg/m^2 q 3 wks	356	29 (13–34)
Actinomycin D (Act-D)	30	17
Dacarbazine (DTIC	53	17
without leiomyosarcoma and Kaposi's sarcoma		~10
Methotrexate (MTX)	49	18
Iphosphamide	18	38
Activity < 10%		
Cis-platinum (DDP)		
Cyclophosphamide (CTX)		
5-Fluorouracil (5-FU)		
Vindesine, vincristine (VCR)		
Amsacrine (*m*-Amsa)		
High-dose MTX-citrovorum factor (CF)		

Comment. ADM is the most active single agent in soft-tissue sarcoma. Response rate seems to be dose-related.

25.6.2 Multidrug Chemotherapy for Advanced Soft-Tissue Sarcoma

	No. patients	Response (%)
Cyvadic (CTX + VCR + ADM + DTIC)	~600	30–50
Split Cyvadic (ADM + DTIC – CTX + VCR)	52	23
Cyvadact (DTIC replaced by Act-D)	199	40
CAD (CTX + ADM + DTIC)	23	56
ACM (ADM + CTX + MTX)	100	36
MAD [ADM + methyl-CCNU (Me-CCNU)]	41	49
CAP (CTX + ADM + DDP)	20	20
R – ADM/DTIC (Southwest Oncology Group (SWOG) study)	243	22
R – ADM/DTIC/CTX (Southwest Oncology Group (SWOG) study)		35
R – ADM/DTIC/Act-D (Southwest Oncology Group (SWOG) study)		25

Comment. Comparison of results of different combination regimens is difficult because of differences in patient population and types of soft-tissue sarcomas treated. Few randomized trials have been performed. They were not able to demonstrate significant superiority of 3-5 drug combinations over two-drug combinations in terms of response rate, response duration and survival. Leiomyosarcomas tend to have a higher, malignant fibrous histiocytomas a lower, response rate. Kaposi's sarcoma and mesothelioma should not be included in soft-tissue sarcomas. Women tend to survive longer than men.

It is still uncertain, if drug combinations produce longer median survival.

25.7 Recommended Chemotherapy for Advanced Soft-Tissue Sarcoma

The most commonly used combination has been Cyvadic, and the schedule is as follows:

CTX	500 mg/m^2 i.v. push, day 1
VCR	1 mg/m^2 i.v. push, days 1 and 5
ADM	50 mg/m^2 i.v. push, day 1
DTIC	250 mg/m^2 i.v. push, day 1-5

Each 5-day course may be repeated at intervals of 3 or 4 weeks

25.8 Adjuvant Chemotherapy for Soft-Tissue Sarcoma

For this heterogeneous group of tumours, studies need to contain large numbers of patients and a concurrent control group not receiving chemotherapy to eliminate bias introduced by such factors as histological subtype and grade, size of tumour, adequacy of surgery and thoroughness of metastatic workup. No published study fulfils all these criteria; however, there are a number of retrospective studies suggesting that adjuvant combination chemotherapy may be of added value to surgery and radiotherapy. At the present time, adjuvant chemotherapy should not be used on a routine basis. Large randomized trials are currently being conducted by the National Cancer Institute (NCI) and the European Organization for Research and Treatment of Cancer (EORTC).

Further Reading

Bramwell VHC, Pinedo HM (1980) Bone and soft tissue sarcomas. In: Cancer Chemotherapy 1980. Pinedo HM (Ed). Excerpta Medica, Amsterdam
Van Oosterom AT, Muggia FM, Cleton FJ (1980) Therapeutic Progress in Ovarian Cancer, Testicular Cancer and the Sarcomas. Leiden University Press, Leiden
Monfardini S, Gianni C, Lombardi F, Fossati-Bellani F (1979) Chemotherapy and controlled studies in soft-tissue sarcomas. In: Advances in Medical Oncology, Research and Education. Vol 10. Kumar S (Ed). Pergamon Press, Oxford
Sears HF, Hopson R, Inouye W et al. (1980) Analysis of staging and management of patients with sarcoma: a ten year experience. Ann Surg 91: 488

26 Tumours of the Endocrine Organs and Apudomas

I. Thyroid

26.1 Incidence and Epidemiology

Cancer of the thyroid in the general population accounts for approximately 1% of the total cancer incidence.

High risk
- United States white population, Europeans
- Factors: previous neck irradiation
- Conditions: papillary adenoma, auto-immune thyroiditis, Hashimoto's disease

N. B. Medullary cancer of the thyroid can be considered a genetically determined disease. Chromosome analysis has confirmed the existence of a familial incidence.

26.2 Histopathological Classification of Thyroid Cancer

Histological type	Percentage of all thyroid cancers
Differentiated:	
Follicular	20
Papillary	50
Medullary	4
Undifferentiated	26

26.3 Staging

26.3.1 TNM Classification

T *Primary Tumour*

Tis Pre-invasive carcinoma (carcinoma in situ)

T0 No evidence of primary tumour

T1 Single nodule in one lobe with or without deformity of the gland and with no limitation of mobility
T2 Multiple nodules in one lobe with or without deformity of the gland and with no limitation of mobility
T3 Bilateral tumour with or without deformity of the gland and with no limitation of mobility or single nodule of the isthmus
T4 Tumour with extension beyond the gland capsule
TX The minimum requirements to assess the primary tumour cannot be met

N *Regional Lymph Nodes*
N0 No evidence of regional lymph node involvement
N1 Evidence of involvement of movable homolateral regional lymph nodes
N2 Evidence of involvement of movable contralateral, midline or bilateral regional lymph nodes
N3 Evidence of involvement of fixed regional lymph nodes
NX The minimum requirements to assess the regional lymph nodes cannot be met

M *Distant Metastases*
M0 No evidence of distant metastases
M1 Evidence of distant metastases
MX The minimum requirements to assess the presence of distant metastases cannot be met

26.3.2 Clinical Stages

No stage grouping is at present recommended by the UICC, but the following is given for information purposes:

Stage	T	N	M
IA	T0	N0–3	M0
IB	T1	N0–3	M0
II	T2	N0–3	M0
III	T3	N0–3	M0
IV	any T	any N	M1

26.4 Survival in Thyroid Cancer

26.4.1 Survival in Relation to Age and Histological Type

Age of patient in years	Survival rate (%)		
	Undifferentiated 1 year	Undifferentiated 3 years	Differentiated 7 years
0–9			100
10–19			100
20–29			100
30–39			100
40–49	75	23	68
50–59	47	18	73
60–69	39	9	69
70	36	0	50

26.4.2 Survival After 10 and 15 Years from Surgical Treatment in Relation to Histological Type

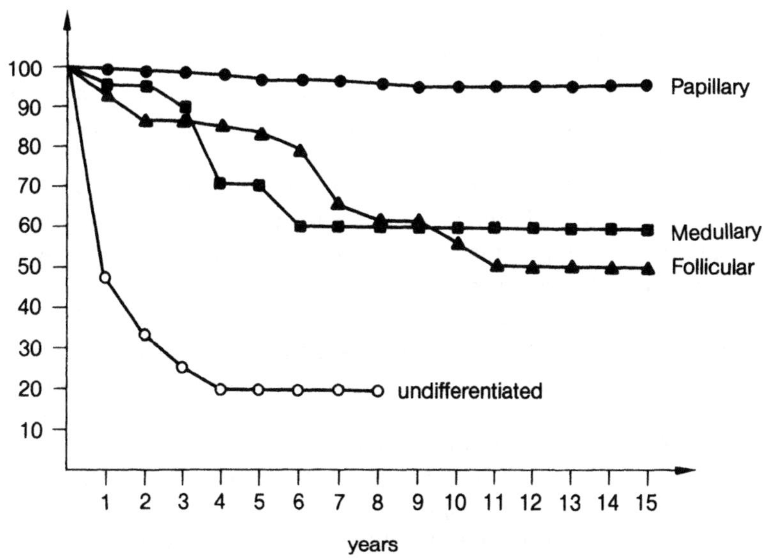

26.4.3 Survival After 10 and 15 Years According to Clinical Stage

Stage	Frequency (%)	Survival after 10 years (%)	Survival after 15 years (%)
T0 N0-3 M0	14	90	88
T1 N0-3 M0	55	89	82
T2 N0-3 M0	15	54	42
T3 N0-3 M0	10	29	16
any T and N, M1	6	10	10

26.5 Chemotherapy in Thyroid Cancer

Cytotoxic agents are reserved for cases that are no longer amenable to local therapy or ^{131}I.
Partial remission has been achieved with Adriamycin (37.45%; for drug dosage, see Chap. 6).
Only isolated cases benefit 5-flourouracil (5-FU), cyclophosphamide or bleomycin.

26.6 Suggested Therapeutic Strategy in Thyroid Cancer

1. Surgical resection is treatment of choice: sub-total or total thyroidectomy, with or without lymph node dissection, depending on the extent of the disease and the histology. Thyroxine or tri-iodothyronine should be given systematically after surgery for replacement purposes and to suppress thyrotrophin (TSH) secretion.
2. Operable undifferentiated anaplastic thyroid carcinoma, which has a very poor prognosis and bears a very high risk of early haematogeneous metastasis (lung), may be treated by adjuvant post-operative chemotherapy with Adriamycin.
3. If tumour cannot be completely resected, as much as possible should be excised to prevent or alleviate oesophageal or tracheal compression. This should be followed by post-operative irradiation or ^{131}I, depending on histology.
4. Inoperable disease can be treated with suppressive therapy using thyroxine if the tumour is of the papillary variety. Radioactive iodine is sometimes effective in papillary and follicular cancers, but not in medullary or anaplastic thyroid cancer. Irradiation of the primary neck tu-

mour is indicated (even if it is inoperable and distant metastases are present) to reduce or prevent compression phenomena. Chemotherapy should be reserved for patients with refractory recurrent disease and for all rapidly progressing tumours. Adriamycin is the first-choice drug.

II. Pituitary Gland

26.7 Epidemiology and Incidence

Risk factors associated with pituitary tumours have not yet been identified. These tumours account for around 10% of all brain tumours.

26.8 Histopathology of Pituitary Tumours

1. Adenoma (may be of mixed type):
   Chromophobe adenoma 79%
   Eosinophil adenoma 15%
   Basophil
2. Craniopharyngioma: commonest tumour in pituitary area in children and adolescents
3. Pituitary carcinoma, sarcoma (extremely rare)

26.9 Presentation of Pituitary Tumours

1. Local Consequences of space-occupying lesion:
   Headache - frequent
   Visual disturbances - common
   Cranial nerve palsies - uncommon
   Hypothalamic syndromes - obesity, sleep disturbances, diabetes insipidus
   Pituitary apoplexy - haemorrhage into tumour
2. Hormone hypersecretion:
   Growth hormone ⟶ Acromegaly, gigantism
   Associated with chromophobe or eosinophil tumours
   Prolactin ⟶ Amenorrhoea, galactorrhoea
   Associated with chromophobe or eosinophil tumours
   ACTH ⟶ Cushing's syndrome
   Associated with basophil or chromophobe adenomas
   TSH ⟶ Thyrotoxicosis (very rare)

3. Hormone hyposecretion:

Growth hormone →	Short stature if prior to epiphysial fusion
Prolactin →	Inability to breast-feed post-partum
ACTH →	Secondary hypoadreanalism
TSH →	Secondary hypothyroidism
Gonadotrophins →	Hypogonadism

26.10 Therapeutic Alternatives for Pituitary Tumours

1. Surgical hypophysectomy:
   a) Transfrontal - primarily indicated if visual field loss
   b) Transnasal
   c) Trans-sphenoidal
2. External radiation
3. Internal radiation - yttrium-90 rods implanted in pituitary.
   No place for cytotoxic agents

26.10.1 Alternative Treatments for Acromegaly

1. Surgical hypophysectomy
2. Surgical hypophysectomy + radiation
3. Surgical hypophysectomy + radiation + bromocryptine
4. External radiation
5. External radiation + bromocryptine
6. Internal radiation
7. Internal radiation + bromocryptine
8. Bromocryptine

26.10.2 Alternative Treatments for Pituitary Adenoma with Prolactin Hypersecretion

1. Surgical hypophysectomy
2. Surgical hypophysectomy + external radiation
3. Surgical hypophysectomy + external radiation + bromocryptine (used in doses of 5-7.5 mg/day)
4. External radiation
5. External radiation + bromocryptine
6. Bromocryptine

26.10.3 Alternative Treatments for Cushing's Syndrome with Pituitary Adenoma

1. Surgical hypophysectomy
2. Surgical hypophysectomy + radiation
3. Radiation: either external or internal alone.
   Additional therapy may be directed at adrenal using either surgical or medical means, i.e. adrenalectomy or use of metyrapone and aminoglutethimide

26.10.4 Alternative Treatments for Non-Secretory Pituitary Adenoma

1. Surgery + external irradiation
2. External irradiation

26.11 Elements fo Be Considered for the Choice of the Strategic Approach of Pituitary Tumours

1. Signs of extrasellar extension generally are an indication for surgery.
2. In the absence of signs of extrasellar involvement, radiation therapy may be employed. In those patients who do not respond to radiation, operative treatment may be undertaken.
3. Radiation therapy after non-radical surgery may be indicated.
4. Bromocryptine has a relevant place in the initial treatment of acromegaly and galactorrhoea without signs of extrasellar extension, but can also be associated to other therapeutic measures.
5. Yttrium-90 rod implants have been employed; however, this procedure may result in spinal fluid rhinorrhoea, and meningitis may occur.

26.12 Further Management of Patients with Pituitary Tumours (Replacement of Deficient Hormones)

1. Assess full pituitary function prior to treatment and replace with thyroxine (0.1-0.2 mg/day), cortisone acetate (25-50 mg/day), and androgens/oestrogens as required depending on the results.
2. After definitive treatment, assess full pituitary function at 3-monthly intervals for the 1st year and then at yearly intervals and replace deficient hormones as indicated above. At the same time check visual fields, clinical state and size of pituitary fossa.

3. In children, assess growth hormone status and growth rate after treatment. If both growth hormones are deficient and growth rate is poor, then human growth hormone should be administered intramuscularly in a dose of 5 mg three times weekly.
4. Where there is hypersecretion, check growth hormone and prolactin levels at three-monthly intervals for the first year in acromegaly or galactorrhoea-amenorrhoea states respectively, and subsequently at yearly intervals.
5. In Cushing's syndrome, check plasma cortisol levels, urinary 17-oxogenic steroids and urinary free-cortisol levels at three-monthly intervals for 1st year, then at yearly intervals subsequently.

III. Adrenals

26.13 Presentation of Adrenal Carcinoma

Cushing's syndrome
Virilization
Feminization
Non-functioning mass

26.14 Therapeutic Strategy for Adrenal Carcinoma

1. Surgical resection is the treatment of choice.
2. Recurrence in the adrenal bed may also be treated surgically.
3. Rising steroid levels and clinical evidence of hormone excess are indications of recurrence of metastases.
4. Chemotherapy with o,p, DDD (mitotane, Lysodren), the ortho-para-derivative of the commercial insecticide DDD, is now of established value in inoperable or recurring disease with both functioning and unfunctioning adrenal carcinoma. Dosage starts with 1.5–2 g daily and should be increased gradually up to 8–10 g daily, according to individual gastrointestinal tolerance. Steroid replacement with dexamethasone is necessary, because of unavoidable damage to normal adrenocortical tissue.

IV. Pancreas (Islet Cell Carcinoma)

26.15 Classification of Endocrine Pancreatic Tumours

Cell type	Hormone	Clinical features
α-cell	Glucagon	Hyperglycaemia and dermatitis
β-cell	Insulin	Hypoglycaemia
Non-β-cell	Gastrin	Gastric, duodenal and jejunal ulceration. Diarrhoea, steatorrhoea
Non-β-cell	Vasoactive intestinal peptide (VIP)	Watery diarrhoea
Non-β-cell	Ectopic hormones such as ACTH, serotonin	Cushing's syndrome Carcinoid syndrome

ACTH, adrenocorticotrophic hormone

26.16 Frequent Forms of Endocrine Pancreatic Tumours (Islet Cell Carcinoma)

1. Insulinoma:
   β-cell insulinoma is the most commonly recognized functioning islet cell neoplasm. Of these, 90% behave as benign adenomas and 10% show metastases.
2. Gastrin-Producing Tumours (Zollinger-Ellison syndrome).
3. VIPoma, Glucagonoma and other tumours which produce ectopic hormones.

26.17 Suggested Therapeutic Strategy for Endocrine Pancreatic Tumours

26.17.1 Surgery

For tumours confined to pancreas. For gastrin-producing tumours, total gastrectomy may be helpful even in patients with metastases.
In tumours producing ACTH, surgical adrenalectomy may be required or medical treatment with metyrapone 3 g daily or aminoglutethimide.

26.17.2 Results of Chemotherapy and Recommendation

Besides 5-FU, which is of limited therapeutic activity in these tumours, streptozotocin is the only drug which has been meaningfully evaluated. More recently dacarbazine (DTIC) was found to be effective.

In functional tumours, biochemical response was observed in 64% (41 patients) and tumour regression in 50%. All patients with biochemical response had amelioration of hypoglycaemia symptoms. Average duration of response: 10 months for biochemical response and 13 months for measurable tumour decrease. Streptozotocin combined with 5-FU seems to produce even better results. The suggested schedules are therefore the following:

1. 5-FU,	325 mg/m^2 i.v. daily for 5 days
streptozotocin	500 mg/m^2 i.v. daily for 5 days
2. Streptozotocin	1 g/m^2 i.v. weekly
3. DTIC	200-300 mg/m^2 i.v. daily for 5 days, repeated every 3-4 weeks

Further Reading

Harrison JM, Mahoney EM (1973) Adrenal cortex and medulla. In: Cancer Medicine. Holland JF, Frei E (Eds). Lea & Febiger, Philadelphia

Moertel CG (1973) Endocrine pancreas. In: Cancer Medicine. Holland JF, Frei E (Eds). Lea & Febiger, Philadelphia

Ney RL (1973) Pituitary tumors and pituitary hormones. In: Cancer Medicine. Holland JF, Frei E (Eds). Lea & Febiger, Philadelphia

Stratton Hill C (1973) Thyroid gland. In: Cancer Medicine. Holland JF, Frei E (Eds). Lea & Febiger, Philadelphia

27 Adult Central Nervous System Tumours

27.1 Epidemiology and Incidence

CNS tumours account for 2%-5% of all tumours in man.

Two age peaks: 3-12 years and 50-70 years.

Two-thirds of adult brain tumours are supratentorial (Childhood brain tumours: two-thirds infratentorial). In adults cortical and hemispheric tumours are more frequent.

Sex ratio is about 1:1 for most types, but astrocytomas are more common in male, meningiomas in female patients.

Certain mesenchymal tumours have a familial tendency.

27.2 Diagnosis

1. Non-localizing clinical signs:
   a) Progressive intracranial hypertension: vomiting, clouding of consciousness, hypertension, etc.
   b) Papilloedema
   c) Coma with hyperthermia, sudden death
2. Localizing clinical signs:
   Depends on site of tumour (hemianopsia, nystagmus, anosmia, cranial nerve paralysis, dysarthria, disturbance of deep sensation and orientation, hemisyndromes, mild psychic disturbances, deafness, etc.)
3. X-Ray signs - often lacking:
   Spreading of sutures, osseous erosions of sella or vault, hyperostotic reactions along a lacuna in meningeoma, calcifications of pinealoma and oligodendroglioma
4. Diagnostic tests:
   a) Computed tomographic (CT) scan
   b) Echoencephalography
   c) Ventriculography
   d) Encephalography
   e) Carotid angiography
   f) Open biopsy through a small burrhole

27.3 Histopathological Types

1. Gliomas: 40%–50% of all CNS tumours:
   a) Astrocytoma: may originate from any part of the brain, occur in adults and children
   Grade I: "benign"
   Grade II: low-grade malignant
   Grades III and IV: progressively more malignant
   b) Glioblastoma multiforme: in adults, frequently in cerebral hemispheres.
   May resemble anaplastic astrocytoma
   c) Medulloblastoma: the most rapidly growing and most radiosensitive brain tumour
2. Tumours of the membranes:
   a) Meningiomas: 20% of all brain tumours
   Tumours of the sheaths of Schwann (schwannoma): usually benign
3. Embryoplastic Tumours:
   a) Craniopharyngioma: often cystic, slow-growing
   b) Pinealoma
4. Mesenchymal tumours:
   a) Haemangioblastoma: familial tendency
   b) Haemangiosarcoma, reticulosarcoma, malignant lymphoma: rare

27.4 Histopathological Types and Age

1. Below 20 years:
   a) Cerebellar astrocytoma
   b) Medulloblastoma
   c) Craniopharyngioma
   d) Brain stem glioma
   e) Choroid plexus papilloma
2. All ages:
   a) Ependymoma (peak 10–30 years)
   b) Oligodendroglioma (peak 35–45 years)
3. Adults (above 20 years):
   a) Glioblastoma multiforme
   b) Cerebral astrocytoma
   c) Meningioma
   d) Schwannoma

e) Pituitary adenoma
f) Haemangioblastoma
g) Metastatic tumours

27.5 Treatment and Prognosis

Prognosis depends upon the histological malignancy and the chance of radical removal (site of the tumour).

a) Radical removal with good results:
   - Localized meningioma
   - Neurinomas
   - Cerebellar haemangioma
   - Colloid cysts
   - Cholesteatomas

b) Radical removal rarely possible with less satisfactory results:
   - Cerebellar astrocytoma (childhood)
   - Craniopharyngioma

c) Palliative surgical procedures:
   - Partial removal
   - Decompression operations
   - Ventriculocisternostomy
   - Ventriculovenous shunt

2. Radiotherapy:
   a) In all medulloblastomas: primary site and entire neuraxis
   b) In all partially removed malignant brain tumours:
      - Prolongs survival for 3-5 months
      - Poor effect in glioblastoma
3. Place of chemotherapy: remains to be defined

27.6 Chemotherapy of CNS Tumours

Chemotherapy of brain tumours in the adult is still in the experimental stage. The most significant effects have been observed in glioblastomas and high-grade astrocytomas (III-IV). Objective and subjective remissions have been documented with a number of drugs (see Sect. 27.6.2), but comparability of results of various investigators is still a problem, due to difficulties in defining criteria for remission and due to prognostic variables in this disease. It is still uncertain if the use of cytostatic drugs in conjunction with surgery and/or radiotherapy (adjuvant chemotherapy) is superior to the use of these drugs at the time of recurrence and symptomatic disease.

27.6.1 Requirements for Effectiveness of Chemotherapy in Brain Tumours

1. Drugs have to cross "blood-brain barrier" (physiological-pharmacological entity located in the endothelium of the majority of the cerebral capillaries):
   - High lipid solubility
   - No ionization
   - Molecular weight below 200 daltons
2. Drugs have to be effective in experimental brain tumour models.
3. Drugs should be effective in other human neoplasms.
4. Cytostatic drugs are most effective in high-grade malignant brain tumours, especially high-grade astrocytomas (cellular kinetics).

27.6.2 Single Drugs and Drug Combinations Active in Inoperable or Recurrent Malignant Gliomas

Drug	Reported response rate (%)
Procarbazine	27-50
Teniposide (VM-26)	63
Carmustine (BCNU)	48-51
Lomustine (CCNU)	43-47
Methyl-CCNU (Me CCNU)	56
BCNU, vincristine	31-41
Procarbazine, CCNU, vincristine	60
Cyclophosphamide, CCNU, vincristine	38
Methotrexate, CCNU, vincristine	40

27.6.3 Adjuvant Chemotherapy After Surgery with or Without Radiotherapy: [Brain Tumor Study Group (BTSG)]

	No. of patients	Median Survival (weeks)	alive at 18 months
Surgery + Me-CCNU	81	24	10
Surgery + radiotherapy	94	36	15.1
Surgery + radiotherapy + BCNU	92	51	27.2
Surgery + radiotherapy + Me-CCNU	91	42	23.3

Walker et al. N. E. J. M. 303: 1323, 1980

Comments. Radiotherapy is significantly better than no radiotherapy. Radiotherapy + BCNU is better than radiotherapy alone, but this does not quite reach statistical significance.

27.6.4 Prognostic Factors for Survival After Primary Treatment

1. Age: below 45 years better survival than > 45 years.
2. Personality change: higher death rate.
3. Duration of symptoms before first treatment:
   > 6 months before operation: patients live twice as long as those with symptoms less than 6 months.
4. Performance status before operation.
5. Histopathology: glioblastomas have twice the death rate per time than other grade III gliomas.

27.6.5 Value of Adjuvant Nitrosoureas in Malignant Gliomas

1. Since surgery and radiotherapy do not influence the ultimate course of glioblastomas, adjuvant chemotherapy is a potentially promising approach.
2. Multiple-agent combinations for inoperable or recurrent disease have not given better results than nitrosoureas.
3. At present, nitrosourea compounds seem to be more effective as palliative treatment than as adjuvant chemotherapy.
4. Available results would indicate that adjuvant nitrosoureas have slightly improved both the disease-free and the overall survival.
5. The apparent discrepancy in survival among available series treated with combined modality is most probably due to patient selection and extent of surgery.

27.6.6 Suggested Dose Schedules for Nitrosoureas Administered as Single Agents

BCNU	80 mg/m^2 day × 3 days i.v.	every 6–8 weeks
CCNU	130 mg/m^2 p.o.	every 6–8 weeks
Me-CCNU	150–200 mg/m^2 p.o.	every 6–8 weeks

27.7 Metastatic Brain Tumours

1. Metastatic brain lesions are more frequent than primary brain tumours.
2. Frequent primary tumours which metastasize into the brain are:
   Breast
   Lung
   Melanoma
   Hypernephroma
   Acute lymphoblastic leukaemia
   High-grade malignant lymphoma
3. May develop in complete remission of the primary disease, but are the cause of death in less than one-third of the patients: most patients with brain lesions die of systemic complications.
4. Differential diagnosis: Metabolic encephalopathy
   Hypercalcaemia
   Infection

Treatment. Depends upon the primary tumour, the number and location of brain metastases (intracerebral, meninges, etc.).

a) Radiotherapy is the mainstay of treatment of metastatic brain tumours: it improves symptoms in two-thirds of the patients.
b) Solitary lesions: surgical treatment may be considered in patients with otherwise good prognosis (testicular cancer, etc.).
c) Systemic chemotherapy is rarely effective.
d) Meningeal carcinomatosis may be treated with intrathecal methotrexate and cytosine arabinoside.
e) Excellent symptomatic relief is often observed with high-dose corticosteroids ($\geqslant$100 mg per day).

Further Reading

Bingham WG (Ed) (1972) Recent Advances in Brain Tumor Research. Karger, Basel

Hildebrand J (1978) Lesions of the Nervous System in Cancer Patients. Raven Press, New York

Laerum OD, Bigner DD, Rajewsky MF (Eds) (1978) Biology of Brain Tumours. UICC Technical Report Series, Vol. 30. UICC, Geneva

Monfardini S, Brambilla C, Solero GL et al (1979): Adjuvant chemotherapy with nitrosourea compounds following surgery plus radiotherapy in glioblastoma multiforme. In: Adjuvant Therapies and Markers of Post-surgical Minimal Residual Disease. Bonadonna G, Mathé G, Salmon SE (Eds). Springer-Verlag, Berlin-Heidelberg-New York

Shapiro WR (1980) Brain tumors. In: Cancer Chemotherapy 1980. Pinedo HM (Ed). Excerpta Medica, Amsterdam

Walker MD, Green SB, Byar DP et al (1980) Randomized comparisons of radiotherapy and nitrosoureas for the treatment of malignant gliomas after surgery. New Engl J Med 303: 1323

Wilson CB (Ed) (1975) Brain tumours. Semin Oncol, March

Part III

Management of Paediatric Malignancies by Site

28 General Characteristics of Paediatric Tumours

28.1 Incidence, Types and Age Distribution of Cancer in Childhood

Incidence of cancer in childhood (i.e. number of children newly diagnosed with a cancer per number at risk in the population within a given time period) is given by registries established either in Europe or in United States (USA Third National Survey). Data from Manchester Children's Tumour Registry give an average annual incidence of 100 new cases per year out of a total population of 5 million. Whereas 20% of this population is less than 15 years of age, malignant tumours form less than 1% of the cancers of the total population.

In this registry, the incidence of different types of cancer in childhood is as follows:

Type of cancer	Average annual incidence (%)
Leukaemia	29.5
Lymphomas	9.0
Tumours of CNS	17.0
Retinoblastomas	3.0
Neuroblastomas	7.5
Wilms' tumours	5.5
Bone and soft-tissue sarcomas	14.0
Teratomas	4.0
Ovary	0.5
Testis	1.0
Liver	0.5
Miscellaneous	8.5

(Manchester Registry, 1954-1968, assessed 1972)

Childhood cancer rates and cancer types vary markedly according to:

1. Age – 0-4 years: 50% (mostly embryonal tumours), 5-9 years: 25%, 10-14 years: 25%

2. Sex - 1.2 M : 1 F
3. Geographical and ethnic factors

Accidents, infections, congenital malformations and cancer are the four causes of death in children, the order of frequency depending on the country (malnutrition) and the age.

28.2 Major Malignant Tumours According to Site

28.2.1 Head and Neck

1. Brain	See under Chap. 33
2. Orbit and eye	Rhabdomyosarcoma Non-Hodgkin lymphoma Optic nerve glioma Neuroblastoma (metastatic) Retinoblastoma
3. Nasopharynx	Rhabdomyosarcoma Non-Hodgkin lymphoma Undifferentiated carcinoma
4. Oropharynx and mouth	Non-Hodgkin lymphoma Rhabdomyosarcoma Tumour of retinal anlage
5. Cervical origin (lymph nodes and soft tissues)	Hodgkin's disease and non-Hodgkin lymphoma Rhabdomyosarcoma Neuroblastoma
6. Jaw	Non-Hodgkin lymphoma (Burkitt) Neuroblastoma Rhabdomyosarcoma Osteosarcoma Ewing's sarcoma Fibroblastic tumours
7. Ear	Rhabdomyosarcoma
8. Salivary glands	Rhabdomyosarcoma Non-Hodgkin lymphoma Carcinoma
9. Thyroid	Carcinoma Non-Hodgkin lymphoma

28.2.2 Thorax

1. Parietal origin	Ewing's sarcoma Rhabdomyosarcoma
2. Anterior mediastinum	Small round-cell tumour Acute lymphoblastic leukaemia Hodgkin's disease and non-Hodgkin lymphoma Rhabdomyosarcoma Thymic tumour
3. Central mediastinum	Lymphoma and leukaemia Rhabdomyosarcoma Teratoma Malignant histiocytosis
4. Posterior mediastinum	Neuroblastoma and ganglioneuroblastoma Schwannoma
5. Metastatic lung tumours	Nephroblastoma and ganglioneuroblastoma Osteosarcoma Ewing's sarcoma Soft-tissue sarcoma
6. Breast	Non-Hodgkin lymphoma

28.2.3 Abdomen, Pelvis, Perineal Region, Gonads

	Nephroblastoma Neuroblastoma Non-Hodgkin lymphoma Rhabdomyosarcoma Primary liver tumours Ovary and vaginal tumours Testis tumours Teratomas

28.2.4 Limbs

1. Primary bone tumours	Osteogenic sarcoma Ewing's sarcoma
2. Bone metastases	Neuroblastoma Leukaemia and lymphoma
3. Soft tissue	Rhabdomyosarcoma and other mesenchymal malignant tumours

28.3 General Remarks

1. Common epithelial tumours of adults are very rare in childhood, where the most frequent malignant diseases are acute leukaemias, embryonal tumours and sarcomas.
2. Some of the childhood cancers are genetically determined: mendelian inheritance of one type of tumour (e.g. retinoblastoma), or of predisposing situation (chromosomal instability syndromes, immunodeficiencies, hamartomatous syndromes ...), chromosomal abnormalities, congenital defects, familial aggregations of cancer. The role of environmental factors (sometimes in addition to genetic predisposition) is under study:
   - Pre- or post-natal irradiation
   - Some chemical factors (e.g. diethylstilboestrol during pregnancy)
   - Viruses (e.g. Epstein-Barr virus and Burkitt's lymphoma or undifferentiated nasopharyngeal carcinoma, HTLV I, and T-lymphoma-leukaemia).
3. The effectiveness of chemotherapy in childhood cancers is due to the histological and kinetic characteristics of the tumours; consequently, chemotherapy plays an increasing role in the treatment planning; indications and timing of surgery and radiotherapy have to be discussed in relation to results obtained with chemotherapy. Immunotherapy is controversial.
4. Many attempts have been made to classify childhood tumours, but as yet no method has been accepted. The adaptation of the TNM nomenclature to paediatric tumours is under study and has already been applied to nephroblastomas, neuroblastomas and soft-tissue sarcomas.
5. Age, stage, site of origin, histological type and grade are important in assessing the risks of local recurrence and distant dissemination and subsequently in choosing the best treatment. Constant consideration must be given to the major risk of immediate acute complications and late sequelae due to the use of radiotherapy and/or chemotherapy in growing human beings. Cure is not enough; quality of survival is a factor of prime importance, and it is necessary to have a long-term follow-up of these children.
6. There is a need for specialized units, either located in a children's hospital or in a separate cancer research centre, working in close collaboration with medical oncologists, haematologists, surgeons, radiotherapists, pathologists and psychologists.

7. Current results show:
   a) An increase in the percentage of remissions (metastatic tumours)
   b) An increase in the survival time
   c) Cure in some 60% of cases

28.4 Psychological Care of the Child with Cancer and of the Child's Family

28.4.1 When Diagnosis Is First Made

Explain:

1. *To both parents:* diagnosis, with therapeutic planning and expected results. Repeat interviews may be necessary to be sure that the parents have a correct knowledge of the situation.
2. *To the child:* the necessity of hospitalization, the severity of the disease and the modalities of necessary diagnostic examinations and therapeutic approaches.

28.4.2 Before Starting Treatment

Explain to the child the different steps of therapy and the consequences of:

a) Surgery (e.g. mutilations)
b) Chemotherapy (e.g. risk of alopecia, digestive troubles, etc.)
c) Radiotherapy (the improbability of any immediate effects)

28.4.3 During the Maintenance Treatment and the Follow-Up.

Do not underestimate the child's underlying anxiety, his difficulties in accepting treatment, his aggressivity, his problems at school and within the family.

1. *If a relapse occurs:*
   a) Try to reassure the parents about the future possibilities of treatment.
   b) Try to relieve the child's anxiety, especially as death approaches.
2. *If a cure is obtained:* The child must be made to accept the possibility of sequelae of treatment; thus an adolescent who was treated in infancy for a malignant tumour must know the diagnosis, the treatment he has undergone, and the risks involved.

29 Wilms' Tumour

29.1 Incidence and Epidemiology

1. Incidence: 8%–10% of solid tumours, throughout the world,
2. Host factors:
   a) Sex: equal incidence in both sexes,
   b) Age: peak under 4 years.
   c) Genetic predisposition: congenital anomalies are observed in 12%–15% of cases: sporadic aniridia (deletion *11p*), focal gigantism, Wiedemann-Beckwith syndrome, neurofibromatosis, horseshoe kidney, cryptorchidy, sexual ambiguity, haemangiomas. Uni- but mainly bilateral, multifocal, Wilms' tumours may arise form renal dysplasia: nodular or diffuse nephroblastomatosis.
      Familial cases are rare, usually multifocal and/or associated with above congenital anomalies.
3. Environmental factors: no information.

29.2 Pathological Classification

1. Favourable common pathological features:
   Three cell types more or less mixed: blastemal (metanephric origin), epithelial, stromal pattern.
2. Unfavourable pathological features (12%–15% of cases):
   a) Anaplastic: threefold nuclear enlargement, hyperpolyploidy, atypical mitotic figures.
   b) Sarcomatous: rhabdomyosarcomatoid; clear-cell.
3. Allied tumoral conditions in infants less than 6–12 months:
   a) Mesoblastic nephroma is theoretically a benign tumour.
   b) Nodular subcapsular renal blastemas in diffuse nephroblastomatosis are potentially malignant lesions.

29.3 Main Clinical Features

1. Major:
   Abdominal mass
   Abdominal pain
   Haematuria
2. Possible:
   Vomiting
   Fever
   Anaemia
   Hypertension
   Acute surgical abdomen
   Varicocele
   Malformations
3. Unusual:
   Hypercalcaemia
   Hypoglycaemia
   Cushing's syndrome

29.4 Staging Procedures

1. Compulsory examinations
   Ultrasonography
   Abdominal x-ray, i.v. pyelogram
   Complete blood count
   Renal function
   Urinary catecholamine metabolizes
   Chest x-ray
2. Optional examinations
   Abdominal and chest computerized axial tomography[1]
   Chest tomography
   Vena cavogram
   Arteriogram (in the case of bilateral tumours or doubtful diagnosis)
   Bone isotope scan and skeletal survey (clear-cell type)
   Brain computed tomography (CT) (rhabdomyosarcomatoid type)

---

[1] CT scan is the best diagnostic and staging procedure and may be considered as the only compulsory examination, if it is available.

29.5 Staging Systems

29.5.1 Surgical and Histological Grouping (National Wilms' Tumour Study - NWTS)

Group I	Tumour limited to the kidney and completely excised
Group II	Tumour extends beyond the kidney, but is completely resected: penetration beyond the capsule into perirenal soft tissues or peri-aortic lymph nodes, infiltration of renal vessels
Group III	Residual non-haematogenous tumour confined to abdomen: tumour biopsy, tumour rupture before or during surgery, peritoneal implants, positive lymph nodes beyond peri-aortic chain, tumoral infiltration into vital structures
Group IV	Haematogenous metastases (20% at diagnosis): lungs (80% of whole metastases), liver, bone, brain
Group V	Bilateral renal tumours (5%-10% of cases), either initially or subsequently

29.5.2 Recent Staging System (Based on NWTS Trials 1 and 2)

Stage I:	No change.
Stage II:	Tumour may have been biopsied or there has been local spillage.
Stage III:	- Positive lymph nodes in the hilus, peri-aortic chains, or beyond. - Microscopic or macroscopic tumoral extension beyond the surgical margins.
Stage IV:	No change.
Stage V:	Bilateral renal involvement at diagnosis. An attempt should be made to stage each side according to the above criteria.

Moreover, each patient should be characterized according to favourable or unfavourable histology.

29.5.3 Other System of Nomenclature: TNM

1. TNM clinical classification

T1	Unilateral $\leqslant 80\ cm^2$ area on i. v. pyelogram
T2	Unilateral $> 80\ cm^2$ area on i. v. pyelogram
T3	Unilateral, ruptured before treatment
T4	Bilateral
N0	No evidence of regional lymph node involvement
N1	Evidence of regional lymph node involvement
M0	No evidence of distant metastases
M1	Evidence of distant metastases

2. Post-surgical histopathological TNM classification

p T0 No evidence of tumour found on histological examination
p T1 Encapsulated, complete excision
p T2 Invasion beyond capsule, complete excision
p T3 Incomplete excision:
  a - microscopic residue
  b - macroscopic residue or spillage
  c - unresectable at surgery
p T4 Bilateral tumour
p N0 No evidence of tumour at histological examination of regional lymph node
p N1 Invasion of regional lymph node
  - pN1 a completely resected
  - pN1 b incompletely resected
pM0 No evidence of distant metastases
pM1 Evidence of distant metastases

N. B. The letter y is added when surgery has been done after other primary treatment.

29.6 Prognostic Factors

29.6.1 According to Their Importance

Major factors	Minor factors
Stage and surgical removal	Age (<2 yrs)
Tumour size and weight	Tumour rupture
Histology	Vascular emboli
Regional lymph nodes	Renal vein invasion
	Capsular invasion
	Laterality

29.6.2 Positive Prognostic Factors

1. Stages I and II
2. Tumour size: <80 cm^2 on i.v. pyelogram; or <250 g in cases of primary surgery
3. Negative para-aortic lymph nodes (meticulous surgical technique with biopsy of suspicious lymph nodes)
4. Absence of anaplastic or sarcomatous component
5. Absence of tumoral rupture

6. Site of metastases: lung is far better than abdomen
7. Time of relapses: late relapses are better than early (> 12 months from diagnosis)

29.7 Common Chemotherapeutic Practice in Wilms' Tumour

1. Useful drugs:
   a) Major drugs: actinomycin-D, vincristine, Adriamycin
   b) Drugs under study: cyclophosphamide, *cis*-platinum, etoposide (VP-16-213), iphosphamide
2. Pre-operative therapy:
   This is useful to reduce a large tumour and to decrease the risk of its rupture.
   a) Actinomycin D - 15 μg/kg/day for 3-5 days (one or two courses with a 2-week treatment-free interval): and/or
   b) Vincristine - 1.5 mg/m^2/week - three to four injections
      Duration: 3-4 weeks, except in bilateral cases (see also 29.9)
3. Post-operative therapy:
   Use of actinomycin and vincristine in combination is more effective in preventing metastases than the use of either agent alone.
   a) Vincristine - 1.5-2 mg/m^2/week: once a week, starting 1 week after surgery for 4-6 weeks
   b) Actinomycin D - 15 μg/kg/day for 3-5 days; timing varies according to modalities of pre-operative treatment
4. Maintenance therapy:
   a) Actinomycin D - 15 μg/kg/day for 5 days
   b) Vincristine - 1.5 mg/m^2/day, days 1 and 5
      Every 6-8 weeks
      Total: 5-6 courses; in stage I, the maintenance treatment may be of shorter duration
5. Therapy of relapses and initial stages IV:
   Adriamycin (60 mg/m^2/course) or combined with the previous drugs given as an alternating schedule (do not exceed 350 mg/m^2 when combined with chest radiotherapy):
   a) Vincristine 1.5 mg/m^2, day 1 + Adriamycin 60 mg/m^2, day 2. Interval: 3 weeks
      then
   b) Vincristine 1.5 mg/m^2, days 1 and 5 + actinomycin D 15 μg/kg, days 1-5.
      Interval 3 weeks

Under study: alkylating drugs, VP-16-213
N.B. Doses should be reduced by 30%-50% in infants < 1 year

29.8 Therapeutic Strategy for Non-Metastatic Wilms' Tumour

1. Pre-operative treatment:
   Chemotherapy for 2-4 weeks is recommended for very large tumours; this pre-operative treatment may be omitted in standard tumours and if diagnosis is doubtful; the risk of diagnostic errors is 5%-10%. For this reason, and to facilitate histological examination, some teams perform surgery at first in all cases. In infants less than 6 months, primary surgery is recommended, due to the high frequency of benign mesoblastic nephromas.
2. Nephrectomy.
3. Post-operative and maintenance treatment (8 days after surgery):
   a) Radiotherapy: to the tumour bed, except in stage I (even if the staging is obtained after pre-operative chemotherapy) and in stage II with negative lymph nodes and favourable histology
   b) Adjuvant chemotherapy in all stages, using actinomycin D and vincristine in multiple courses for 6-15 months; Adriamycin may be added in unfavourable cases
4. Current recommended schedules (adapted from results obtained by NWTS and Société Internationale d'Oncologie-Pédiatrique - SIOP):
   A. *First schedule, including primary chemotherapy* - recommended for large tumours

Pre-operative chemotherapy
Actinomycin D
15 μg/kg/d
Vincristine
1.5 mg/m^2/wk

Post-operative chemotherapy

Maintenance chemotherapy
Total = 5 courses
every 6 weeks

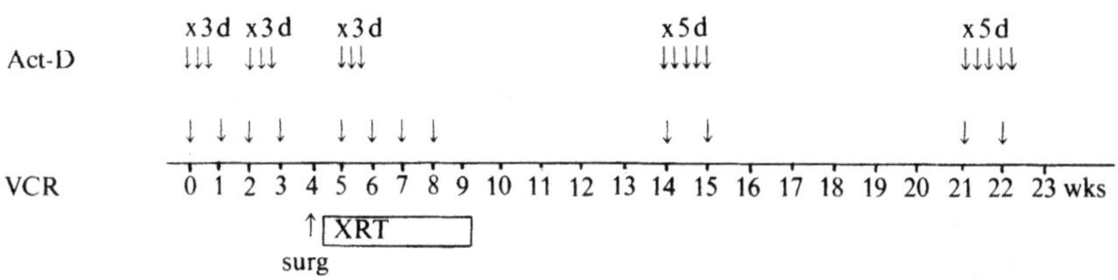

B. *Second schedule, including primary surgery* – recommended for infants < 6 months, small tumours any age, doubtful diagnosis (same dosages as above)

Post-operative chemotherapy
Actinomycin D
15 µg/kg/d
Vincristine
1.5 mg/m^2/wk

Maintenance chemotherapy
Total = 5 courses every 6 weeks

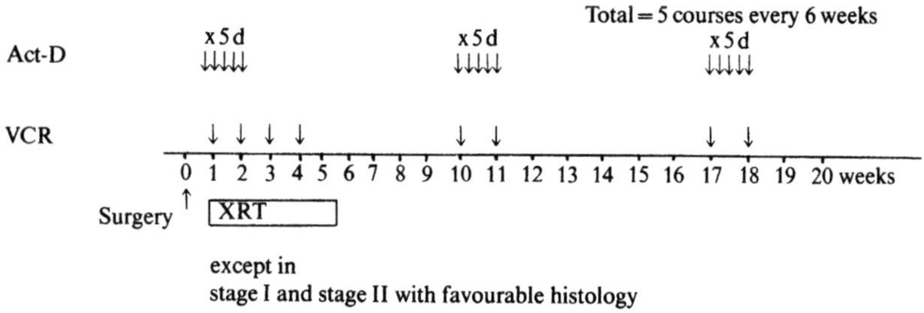

XRT, radiation treatment

5. Problems under study:
   Addition of Adriamycin in high-risk cases (unfavourable histology, positive lymph nodes, stages III and IV); duration and reduction of maintenance chemotherapy (mainly in stage I); reduction of radiotherapy (indications and doses in stage II)

29.9 Recommended Therapy of Wilms' Tumour in Patients with Metastases and Bilateral Tumours (5%–10%)

29.9.1 Pulmonary Metastases at Diagnosis or After Diagnosis

Primary chemotherapy using vincristine and actinomycin D and/or Adriamycin, for 6–12 weeks, followed by:

1. Excision (wedge, segmental or lobar excision), in case of incomplete regression of a solitary metastasis
2. or XRT to both lungs in case of incomplete resection and multiple or bulky metastases
3. then maintenance chemotherapy with actinomycin D, vincristine and/or Adriamycin.
   Great care must be taken in repeating actinomycin D and/or Adriamycin courses to avoid cardiac and pulmonary complications.

29.9.2 Hepatic Metastases

1. Single metastases in one lobe:
   Primary chemotherapy; then partial hepatic resection followed by radiotherapy if residual disease. These should not be instituted until full liver regeneration has occurred.
2. Wide-spread metastases:
   Liver radiotherapy and chemotherapy

29.9.3 Abdominal Recurrence After Nephrectomy

Chemotherapy to reduce the tumour mass, maximal tumour resection, post-operative irradiation (if necessary and possible), chemotherapy

29.9.4 Bilateral Wilms' Tumour

1. Pre-operative chemotherapy (vincristine and actinomycin D and/or Adriamycin).
2. Surgery: to be decided when maximal tumoral reduction is obtained (sometimes after 2–3 months).
3. Post-operative chemotherapy (vincristine, actinomycin D, Adriamycin) has to be adapted to renal function abnormalities,
4. Radiotherapy may be used with care according to tumour stage and the extent of surgical excision.

29.10 Complications of the Therapy of Wilms' Tumour

29.10.1 Early Complications

1. Digestive disturbances:
   Vomiting and diarrhoea are observed mainly during irradiation
   An elementary diet without gluten, lactose, saccharose or cow's milk proteins may be necessary and has sometimes to be given by continuous drip-feeding to prevent malnutrition.
2. Haematological disorders (leukopenia, thrombocytopenia):
   Usually observed 8–10 days after the end of a course, sometimes sooner.
   a) Do not commence with full dosage of chemotherapy, if WBC is $<$ 4000 mm^3 and/or platelets $<150\,000/mm^3$,
   b) Stop the course, if platelets fall $<75\,000/mm^3$.

3. Hepatic complications:
   These are noted in cases of right-sided nephroblastomas, when the liver is included in the radiation field.
   - Chemotherapy (actinomycin D, Adriamycin) has to be stopped until recovery.
4. Pneumonitis:
   May be due to an infection, or to lesions induced by lung irradiation, potentiated by chemotherapy (actinomycin D, Adriamycin).
5. Heart toxicity:
   May occur when Adriamycin is used, and mainly when it is preceded or followed by chest radiotherapy.

29.10.2 Late Complications (Mainly Due to Irradiation)

1. Bone growth retardation, scoliosis
2. Functional disturbances of lung, digestive tract, liver, kidney, heart
3. Gonadal injury
4. Second malignancy
5. Genetic consequences

29.11 Results of Treatment of Wilms' Tumour

Assessment of survival without evidence of disease at 2 years from initial diagnosis or from the treatment of the last metastasis, appears to be a valuable guide to the prospects of cure. At present time, 2-year survival rate is 80% in localized disease and about 50% in metastastic disease.
Historical progress of treatment is as follows:
Until 1940 - surgery alone: 15%-20% cure rate
1940-1960 - surgery + radiotherapy: 25%-45% cure rate
1957-1985 - surgery + radiotherapy + chemotherapy: 80% cure rate

29.12 Current Investigations

1. To refine prognostic factors
2. To improve survival rate in unfavourable patients
3. To decrease acute and long-term complications
4. To establish precise epidemiology

30 Neuroblastoma

30.1 Epidemiology and Incidence

1. Incidence: 10% of solid tumours in children and 50% of neonatal malignant conditions. Annual incidence of 10 per million live births
2. High-risk areas: United States, Western Europe. Low rates in black Africans, but not in United States black population
3. Host factors:
   Sex: M/F: 1.3/1
   Age: peak incidence at 2 years
   Genetic predisposition: neural-crest pathology (association with Hirschsprung' disease, von Recklinghausen's disease, adenomatosis)
4. Environmental factors:
   Possible association with foetal hydantoin syndrome and foetal alcohol syndrome.

30.2 Pathological Features

Neuroblastomas are composed of undifferentiated neuroblasts; ganglioneuroblastomas contain mixtures of neuroblasts and ganglion cells in varying stages of differentiation. Degree of maturation, mitotic rate, lymphocyte infiltration are possible indicators of prognosis.

30.2.1 Methods Used to Characterize Neuroblastoma Cells

1. Histological study
2. Ultrastructural study
3. Biochemical study
4. Kinetic studies
5. In vitro culture:
   - To observe: Neuroblastic differentiation
     Secretion of catecholamines
   - To test: Sensitivity of drugs

- To study: Cytogenetic abnormalities and DNA content (*1p*⁻, *11q*⁻, double minute sphere chromosomes)
- To study: The role of oncogenes

6. Monoclonal antibodies
7. Injection to nude mouse
8. Animal models

30.3 Main Clinical Features

Clinical signs depending on primary site (metastases at onset in 75% of cases):
Abdominal pain and distension, weight loss
Diarrhoea, hypertension
Fever, pallor, asthenia, bone pains (lumps)
Proptosis, peri-orbital ecchymoses
Subcutaneous nodules, massive hepatomegaly; adenopathies; neurological signs: paraplegia, myoclonic encephalopathy, cervical enlargement, rectal or bladder compression

30.4 Staging Procedures

1. Compulsory examinations:
   a) X-Ray examinations according to primary site: cervical and chest, i.v. pyelogram, oblique views of spine, complete skeletal survey
   b) Ultrasonography (chest, abdomen)
   c) Urinary catecholamine levels, expressed as a ratio of creatinine
   d) Complete blood count
   e) Coagulation tests
   f) Multiple bone marrow aspirates and biopsy
   g) Cerebrospinal fluid examination
   h) Biopsy of peripheral tumoural lymph nodes or subcutaneous nodules
2. Optional examinations (or under study):
   a) Computerized axial tomographic (CAT) scan (chest or abdomen)
   b) Isotope scanning: bone (technetium-99); any tumoural site (I^{131} methyliodobenzylguanidine, radiolabelled monoclonal antibodies)
   c) Myelography
   d) Lymphangiography
   e) Serum ferritin level
   f) Vasoactive intestinal vasopeptide

g) Urinary cystathionine
h) Neuron-specific enolase

3. Frequency of various stages at diagnosis (Evans' staging):

Stage I	10%-15%
Stage II	10%-15%
Stage III	10%
Stage IV	50%-60%
Stage IV_S	10%

The percentage of stage IV cases increases with the age of the patients from 10%-15% in children <6 months to 75% >24 months.

4. Frequency by site of primary tumour:

Abdominal	70%-75% of cases
Thoracic	20%-25%
Pelvic Cervical Others and unknown	5%-10%

30.5 Staging Systems

30.5.1 Evans' Staging System

Stage I	Tumour limited to the organ or structure of origin.
Stage II	Tumour extending in continuity beyond the organ or structure of origin, but not crossing the midline. Regional lymph nodes, on the homolateral side may be involved.
Stage III	Tumour extending in continuity beyond the midline. Regional lymph nodes may be involved bilaterally.
Stage IV	Distant metastases.
Stage IV_S	Patients who would otherwise be stage I or II, but who have remote disease confined only to one or more of the following sites: liver, skin or bone marrow (without radiographic or scanning evidence of bone metastases).

30.5.2 TNM Classification

1. TNM clinical classification:

T0	No evidence of primary tumour
T1	Single tumour <5 cm
T2	Single tumour >5 cm <10 cm

T3	Single tumour > 10 cm
T4	Multicentric
N0	No evidence of regional lymph node involvement
N1	Evidence of regional lymph node involvement
M0	No evidence of distant metastases
M1	Evidence of distant metastases

2. Post-surgical-histopathological TNM classification:

pT0	No evidence of tumour found on histological examination
pT1	Complete excision, margins free
no pT2	in neuroblastoma
pT3	incomplete excision
pT3a	- microscopic
pT3b	- macroscopic
pT3c	- unresectable
pT4	Multicentric
pN0	No evidence of tumour histological examination of regional lymph nodes
pN1	Invasion of regional lymph nodes
pN1a	- completely resected
pN1b	- incompletely resected
pM0	No evidence of distant metastases
pM1	Evidence of distant metastases

30.6 Prognostic Factors

1. Major:
   Age (< 1 yr; > 6 yrs)
   Stage and lymph node extension in localized disease
   Primary site
2. Minor or under study:
   Vanilmandelic acid (VMA), homovanillic acid levels
   Maturity of tumour enzyme system
   Degree of histological and ultrastructural differentiation
   Ferritin and enolase level
   Immunological status
   Amplification of oncogenes *(N-myc)*

30.7 Recommended Drugs and Therapeutic Schedules for Neuroblastoma

30.7.1 Single Agents Effective in Neuroblastoma

Drug	% CR or PR (4 weeks)
Cyclophosphamide (CTX)	60 (conventional or high-dose)
Adriamycin (ADM)	20–40
Vincristine (VCR)	30–40
Peptichemio	70–80
Cis-platinum (DDP)	30
Teniposide (VM-26)	20–30
Daunomycin	15
Dacarbazine (DTIC)	15
Melphalan (L-PAM)	15

CR, complete remission; PR, partial remission

30.7.2 Drug Combinations

	CR	PR	No. of patients
VCR + CTX	33	42	160
VCR + DTIC	–	3	128
VM-26 + DDP	6	9	22
CTX + ADM	32	13	65
VCR + CTX + ADM	42	35	121
VCR + CTX + DTIC	23	25	60
VCR + CTX + DTIC + ADM	19	17	44
VCR + CTX + VM-26 + DDP ± ADM		25	35

30.7.3 Suggested Chemotherapy Schedules

1. *Two-drug schedule:* (every 3 weeks):
   a) CTX 10–15 mg/kg/day i.v. or orally: for 5–7 days
      VCR 1.5 mg/m^2/day on days 1 and 8 of the course (maximum 2 mg/dose)
   b) CTX 150 mg/m^2/day i.v. or orally for 7 days
      ADM 35 mg/m^2 i.v. day 8

2. OPEC regimen: VCR 1.5 mg/m^2 and CTX 600 mg/m^2, day 1
   DDP 60 mg/m^2, day 2
   VM-26 150 mg/m^2, day 4
   every 3 weeks
3. MADDOC regimen: Nitrogen mustard 4 mg/m^2
   ADM 40 mg/m^2
   DDP 45 mg/m^2
   VCR 2 mg/m^2
   CTX 250 mg/m^2
   DTIC 250 mg/m^2
   every 3 weeks

30.8 Therapeutic Strategy by Stage in Neuroblastoma

Stage I — Total resection is usually feasible. No further treatment seems necessary.

Stage II — Total or partial resection followed by chemotherapy. Usefulness of radiotherapy is controversial.

Stage III
a) *First situation:* tumour judged resectable (e.g. lateral abdominal tumour):
   1. *Complete or partial excision.*
   2. Radiotherapy: to the tumour bed, defined surgically.
   3. Chemotherapy: two- or three-drug schedules (see Sect. 30.7.3); duration: 12–18 months.

b) *Second situation:* tumour judged unresectable (e.g. median abdominal tumour):
   1. Pre-operative chemotherapy: rather than radiotherapy; duration of chemotherapy depends on tumour response.
   2. Partial removal of the tumour, if possible.
   3. Post-operative treatment: radiotherapy and chemotherapy, with two or four drugs; duration: 12–18 months.

Stage IV — At diagnosis, chemotherapy is the only feasible treatment, giving short- or long-lasting remissions. After 3–6 months, if remission is judged to be complete, tumour resection with or without radiotherapy.

Palliative radiotherapy may also be used to decrease bone pain or proptosis.

Treatment under study in stages III and IV: in CR or good PR consolidation by high-dose chemotherapy with or without total-body irradiation, followed by bone marrow allograft or autograft (the value of bone marrow purge using immunological or chemical tools is under study).

Stage IV_S a) Pepper's syndrome (liver involvement):

1. Pre-operable treatment: Chemotherapy alone (VPR-CTX) or combined with low-dose liver irradiation.
2. Exploratory abdominal surgery: May be indicated to remove the residual primary tumour, and should be decided 3-6 months after the beginning of treatment.
3. Post-operative treatment: Chemotherapy in case of relapse that is judged clinically or by biochemical parameters (catecholamines); duration: 6-12 months.

b) Other stage IV_S:

1. Excision of primary tumour:
   - Immediately.
   - Delayed until after chemotherapy.
   - Sometimes not useful if the primary tumour is spontaneously calcified with normal catecholamine levels.
2. Chemotherapy: Before and/or after surgery (6-12 months mainly in the case of bone marrow involvement).
3. Radiotherapy: Usually not useful.

30.9 Current Results

Overall 3-year survival rate: 30% (= cure rate):

Actuarial survival rate:

1. According to stage and age (O. Hartmann, Arch. Fr. Ped. 1983, 40, 15-21)

   Stage I-II (any age): 95%

   Stage III <1 yr: 77%

   >1 yr: 63%

   Stage IV <1 yr: 57%

   >1 yr: 12%

2. According to primary site: Thorax 84%

   Abdomen 37%

31 Rhabdomyosarcomas

31.1 Incidence and Epidemiology

1. Incidence: 10%–12% of malignant solid tumours in childhood
2. Host factors:
   a) Sex ratio: 1.1 M/1 F
   b) Mean age: 6 years
   c) Race: 4.4 per million white children and 1.3 per million black children in United States
   d) Genetic factors: some cases are associated with von Recklinghausen's disease, basal cell naevomatosis, lung adenomatosis, nervus sebaceous of Jadassohn; and with a history of familial multiple malignancies: breast, soft tissue, brain, adrenocortical tumours, osteogenic sarcomas
3. Environmental factors: role of chemical agents is under study (herbicides)

31.2 Pathological Classification (Intergroup Rhabdomyosarcoma Study)

1. Embryonal type (57% of cases)
2. Alveolar cell type (18%)
3. Botryoid cell type (7%)
4. Pleiomorphic adult type (2%)
5. Undifferentiated cell type (16%)

More sophisticated methods are needed to better define tumoral cells: microscopy, immunocytochemistry, cytogenetics, oncogene expression, potential for differentiation in culture.

31.3 Staging Procedures

1. Examinations depending on site:
   a) Head and neck:
      - Ear, nose and throat examination (under anaesthesia)
      - Ophthalmological examination
      - Tomograms of the primary site
      - Brain computed tomographic (CT) scan
      - Head CT scan
      - Spinal fluid cytology
   b) Genito-urinary and abdominal:
      - Intravenous urogram
      - Cystoscopy, vaginoscopy
      - Ultrasonography
      - CT Scan
      - Lymphangiography (optional)
   c) Thorax:
      - Chest x-rays and tomograms
      - Ultrasonography
      - CT scan
   d) Limbs:
      - Bone x-rays
      - CT scan
      - Lymphangiography
      - Arteriography (optional)
2. Common examinations to detect metastases:
   a) Chest x-rays and CT scan
   b) Bone marrow aspiration
   c) Bone x-rays or isotope scanning
   d) Biopsy of suspicious lymph node

31.4 Staging Systems

31.4.1 Stage Grouping of Intergroup Rhabdomyosarcoma Study (Post-Surgical Staging)

Group I (16% of cases):	Localized disease; microscopic confirmation of complete resection. No lymph node involvement
Group II (28% of cases):	A. Grossly resected tumour with microscopic residue and negative lymph node B. Regional disease, completely resected (negative or positive nodes)

	C. Regional disease, grossly resectable with microscopic residue and positive lymph nodes
Group III (36% of cases):	Biopsy or incomplete resection of local or regional disease with gross residual tumour
Group IV (20% of cases):	Distant metastatic disease: lung, liver, bones, bone marrow, brain or extraregional lymph nodes

31.4.2 TNM Classification

a - TNM Clinical classification
- T1 Tumour confined to organ or tissue of origin
  T1 a $\leqslant$ 5 cm
  T1 b $>$ 5 cm
- T2 Tumour involves contiguous organs or tissues
  T2 a $\leqslant$ 5 cm
  T2 b $>$ 5 cm
- no T3
- no T4

N0 No evidence of lymph node involvement
N1 Evidence of lymph node involvement
M0 No evidence of distant metastases
M1 Evidence of distant metastases

b - Post-surgical TNM histopathological classification
pT0 No evidence of tumour found on histological examination
pT1 Limited to organ of origin. Complete excision, margins free
pT2 Invasion beyond organ, complete excision
pT3 Invasion beyond organ, incomplete excision
  a - Microscopic residue
  b - Macroscopic residue
  c - Unresectable tumour

no pT4
pN0 No evidence of lymph node involvement
pN1 Evidence of lymph node involvement
pM0 No evidence of distant metastases
pM1 Evidence of distant metastases

31.5 Prognostic Factors in Rhabdomyosarcoma

1. Stage:
   Survival durations for patients in different clinical groups (I–IV). (Survival duration equal to the interval between treatment start and death or last follow-up date.) (Maurer et al.)

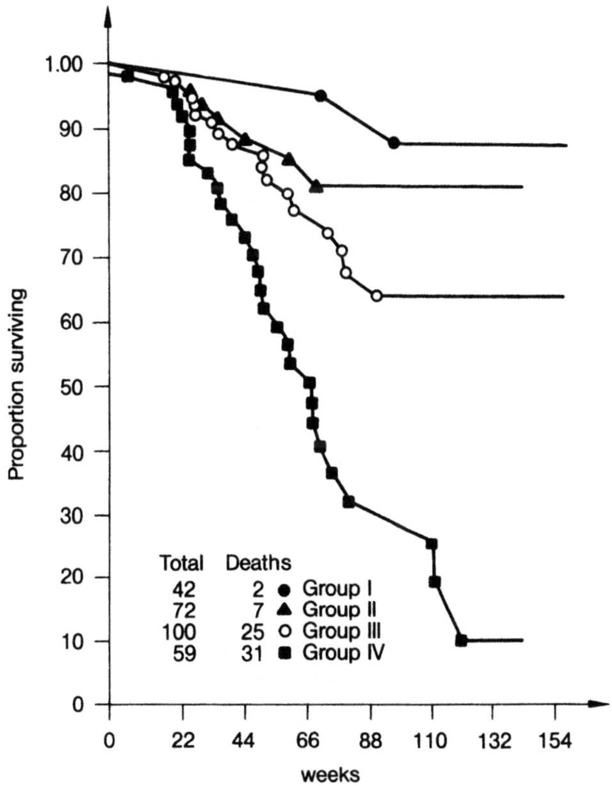

2. Primary site:
   a) Best prognosis: orbit, vagina, bladder, paratesticular site
   b) Intermediate: vesico-prostatic, limbs, trunk
   c) Poor: nasopharynx, middle ear
3. Histological and cytological type:
   a) Alveolar type is considered as having a worse prognosis than other types.

b) Unfavourable cytology: monomorphous and anaplastic types.
4. Lymph node involvement

31.6 General Principles of Treatment of Rhabdomyosarcoma

31.6.1 Aims:

a) Local control
b) Maintenance of function of the affected part
c) Prevention of metastases

31.6.2 Methodology:

1. *Surgery* is the most effective method of eradicating a localized tumour when it can be removed without significant residual defect ($\leqslant$30%–40% of cases). In the other cases, biopsy is performed; then, some weeks or months later, a resection may be easier after tumoral shrinkage by chemotherapy with or without radiotherapy.
2. *Radiotherapy* is used after partial resection or simple biopsy, to eradicate macroscopic or microscopic residual disease. But, with an effective chemotherapy, indications and dose of radiotherapy might be reduced to avoid late sequelae.
3. Chemotherapy is used for:
   a) Treatment of metastases
   b) Local control after excision, with or without radiotherapy
   c) Eradication of micrometastases; without chemotherapy, metastases occur usually in 70% of patients during the 1st year
   d) Tumour shrinkage, as primary treatment (after biopsy)
   e) Under study: massive chemotherapy followed by bone marrow graft in high-risk patients

31.7 Single Agents and Drug Combinations Effective in Rhabdomyosarcoma

More active	*Less active* or under study
Actinomycin D	Dacarbazine (DTIC)
Vincristine (VCR)	Vinblastine
Cyclophosphamide (CTX)	Teniposide (VM-26)
Adriamycin (ADM)	Bleomycin
Iphosphamide	Cytosine arabinoside
	High-dose methotrexate (MTX) and citrovorum factor (CF)
	Lomustine
	Etoposide (VP-16-213)
	5-Azacytidine
	Cis-platinum (DDP)
	L-PAM

31.7.1 Recommended Drug Combinations for Rhabdomyosarcoma

Using VCR - actinomycin D - CTX, either sequentially or intermittently (VAC-pulse), increase of percentage and duration of complete remission has been obtained. ADM may be added to these drugs in unfavourable cases. However, comparison between many varying multi-drug schedules does not show differences on disease-free survival.

Actinomycin D und ADM have to be avoided during irradiation, especially in orbital, abdominal and pelvic tumours.

1. *Standard VAC regimen:*

VCR	2 mg/m^2/week × 12 doses (max. dose 2 mg)
Actino-mycin D	0.015 mg/kg/day × 5 days (max. 500 μg/injection) every 3 months (5-6 courses)
CTX	2,5 mg/kg given orally starting on day 42 through 24 months

2. *Pulse-VAC regimen:*

VCR	2 mg/m^2 i.v. days 1 and 5 (max. dose 2 mg/inj)
Actino-mycin D	0.015 mg/kg/day i.v. days 1 to 5 (course repeated 12, 24, 36 and 38 weeks)
CTX	10 mg/kg/day i.v. days 1 to 5

3. *VAC-VAD regimen:*

VAC	VCR	1.5 mg/m^2 day 1
	Actino-mycin D	0.015 mg/kg/days 1–5
	CTX	300 mg/m^2 days 1–5

   Course alternated every 3 weeks with:

VAD	VCR	1.5 mg/m^2 day 1
	ADM	60 mg/m^2 day 1 (max. cumulative dose: 350–500 mg/m^2)

4. *Under study:*
   DDP - ADM regimen; VP-16-213 - DDP regimen

31.8 Therapeutic Strategy by Stage

1. Stage I:
   a) Surgery
   b) Chemotherapy (1 year); irradiation is unnecessary
2. Stage II:
   a) Surgery
   b) Irradiation on residual microscopic tumour
   c) Chemotherapy (1 year)
3. Stage III:
   a) Biopsy or partial resection
   b) Chemotherapy to obtain maximal tumoral shrinkage, trying to avoid an important initial mutilation
   c) According to its effect, primary chemotherapy is followed by irradiation or tumoral excision or both
   d) Maintenance chemotherapy: 12–18 months
4. Stage IV:
   a) Primary chemotherapy
   b) Surgery and/or irradiation may be indicated if partial or complete remission
   c) Under study: consolidation using massive chemotherapy followed by autologous bone graft

31.9 Current Therapeutic Strategy by Main Sites (Stages I, II, III)

1. Orbital Rhabdomyosarcoma:
   a) Complete or partial removal.
   b) Orbital XRT (radiation treatment).
   c) Chemotherapy: VAC-pulse regimen; duration: 12–18 months, according to stage.
2. Nasopharynx and middle-ear rhabdomyosarcoma:
   a) Biopsy.
   b) Induction chemotherapy: VAC-pulse regimen or VAC-VAD,
   c) Surgery and/or XRT on residual tumour.
   d) Maintenance chemotherapy 18 months.
   e) Prevention or treatment of meningeal and brain stem extension: loco-regional or whole-brain irradiation.
3. Trunk Rhabdomyosarcoma (thorax, retroperitoneal):
   a) Partial excision or biopsy.
   b) Chemotherapy: VAC-pulse or VAC-VAD.
   c) Second-look surgery and/or XRT.
   d) Maintenance chemotherapy, duration 18 months.
4. Bladder, vaginal rhabdomyosarcoma:
   a) Biopsy.
   b) Chemotherapy: VAC or VAC-VAD until maximum shrinkage.
   c) Conservative surgery and/or
   d) Interstitial XRT to residual tumour.
   e) Chemotherapy: duration/18 months.
5. Prostate, vesico-prostatic, vesico-vaginal rhabdomyosarcoma:
   a) Biopsy.
   b) Chemotherapy: VAC or VAC-VAD until maximum shrinkage.
   c) Less mutilating surgery and/or XRT.
   d) Chemotherapy: 18 months.
6. Paratesticular rhabdomyosarcoma:
   a) Excision with high cord ligation.
   b) Systematic lumbar-aortic lymphadenectomy is controversial in localized tumours completely resected with negative cord section, negative lymphangiography and ultrasonography (or CT scan).
      It is compulsory in tumours with loco-regional extension.
   c) XRT: in case of local extension and of positive lumbar-aortic lymph nodes.
   d) Maintenance chemotherapy: 12–18 months, according to stage (VAC).

7. Limb rhabdomyosarcoma:
   a) Resection: it may be preceded by chemotherapy.
   b) Regional lymph node dissection: either systematically or only if suspicious lymph nodes, according to teams.
   c) Chemotherapy, combined with XRT on tumour residue: VAC + VAD.
8. Metastatic rhabdomyosarcoma at onset (any site):
   Multiple chemotherapy followed by standard treatment according to site. Massive chemotherapy is under study.

31.10 Current Results of Treatment of Rhabdomyosarcoma and Problems Under Study

With surgical approach alone, 3-year survival rate was about 10%. It was 20%-35% after excision and irradiation. With intensive chemotherapy regimens, it has gone up to 60%. Moreover, chemotherapy has permitted modification of treatment planning and thus, the reduction of complications of surgery and radiotherapy.

31.10.1 Problems Under Study

1. Is it possible to avoid XRT and/or surgery in cases of complete remission obtained by chemotherapy to avoid late sequelae?
2. Is it possible to prevent or to treat meningeal and brain extension in parameningeal rhabdomyosarcoma, using chemotherapy alone, notably in patients less than 5 years of age?
3. How to improve the survival rate in stage IV patients: place of high-dose chemotherapy and bone marrow graft?

32 Paediatric Bone Tumours

I. Osteogenic Sarcoma (or Osteosarcoma)

32.1 Incidence and Epidemiology

1. Incidence – 1.5/million/year before the age of 15 years (United States); 5% of malignant solid tumours in children
2. No geographic variation
3. Host factors;
   Sex: slightly higher risk for males: 1.6–2 M/1 F.
   Age: a first peak related to adolescent growth spurt; 12 years in female, 16 years in male patients. A second peak in older age is related to Paget's disease.
   Genetic predisposition: hereditary retinoblastoma is associated with an increased risk both of radiation-induced and spontaneous osteogenic sarcoma; multiple primary neoplasms may occur in some of these cases. Familial aggregations of osteogenic sarcomas are observed, either associated with bony malformations (e.g. osteogenesis imperfecta, fibrous dysplasia, multiple osteochondromatosis, Maffucci's syndrome, multiple hereditary exostoses), or with other tumours (brain, breast, soft-tissue).
   Radiation: increased risk from high-dose radiation therapy either after treatment of a tumour in childhood, or following exposure to internal bone-seeking radioisotopes (period of latency: 5–40 years).

32.2 Pathological Classification

1. Before any treatment:
   a) *Conventional osteosarcomas* (occurring in normal bone) are subdivided on the basis of the predominant histological pattern into osteoblastic (about 50%), chondroblastic (25%), and fibroblastic (25%).
   b) *Other types:* telangiectatic, para-osteal, peri-osteal, multicentric post-irradiation osteosarcomas and tumours allied to benign conditions.

2. Histopathological grading after primary chemotherapy: to evaluate tumour chemosensitivity and to classify patients in responders (grades I-II) and poor responders (grades III-IV), according to importance of tumour necrosis and presence of viable tumoral cells.

32.3 Main Clinical Features

1. Incidence according to primary site:
   Femur: 40%-50% } distal femur and proximal
   Tibia: 20% } tibia account for 50%-60% of osteosarcomas
   Humerus: 10-15%
   Mandible and maxilla: 7%
   Pelvis: 7%
   Fibula: 4%
2. First symptoms and signs:
   Pain, swelling, limitation of movement in adjacent joint, pathological fracture

32.4 Diagnostic and Staging Procedure

1. Primary site X-rays and tomography
2. x-Rays and tomography of lungs
3. Computerized axial tomographic (CAT) scan (bone and chest)
4. Isotopic bone scanning and/or X-rays
5. Serum alkaline phosphatase
6. Biopsy on primary site

32.5 Prognostic Factors

32.5.1 Conventional Factors

1. Histology:
   5-year-survival (Dahlin)

Osteoblastic	Chondroblastic	Fibroblastic
17.1%	22.3%	25.5%

2. Primary site:
   Limbs > Axial, shoulder, clavicular
   Tibia > Femur
   Distal > Proximal

3. Tumour size at diagnosis:

5-year survival (McKenna)		2-year survival (Winkler)	
< 5 cm	40%	⅓ length	59%
5–10 cm	17%	⅓ length	84%
10–15 cm	4%		
> 15 cm	0		

4. Metastases

32.5.2 New Prognostic Factors

1. Histological post-CT grading
2. Quality of the team

32.5.3 Controversial Prognostic Factors

1. Age
2. Sex

32.6 Single Agents Active in Osteogenic Sarcoma

Evaluated in lung metastases or primary tumour:

	CR + PR %
Cyclophosphamide (CTX)	
Melphalan (L-PAM)	15
Mitomycin C	
Dacarbazine (DTIC)	22
ADM	43
High-dose methotrexate	
(HDMTX)/3 weekly	35
HDMTX weekly	68
Cis-platinum (DDP)	60
Iphosphamide	33

CR, complete remission; PR, partial remission

32.7 Drug Combinations

Tested in evaluable tumours: lung metastases, and then as adjuvant and neoadjuvant (before surgery) chemotherapy:

	CR + PR %
ADM + DTIC + Vincristine (VCR)	35
DTIC + CTX + VCR + ADM	24
VCR + HDMTX (weekly)	66
HDMTX + ADM	54
VCR + HDMTX + ADM + CTX	77
Bleomycin (BLM) + CTX + Act-D	62
DDP + HDMTX	35
ADM + DDP	50

	2-year disease-free survival rate %
COMPADRI (I - II - III)	42-55
CYVADIC	60
HDMTX - VCR - ADM	62
DDP - ADM	50
T 10 (Rosen)	92

32.7.1 T 10 Protocol of Rosen

The place of chemotherapy is no longer debatable: using pre- and post-operative chemotherapy, the 3-year survival rate has increased to 70%-90% vs 20% with surgery or radiotherapy. Recent randomized trials have definitely proven the need for chemotherapy and at the same time the possibility of proposing conservative surgery has been demonstrated in more than half of the patients. Nevertheless, the toxicity of these schedules has to be emphasized.

32.8 Therapeutic Strategy

32.8.1 Non-Metastatic Osteogenic Sarcoma (Fig. see on page 340)

1. Biopsy
2. Indications of primary radical surgery:
   a) Initial fracture (lower limb), major vascular lesions
   b) Infection of the site of biopsy
   Methods:

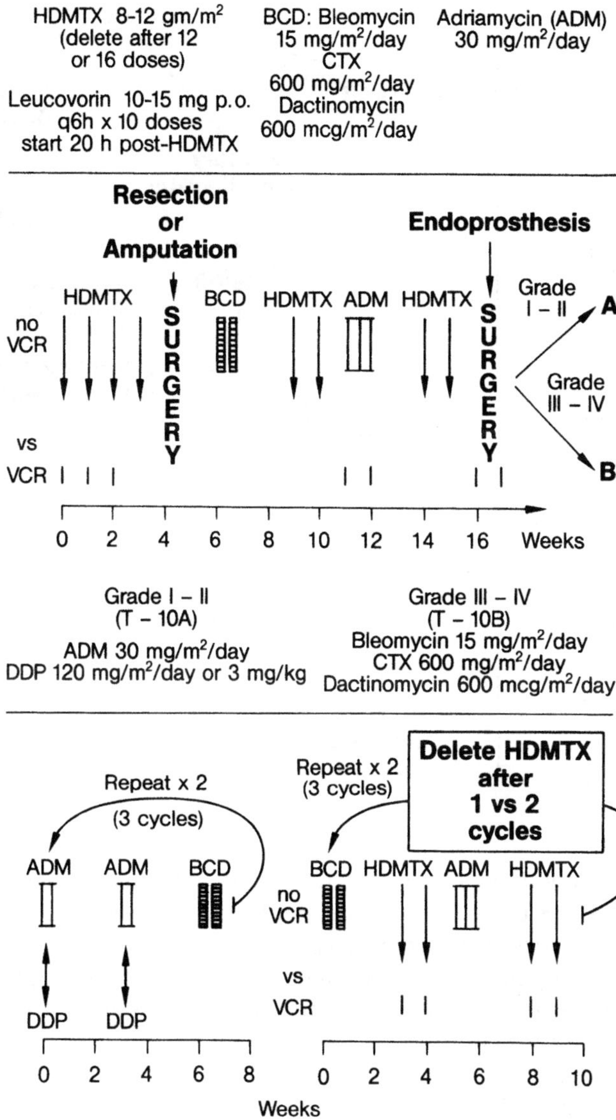
HDMTX 8-12 gm/m²
(delete after 12
or 16 doses)
Leucovorin 10-15 mg p.o.
q6h x 10 doses
start 20 h post-HDMTX
BCD: Bleomycin
15 mg/m²/day
CTX
600 mg/m²/day
Dactinomycin
600 mcg/m²/day
Adriamycin (ADM)
30 mg/m²/day
Resection
or
Amputation
Endoprosthesis
HDMTX
SURGERY
BCD
HDMTX
ADM
HDMTX
SURGERY
Grade
I – II
A
Grade
III – IV
B
no
VCR
vs
VCR
0 2 4 6 8 10 12 14 16 Weeks
Grade I – II
(T – 10A)
ADM 30 mg/m²/day
DDP 120 mg/m²/day or 3 mg/kg
Grade III – IV
(T – 10B)
Bleomycin 15 mg/m²/day
CTX 600 mg/m²/day
Dactinomycin 600 mcg/m²/day
Repeat x 2
(3 cycles)
ADM
ADM
BCD
DDP
DDP
Repeat x 2
(3 cycles)
Delete HDMTX
after
1 vs 2
cycles
BCD
HDMTX
ADM
HDMTX
no
VCR
vs
VCR
0 2 4 6 8
0 2 4 6 8 10
Weeks

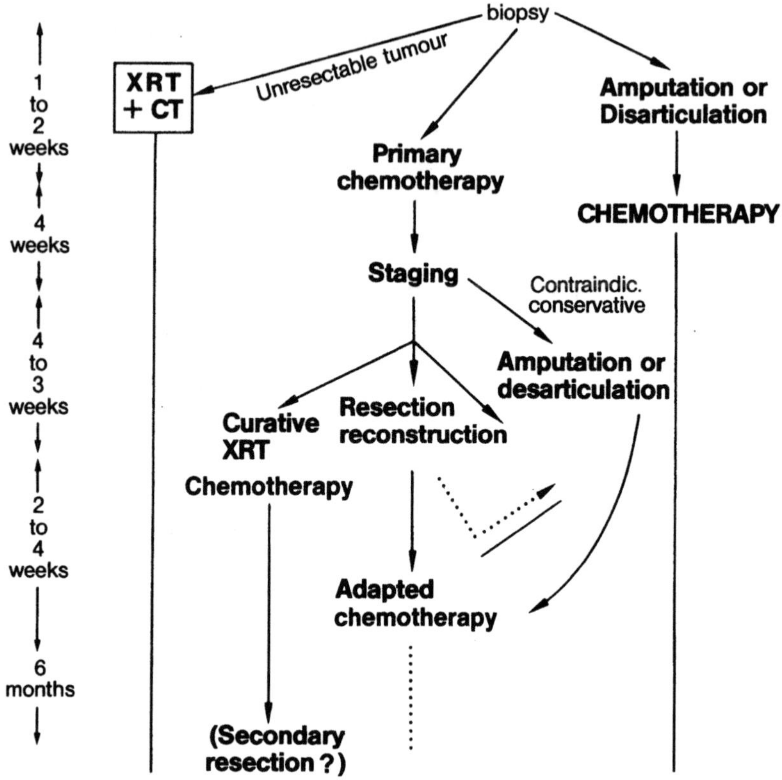

Amputation or disarticulation according to tumoral extension (skip metastases on computed tomography (CT) scan and isotope scanning)
Post-operative chemotherapy

3. Primary pre-operative chemotherapy, with careful sequential evaluation of the tumour response (clinical signs, x-rays and CT scan); mean duration: 10–12 weeks
4. Surgery:
   a) Radical surgery –
   Indications: important soft-tissue and skin involvement, sepsis after biopsy, fracture, previous XRT ≥ 2000–3000 rads, previous orthopaedic treatment, doubtful functional result
   b) Conservative surgery – En bloc resection, followed by reconstruction
5. Post-operative chemotherapy, taking into account histological grading. Duration from diagnosis: 12 months

32.8.2 Metastatic Osteogenic Sarcoma

1. Primary chemotherapy
2. If tumoral regression, radical surgery:
   a) On primary tumour
   b) And on metastases
      Then post-operative chemotherapy
3. If no response: second-line antimitotics or phase II agents, palliative treatment

32.9 Current Results and Problems under Study

Dramatic improvement of disease-free survival rate (70%–90% at 2 years), and increase of non-mutilating surgical procedures.
Under study: indications and modalities of intra-arterial chemotherapy.

II. Ewing's Sarcoma

32.10 Incidence and Epidemiology

1. Incidence: 0.8/million/year; about 3% of malignant solid tumours in children
2. Host factors:
   Sex: 1.6 M/F
   Age: 30% in the 1st decade, 50% in the 2nd decade, very rare after 30 years. Very rare in black population, in both Africa and America
   Genetic predisposition: not observed
   Environmental factors: no information

32.11 Main Clinical Features

1. Incidence according to primary site:
   a) Extremities: 60%
   b) Pelvis: 15%–20%
   c) Ribs: 8%
   d) Others: 15%

2. First symptoms and signs:
   a) Pain, swelling, impairment of function (sometimes long-lasting before diagnosis)
   b) Spontaneous fracture
   c) Systemic symptoms with fever
   d) Progressive neurological deficiencies leading to paraplegia
   e) Respiratory distress (haemothorax)

32.12 Diagnostic and Staging Procedure

1. Compulsory examinations:
   a) Primary site X-rays and tomography
   b) Isotopic bone scanning and/or X-rays
   c) Lung x-ray and tomography
   d) Primary site and lung CAT scan
   e) Complete blood count, erythrocyte sedimentation rate
   f) Bone marrow biopsy and aspirations
   g) Serum alkaline phosphatase
   h) Serum lactate dehydrogenase
   i) Urine levels of catecholamine metabolites
2. Optional examinations:
   a) Intravenous pyelography
   b) Lymphangiography
   c) Cerebrospinal fluid examination
   d) Chest, brain CAT scan

32.13 Prognostic Factors

1. Age: prognosis is better after 18 years, worse from 0 to 10 years, intermediate from 10 to 18 years.
2. Primary site: prognosis is better for distal tumours (below the knee and elbow) and the mandible; the worst prognosis is for the "trunk" lesions (pelvis, ribs, sternum, spine, scapula).
3. Disseminated disease at presentation (lung, bone, bone marrow, brain, meninges).
4. Systemic symptoms: fever may be a poor prognostic factor.
5. Tumour response to primary chemotherapy.

32.14 Chemotherapy of Ewing's Sarcoma

Raison d'Etre. Very poor results have been obtained with surgical ablation or radiotherapy to the primary site, 5-year survival rate varying between 10% and 20%. The main therapeutic problem is that, in more than 60% of cases, distant metastases (lungs, bones, bone marrow, lymph nodes, brain) will appear within 2-5 years from diagnosis.

32.14.1 Single Agents Effective in Ewing's Sarcoma

Single drugs have been partly effective in metastatic disease:

More active drugs	Less active drugs
CTX	Bleomycin (BLM)
ADM	Procarbazine
Actinomycin D	Mithramycin
Carmustine (BCNU)	Vincristine (VCR)
Iphosphamide	MTX
	DDP
	5-Flourouracil (5-FU)
	Teniposide (VM-26)
	Etoposide (VP-16-213)

32.14.2 Conventional Recommended Drug Combinations for Ewing's Sarcoma

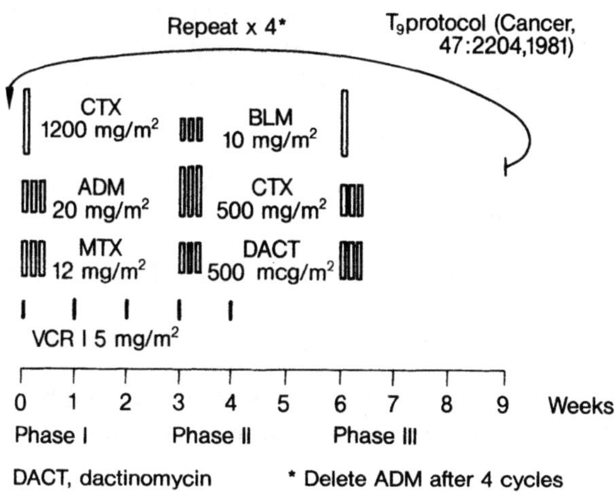

Since 1970, several schedules involving the association of three or four drugs have been used:
First in metastatic disease with an increase in the 2-year survival rate;
Then, as adjuvant therapy, with an increase in the disease-free interval and survival rate (improvement of local control and prevention of distant metastases).

Best results have been obtained with high-dose multidrug chemotherapy: e.g. VAC combined with Adriamycin or T_2, T_5, T_6, T_9 regimens (Sloan Kettering Memorial Hospital, New York)

32.14.3 Protocols Under Study

High-dose chemotherapy followed by bone marrow auto - or allograft, in high-risk patients (metastatic or relapsing).

32.15 Therapeutic Strategy in Ewing's Sarcoma

32.15.1 Local Control

Conventionally, this may be obtained in 80%-90% of cases by irradiating tumoral bone (long bone: 5000 rads on whole bone and a boost of 1000 rads on tumoral site; flat bone: $\geqslant$4500 rads, depending on the local extension and the initial site) and giving simultaneous chemotherapy, indications for surgery being limited to the problem of local recurrence and/or adverse sequelae of irradiation.

At present time, a primary multidrug chemotherapy (for 2-3 months) seems advisable to obtain a tumoral shrinkage, facilitating a curative and conservative surgical approach (e.g. distal tumour, pelvis, rib ...), and/or allowing reduced volume (and perhaps dose) of irradiation, because of the degree of late sequelae.

32.15.2 Eradication of Micro-Metastases by Multidrug Chemotherapy

Preventive lung irradiation is also partly effective, but more toxic.

32.15.3 Treatment of Metastatic and Relapsing Disease

High-dose chemotherapy combined with total-body irradiation, followed by bone marrow auto- and allograft is under study.

32.16 Current Results

When high-dose radiation therapy (or surgery in selected cases) is combined with systemic chemotherapy, the prognosis is improved: the 3-year disease-free survival rate is 50% to 70%. However, a longer follow-up is required, because metastases may be delayed by chemotherapy.

33 Childhood Brain Tumours

33.1 Incidence and Epidemiology

33.1.1 Overall Incidence

20% of malignant diseases in childhood; 17 new cases per year, per million of children less than 15 years of age (Manchester Register).

33.1.2 Incidence of Brain Tumours by Histological Type

The table below is based on reports collected from the literature.

Tumour	Incidence	
	All ages (%)	Children (%)
Glioma	45	70
Astrocytoma	15	30
Glioblastoma	15	5
Oligodendroglioma	8	1
Medulloblastoma	4	20
Ependymoma	4	10
Meningioma	15	1
Neurinoma	6	<0.5
Pituitary adenoma	6	1
Metastases	5-20	<0.5
Craniopharyngioma	3	10
Choroid plexus papilloma	0.5	3
Pinealoma	1	2
Haemangioma	3	1
Epidermoids	2	0.5
Dermoids - teratomas	<0.5	3
Sarcoma	2	4
Optic gliomas	1	4

Note the high frequency of medulloblastoma and astrocytoma in children; in adults nearly half are glioblastoma, followed by astrocytoma. Only 30% of childhood brain tumours are above the tentorium; in contrast, 90% of adult tumours are supratentorial.

33.1.3 Epidemiology

1. Host factors:
   a) Sex: male preponderance for medulloblastoma (2 M/1 F), and pineal gland tumours.
   b) Age: peak incidence at age 5 for medulloblastoma.
   c) Genetic predisposition:
   Association of astrocytoma with neurofibromatosis, tuberous sclerosis, haemangioblastomatosis (multifocal tumours, in some cases).
   Association of medulloblastoma with genodermatoses (basocellular naevomatosis).
   Multiple familial tumours: brain, soft tissues, breast, bones.
   Association with congenital immunodeficiencies.
   d) Environmental factors: no information.
   e) Geographical variations: pineal gland tumours occur six to eight times more frequently in Japan.

33.2 Brain Tumour Characteristics Influencing Response to Chemotherapy

1. Cellular and histological data:
   a) Cellular kinetics: rate of growth, mitotic index.
   b) Spatial distribution of cellular growth fraction; usually three areas may be observed: high peripheral proliferation, central necrosis and low proliferation in the intermediate region.
   c) Natural history of the tumour: risk of local recurrence, risk of seeding to subarachnoid space.
2. Factors influencing drug penetration:
   a) Blood-brain barrier, which theoretically protects the brain from water-soluble drugs $\geqslant$200 daltons of molecular weight; the basis being observations in the treatment of meningeal leukaemia; however, this barrier may be altered by previous radiotherapy.
   b) Better physical and chemical characteristics of drugs: molecular weight, ionization, lipid solubility.
   c) Dose, rate and route of administration of drugs.

d) Cerebrospinal fluid flow obstruction.
e) Modalities of vascularization of tumoral and peritumoral areas.

33.3 Childhood Brain Tumours in Which Prognosis May Be Improved by Chemotherapy

33.3.1 Medulloblastoma and High-Grade Ependymoma

Raison d'Etre. These are malignant tumours, with rapid growth rate, high mitotic index, risk of subarachnoidal space seeding; cure rate is only 30% using surgery and radiotherapy.

1. Partial or complete remissions have been observed in about 50% of recurrent medulloblastomas or ependymomas.
2. The value of adjuvant chemotherapy has been shown in relapsing and high-risk patients.

33.3.2 Glioblastoma Multiforme

In grade IV, (very infrequent in children) adjuvant chemotherapy increases survival duration very slightly: as in adults, prognosis remains very poor.

33.3.3 Brain Stem Glioma

Surgery is not usually feasible (no tumour shrinkage, no pathological data). Brain stem irradiation produces very poor results (5-year survival rate: 10%-15%); combined chemotherapy has not definitely improved these results.

33.3.4 Low-Grade Astrocytoma

Chemotherapy may be of value in case of recurrence.

33.4 Drugs Effective in Childhood Brain Tumours

33.4.1 Single Drugs Effective

1. Lipophilic drugs are probably the best:
   a) Better drug entry and higher drug tumour levels

b) Activity in tumours of low growth fraction
   Nitrosoureas: carmustine (BCNU), lomustine (CCNU), methyl-CCNU (Me-CCNU)
   Procarbazine: (oxidized to a lipophilic intermediate)

2. Therapy optimalization:
   It is expected, but not proven, that lipophilic drugs will have to be combined with cell-cycle-specific and non-lipid-soluble drugs, in spite of their high molecular weight:
   Vincristine
   Dacarbazine (DTIC)
   Teniposide (VM-26)
   Bleomycin
   Cyclophosphamide
   Adriamycin
   Cytosine arabinoside (intrathecally i.t.)
   Methotrexate (intrathecally, intraventricularly, high-dose or intermediate intravenous methotrexate with leucovorin)
   Tetracosactide, dexamethasone or prednisone are frequently combined with x-ray therapy and/or antimitotic drugs.

33.4.2 Drug Combinations

Several two-to-four-drug schedules have been proposed; their results are nearly identical in recurrent tumours (50% of complete or partial remission), with variable toxicity, depending on previous treatment, X-ray therapy, the route of drug administration and drug dosage (e.g. intraventricular methotrexate or high-dose intravenous methotrexate).

1. Useful combinations:
   Vincristine + CCNU or BCNU ± i.t. methotrexate
   Vincristine + CCNU or BCNU ± procarbazine
   MOPP (see Appendix A)
   Vincristine + cyclophosphamide
   Intermediate dose of methotrexate i.v. + CCNU + methotrexate i.t.

33.4.3 Currently Being Researched

Agents potentiating the effectiveness of irradiation and radiosensitizing drugs.

33.5 Staging and Staging Procedure in Medulloblastoma

33.5.1 Operative Staging System of Harisiadis and Chang

T1 Tumour less than 3 cm diameter and limited to the classic midline position in the vermis, the roof of the fourth ventricle and less frequently, to the cerebellar hemispheres.

T2 Tumour 3 cm or greater in diameter further invading one adjacent structure or partially filling the fourth ventricle

T3 This stage is subdivided into T3 a and T3 b:
- T3 a: tumour further invading two adjacent structures or completely filling the fourth ventricle with extension into the aqueduct of Sylvius, foramen of Magendie, or foramen of Luschka, thus producing marked internal hydrocephalus
- T3 b: tumour arising from the floor of the fourth ventricle or brain stem and filling the fourth ventricle

T4 Tumour further spreading through the aqueduct of Sylvius to involve the third ventricle or midbrain, or tumour extending to the upper cervical cord

M0 No evidence of gross subarachnoid or haematogenous metastasis

M1 Microscopic tumour cells found in cerebrospinal fluid (CSF)

M2 Gross nodular seedings demonstrated in the cerebellar, cerebral subarachnoid space, or in the third or lateral ventricles

M3 Gross nodular seeding in spinal subarachnoid space

M4 Metastasis outside the cerebrospinal axis

33.5.2 Staging Procedure

1. Where computerized axial tomographic (CAT) scan is not available: arteriogram followed by pneumoencephalogram and/or ventriculogram
2. Where at present CAT scan is available: this is sufficient for diagnosis
3. CSF cytology
4. Myelography (optional)

33.6 Prognostic Factors in Medulloblastoma

1. Sex: likelihood of cure twice as high in female patients.
2. Stage: 5-year survival is 75% for T1, 50.5% for T2, 32.3% for T3 and 0 for T4.
3. Poor prognostic factors include: invasion of fourth ventricle and/or

brain stem, leading to incomplete removal; gross nodular seeding in the subarachnoid space.

33.7 Therapeutic Strategy for Medulloblastoma and Infratentorial High-Grade Ependymoma

1. Primary surgery:
   To remove the bulk of the tumour within the limits of surgery, and to restore the CSF flow.
2. Post-operative irradiation:
   To eradicate residual disease; it is directed to the whole neuro-axial system, with a booster dose to the posterior fossa; the dosage is adapted to the age.
3. Adjuvant chemotherapy:
   This is recommended; its efficacy has been demonstrated in stages T3 and T4 by two randomized trials where the surgery, radiotherapy and chemotherapy modalities were identical.
   a) Conventional post-operative chemotherapy:
      Vincristine, 2 mg/m^2/week (max. dose 2 mg) × six injections during radiotherapy. 4 weeks after the end of radiotherapy: eight intermittent courses of vincristine and CCNU.
      Intrathecal chemotherapy (methotrexate and/or cytosine arabinoside) are used only in cases of subarachnoidal seeding.
   b) Treatment under study:
      Pre-radiation intensive chemotherapy followed by radiotherapy. Aim: to improve efficiency of drugs and perhaps further to reduce dose of radiotherapy and decrease late sequelae.
4. Metastatic or Recurrent Tumours
   Any drug combination may be used, taking into account previous treatment, and the patient's bone marrow status. Intermediate dose i.v. methotrexate + i.t. methotrexate, MOPP (see Appendix A), *cis*-platinum is currently recommended.
   Low-dose radiotherapy could be of value.

33.8 Present Results in Medulloblastoma and Malignant Ependymoma

Improvement in surgical techniques, the introduction of whole-cerebrospinal-axis radiotherapy and partly, of chemotherapy have markedly increased the 5-year survival rate (which is equivalent to cure) from 10%-15% to 50%-60%. The overall actuarial 4-year survival rate is 54% in the International Society of Paediatric Oncology (SIOP) trial, and 46% in the Children's Cancer Study Group (CCSG) trial.

33.8.1 Prognosis of Recurrences and Metastases (Posterior Fossa, Spinal, Skeletal)

This is always very poor. Comfort and survival duration are improved only by palliative chemotherapy.

33.8.2 Immediate and Long-Term Complications

These are observed in over 50% of patients and include: psychomotor retardation, sensory deficit, leukoencephalopathy; infectious complications; and disturbances of endocrine function (somatotrophic hormone production and gonadal abnormalities).

34 Paediatric Non-Hodgkin Lymphomas

34.1 Incidence and Epidemiology

1. Incidence:
   a) 5%-7% of malignant diseases in childhood (Europe, USA)
   b) Variation within countries: higher frequency in Middle East, Nigeria, Uganda (15/100000 children less than 5-10 years of age)
2. Epidemiology:
   a) Host factors:
      Sex: 2.5 M/1 F
      Age: peak age: 7-10 years
      Genetic predisposition: increased risk in families with immunological defects
   b) Environmental factors:
      Drugs: immunosuppressive therapy and diphenylhydantoin
      Radiation: excess lymphoma in both A-bomb survivors and in spondylitis series
      Virus: Epstein-Barr virus (EBV), human T-lymphocyte virus (HTLV I-II)

34.2 Differences from Adult Non-Hodgkin Lymphomas (NHL)

1. Natural course:
   Rapidly growing malignancy with a tendency to disseminate early to bone marrow and to CNS.
2. Histological characteristics:
   Diffuse type is observed in more than 95% of cases.
3. Staging system.
4. Immediate and delayed complications of combined chemotherapy and radiotherapy:
   These must be taken into account in treatment planning.

34.3 Pathological Classification

Nearly 100% of paediatric NHL are diffuse forms: 90% belong either to lymphoblastic type (Rappaport) or to undifferentiated Burkitt type; 5%-10% are immunoblastic NHL; others are unclassified

Rappaport	Lukes-Collins	Lennert	
Lymphoblastic	Convoluted lymphocyte	Convoluted lymphocyte	} Lymphoblastic
Undifferentiated Burkitt	Small non-cleaved follicular centre cell	Burkitt	
Undifferentiated pleomorphic non-Burkitt	Burkitt non-B		
		Others unclassified	
Histiocytic	Immunoblastic sarcoma Large non-cleaved follicular centre cell Histiocytic	Immunoblastic	
		Unclassified	

34.4 Main Clinical Features of NHL

1. Mediastinal NHL:
   Progressive dyspnoea, cough, vena cava compression, supraclavicular axillary nodes
2. Abdominal NHL:
   Abdominal pains, ileus, diarrhoea, abdominal mass (single or multiple), surgical emergency (intussuception, peritonitis), progressive ascites, hepato-splenomegaly, obstructive icterus
3. Head and neck NHL:
   Cervical node (s), nasal obstruction or rhinorrhoea, hypoacousia, bone tumour (jaw), unilateral tonsil hypertrophy, tumoral parotid gland, cranial nerve palsies (VII)
4. Other primary sites:
   Peripheral node, skin and subcutaneous tissue, orbit, thyroid, bone (± hypercalcaemia), kidney, testis

34.5 Diagnosis and Staging Evaluation

34.5.1 Essential Examinations for Diagnosis and Clinical Staging

1. Detailed history and a complete physical examination
2. Adequate surgical biopsy and/or cytology on:
   Bone marrow aspiration (two to four different sites), CSF, pleural, peritoneal or pericardial effusions.
   Try to avoid useless extensive surgical excision (abdomen, thorax).
3. Radiological studies:
   Chest x-rays.
   Intravenous pyelography.
   Skeletal survey.
   Bilateral lower-extremity lymphangiography (in certain cases of apparently localized NHL).
   Contrast studies of upper and/or lower gastrointestinal tract.
   Myelography (in epidural sites).
4. Ultrasonography and/or computerized axial tomographic (CAT) scan:
   According to initial site and risk of skull and CNS extension.
5. Radionucleide studies:
   Bone scanning (technetium).

34.5.2 Required Examinations for Treatment Monitoring

1. Blood count, coagulation screen.
2. Evaluation of liver function.
3. Evaluation of renal function and metabolic state of the patients: blood urea nitrogen, serum creatinine, serum uric acid, serum electrolytes (Na, Cl, K, Ca, P), urinary output, urine electrolytes.
4. Evaluation of cardiac function: ECG, echocardiography.
5. Evaluation of nutritional status.

34.5.3 Methods for Characterization of Tumour Cells

They are currently becoming a necessary tool in therapy planning:
1. Cytomorphology
2. Cytochemical staining:
   Acid phosphatase, myeloperoxidase, α-naphthylesterases, beta-glucuronidases, periodic-acid-Schiff (PAS), methyl green-pyronine, Sudan black-B
3. Immunological and enzymatic markers as shown in the following table:

T-cell line	B-cell line	
E-rosettes	Surface Ig+ = B-cells	
Anti-T monoclonal antibodies+	Intracytoplasmic Ig (μ, κ, λ) = pre-B-cells	
- Early	Calla+	Early pre-B cells
- Cortex	Ia+	Early pre-B cells
- Medulla	Anti-B monoclonal antibodies	Early pre-B cells
Calla ±		

CALLA, common acute lymphoblastic leukaemia antigen

Burkitt's lymphoma is a monoclonal neoplasm of B-lymphoblasts, which is the most common form of malignancy in children in tropical areas (Africa, South America). It is considered to be a distinct clinical and histological entity: there is a high frequency of jaw and abdominal sites; high risk of bone marrow and CNS involvement, and 98% of cases are associated with Epstein-Barr virus; a correlation with malaria and poor immunological status has been established. At present, following the first observations of so-called "Burkitt-like NHL" in the United States and in Europe, it appears that there is no distinction between endemic and non-endemic Burkitt's lymphoma, on clinical, histological and immunological grounds. The only difference seems related to epidemiology.

4. Cytogenetics:
   Constant presence in malignant B-cells of a translocation involving chromosome 8: t (8; 14) in 70% of cases, t (8;2) or t (8;22) in others. Rearrangements of genes of immunoglobulins (heavy chains on chromosome 14; kappa chains on chromosome 2; lambda chains on chromosome 22) and activation of C-MYC oncogene, located on chromosome 8.

34.5.4 Epidemiological Examinations

1. Burkitt's NHL: Epstein-Barr virus serology, continuous lymphoblastoid cell lines in culture, presence of viral genoma in malignant cells
2. Lymphoma - leukaemia presentation in Japan, Caraibes: HTLVI antibodies and viral genoma in infected cells

34.5.5 Correlations Between Primary Site, Histology, Immunology and Cytogenetics in Paediatric NHL

Primary site frequency (outside Africa)	Histology	Immunology	Cytogenetics
Abdomen 30%-50%	Burkitt[a]	B sIg + μ, κ Ia +, CALLA +	t (8 ; 14) t (8 ; 2) t (8 ; 22)
Mediastinum 25%	Convoluted[b] nuclears	T E +, OKT3 + HTLA +, TdT ± CALLA –	
Others sites	· Convoluted nuclears[b] · Burkitt[a] · Unclassified	T B non-T non-B TdT ± ; Ia ± CALLA ± c IgM	 t (8 ; 14, 2, 22)

TdT, terminal deoxynucleotidyl transferase
[a] Undifferentiated type.
[b] Lymphoblastic type (Rappaport).

34.6 Staging Systems in Childhood NHL

34.6.1 Ann Arbor Staging System

34.6.2 St. Jude Children's Hospital Staging System (S. Murphy)

This currently seems better for predicting prognosis and planning treatment; it takes into account the initial site and the extent of the disease.

Stage I — Single tumour (extranodal) or single anatomical area (nodal), with the exclusion of mediastinum or abdomen.

Stage II — Single tumour (extranodal) with regional node involvement.
Two or more nodal areas on the same side of the diaphragm.
Two single (extranodal) tumours with or without regional node involvement on the same side of the diaphragm.
Primary gastrointestinal tract tumour, usually in the ileocaecal area, with or without involvement of associated mesenteric nodes only.

Stage III — Two single tumours (extranodal) on opposite sides of the diaphragm.

Two or more nodal areas above and below the diaphragm.
All primary intrathoracic tumours (mediastinal, pleural, thymic).
All extensive primary intra-abdominal disease.

Stage IV Any of the above with initial CNS and/or bone marrow involvement. In this presentation, leukaemic cells may be noted in peripheral blood, and/or in bone marrow where their number is less than 25% (arbitrary distinction with acute lymphoblastic leukaemia).

34.6.3 Clinical Staging of Burkitt's Lymphoma (Ziegler)

This staging system has been proposed by Ziegler in non-African Burkitt's lymphoma, taking into account sites, tumour burdens and tumour resectability.

Stage A Localized extra-abdominal site
Stage B Multiple extra-abdominal sites
Stage C Intra-abdominal tumour
Stage D Intra-abdominal tumour with involvement of one extra-abdominal site
Stage AR Resectable primary intra-abdominal tumour (>90%)

34.7 Prognostic Factors

1. Favourable prognostic factors:
   Primary site and stages I and II: head and neck (non-parameningeal), peripheral nodes, abdominal site
2. Unfavourable prognostic factors:
   a) Conventionally: stage III-IV NHL, and parameningeal stages II
   b) If the therapeutic approach is well-adapted to the immunological type the most unfavourable prognostic factors are:
      CNS involvement at diagnosis
      Incomplete initial remission within 2 months

34.8 Chemotherapy Effective in Childhood NHL

34.8.1 Single Drugs Effective

Agents	Response rate - CR + PR (%)
Corticosteroids	50
Cyclophosphamide + Iphosphamide	10-50
Vincristine, Vindesine	15
Vinblastine	20-50
Adriamycin (ADM)	20-40
Cytosine arabinoside	20-40
Bleomycin	20-40
High-dose methotrexate (HDMTX)	20-40
6 Thioguanine-Lomustine (CCNU) - carmustine (BCNU)	20-40
L-Asparaginase (L-Asp)	20-40
Cis-platinum (DDP)	
Melphalan	
Etoposide (VP-16-213)	

CR, complete remission; PR, partial remission

34.8.2 Drug Combinations

1. Outline of LSA_2-L_2

Induction		Consolidation		Maintenance	
LSA_2-L_2					
CTX	1.2 g/m^2 i.v., day 1	Ara-C	100 mg/m^2 i.v., daily × 5 (Mon-Fri) for 4 weeks	1. TG-CTX	TG, 300 mg/m^2, p.o., daily × 4 day, followed by CTX 600 mg/m^2, i.v., single dose, day 5
VCR	2.0 mg/m^2 (max. dose 2.0 mg) i.v., weekly on day 3, 10, 17, and 24	6-TG	50 mg/m^2, p.o., 8-12 after each ara-C injection	2. HU-DNM	HU, 2.4 g/m^2, p.o., daily × 4 days, followed by DNM, 45 mg/m^2, i.v. on day 5.
MTX	6.25 mg/m^2 i.t., day 5, repeat on day 31 and 34 during PDN withdrawal	L-Asp	6000 IU/m^2/ day × 14, i.m., on completion of ara-C + 6-TG	3. MTX-BCNU	MTX, 10 mg/m^2, p.o., daily × 4 day, followed by BCNU, 60 mg/m^2, i.v. on day 5

Induction		Consolidation		Maintenance	
PDN	60 mg/m^2 (max. dose 60 mg), p.o. daily in four divided doses, day 3-30, decremental doses to 0 day 31-37	MTX	6.25 mg/m^2, i.t. twice, 3 days apart, begin 2-3 days after last L-Asp injection	4. ara-C-VCR	ara-C, 150 mg/m^2, i.v. daily × 4 day, followed by VCR 2.0 mg/m^2 (max. dose 2.0 mg), i.v. day 5
DNM	60 mg/m^2, i.v., day 12 and 13	BCNU	60 mg/m^2, i.v., single dose 2-3 days following completion of i.t MTX	5. MTX	6.25 mg/m^2, i.t., 2 doses, 3 days apart
XRT					

PDN, prednisone; CTX, cyclophosphamide; VCR, vincristine; XRT, radiation treatment; TG, thioguanine; HU, hydroxyurea; DNM, daunomycin

2. Outline of COMP protocol

Induction		Consolidation	Maintenance	
COMP				
CTX	1.2 g/m^2, i.v. day 1	...	CTX	1.0 g/m^2, i.v., day 1, repeat every 28 days
VCR	2.0 mg/m^2 (max. 2.0 mg), i.v. weekly on day 3, 10, 17 and 24	...	VCR	1.5 mg/m^2, i.v. (max. dose 2.0 mg), day 1, repeat every 14 days
MTX	i.t. 6.25 mg/m^2, day 5 and on day 31 and 34 during PDN withdrawal	...	MTX	i.t. 6.25 mg/m^2, day 29, repeat every 28 days
MTX	i.v. 300 mg/m^2 on day 12 (60% of dose as i.v. push and 40% as 4-h infusion)	...	MTX	i.v. 300 mg/m^2, i.v., day 15, repeat every 28 days (60% of dose i.v. push, 40% as 4-h infusion)
PDN	60 mg/m^2 (max. 60 mg), p.o. daily, in 4 divided doses, day 3-30, decremental doses to 0 day 31-37	...	PDN	60 mg/m^2 (max. dose 60 mg) p.o., daily × 5 on day 29, repeat every 28 days

PDN, prednisone; CTX, cyclophosphamide; VCR, vincristine; XRT, radiation treatment; TG, thioguanine; HU, hydroxyurea; DNM, daunomycin

3. General outline of LMB French protocol

Induction	Maintenance
Reduction: COP: CTX, VCR, prednisone, i.t. MTX	First course: CTX, ADN, prednisone, HDMTX (+ i.t.)
First course: 1st COPAD-M: CTX, VCR, ADM, prednisone, HDMTX + i.t. MTX	Second course: CCNU, ara-C, 6-TG, L-Asp
Second course: i.d. CTX	Every 1 month
Third course: CAM: CTX, HDMTX (+i.t.), ara-C, L-Asp	Total duration: 1 year
Fourth course: MiniBACT: CCNU, ara-C, 6TG, CTX	
(Every 3-4 weeks)	

4. General outline of BMF group NHL protocil

Prephase	CTX-prednisone (5 days)
Block 1	VM-26 - ara-C, i.d. MTX (+i.t.) - CTX (5 days)
Block 2	i.d. MTX (+i.t.), ADM, CTX
	Low risk: 2 blocks 1-2
	High risk: 4 blocks 1-2

5. Outline of high-dose chemotherapy followed by bone marrow graft. Applebaum BACT protocol:

BCNU	200 mg/m^2, day 1
Cytosine arabinoside	200 mg/m^2, days 2, 3, 4 and 5
CTX	1600 mg/m^2, days 2, 3, 4 and 5
6-TG	200 mg/m^2, days 2, 3, 4 and 5
Autograft	day 7

34.8.3 Choice of Drug Regimen

It has to be decided according to the initial site and stage of NHL and mainly according to immunological findings: (a) repetitive multidrug chemotherapy over 2 years in T-NHL (e.g. LSA_2-L_2); (b) intermittent multidrug chemotherapy over 6-12 months in B-NHL (e.g. COMP, LMB French protocol, BFM group NHL protocol).

34.9 Therapeutic Strategy

34.9.1 General Rules of Treatment

1. Emergency: diagnosis and treatment must be accomplished within a few days. Rapid growth risk of respiratory distress, intestinal occlusion, renal deficiency, CNS extension.
2. Need for an intensive supportive care in advanced diseases due to acute tumour-lysis syndrome.
3. Chemotherapy is the major method.
4. Radiotherapy is controversial. Surgery is of little value.
5. Modalities and duration of therapy have to be adapted to stage and immunological type.

34.9.2 Therapeutic Strategy by Stage

34.9.2.1 Stages I and II (Localized Disease): 20%–25% of Patients

1. Induction of remission:
   Biopsy or partial or complete tumour removal
   Multidrug chemotherapy
   Involved-field radiotherapy: no value
2. CNS prophylaxis:
   Raison d'être: overall risk of CNS spread: 10%–30% of cases; very poor prognosis of CNS relapses
   Timing: early during or just after induction phase
   Modalities: cranial irradiation associated with intrathecal (i.t.) MTX: 6–12 mg/m^2 per week × 4–6 (maximum dose: 12 mg); or HDMTX combined with i.t. methotrexate without irradiation
   Exception: stage I lymphomas and localized abdominal lymphomas, which do not need CNS prophylaxis
3. Maintenance therapy: usual duration 12–24 months
4. Results: cure rate 80%–90%
5. Problems under study:
   What is the best choice to prevent CNS disease?

34.9.2.2 Stage III (30%–50% of Patients) and Stage IV (25%–30% of Patients)

1. Induction of remission:
   Biopsy or partial tumour removal
   Multidrug chemotherapy (debulking procedure)

Irradiation may be indicated to reduce bulky disease, but tolerance is often poor. At present the trend is to abandon it, because it delays intensive chemotherapy

2. CNS prophylaxis or CNS treatment
3. Maintenance therapy: duration 12-48 months
4. Results in stages III and IV; disease-free survival 50%-70% in B-lymphomas (plateau at 1 year); 50%-70% in T-lymphomas (plateau after 3-4 years)
5. Problems under study
   a) More aggressive chemotherapy followed by bone marrow autograft or allograft may give encouraging results in patients in second remission, and in some selected high-risk, stage III-IV patients (incomplete initial remission, CNS involvement at diagnosis)
   b) Is there a clear frontier (and the need for a different therapeutic approach) between stage IV NHL and acute leukaemias?
   c) How to treat relapsing patients?

34.9.3 Therapeutic Strategy by Site in Childhood NHL

1. Abdominal NHL (always B-lymphomas)
   a) Localized disease.
      Surgical resection.
      Chemotherapy.
      Abdominal irradiation and CNS prophylaxis are not of value.
      Maintenance chemotherapy: 6 months.
      Results: cure rate 80%-90% of cases.
   b) For non-resectable tumour:
      Biopsy by laparotomy, if diagnosis cannot be established by more simple methods (notably cytology of pleural or ascites effusion or of bone marrow).
      Intensive chemotherapy: 6-12 months, combined with CNS prophylaxis using chemotherapy (HDMTX) rather than brain irradiation.
      Whole-abdomen irradiation should definitely be abandoned.
      In extensive abdominal disease, second-look surgery may be discussed after tumoral shrinkage by chemotherapy, in case of loco-regional tumoral residue.
      Results: Cure rate of 70% in stages III; 50% in stage IV.
2. Mediastinal NHL (30% of cases nearly always T-lymphomas)
   a) Chemotherapy combined with CNS prophylaxis; duration 2 years.
   b) Local radiotherapy does not improve survival rate.
   c) Results: cure rate of 50%-70% (stages III-IV).

3. Head and neck NHL (15%-20% of cases: T-, B- or non-T-, non-B-lymphomas)
   a) Primary surgery or biopsy.
   b) Chemotherapy.
   c) Involved-field irradiation is unnecessary; CNS prophylaxis is compulsory in parameningeal sites.
   Results: cure rate 50%-90% of patients according to stage.

34.10 Supportive Care in Stages III-IV NHL

Complications	Treatment
Respiratory distress	Emergency corticosteroids and antimitotic drugs
Acute renal failure and metabolic disturbances[a]: ↗K, ↘Ca, ↗P, ↘Na, acidosis	Hyperhydration (3 l/m^2), furosemide urate-oxidase, allopurinol, Na bicarbonate, Ca, ± K, Na.
Hypercalcaemia	Furosemide, thyrocalcitonin
Haematological complications	Haematological and antimicrobial support
Digestive troubles	Enteral continuous drip-feeding; parenteral nutrition; aspiration

[a] Tumour lysis syndrome or kidney invasion.

35 Childhood Acute Lymphocytic Leukaemia

35.1 Incidence and Epidemiology

See Sects. 13.1 and 13.2.

35.2 Main Clinical Features

Pallor, haemorrhages, and fever.
Bone pains.
Adenomegalies, hepato-splenomegaly; renal infiltration, testis and CNS involvement are uncommon at diagnosis.

35.3 Diagnostic and Monitoring Procedures

35.3.1 Examinations Required for Diagnosis

1. Bone Marrow Aspirate:
   a) Cytomorphology (FAB classification)
   b) Histochemical stains: peroxidase, periodic-acid-Schiff (PAS), esterase (α-naphthylacetate and α-naphthylbutyrate), acid and alkaline phosphatase, β-glucuronidase
   c) Immunological markers, allowing classification of leukaemic proliferation along B- or T-pathway of differentiation.
   d) Cytogenetics
   e) Under study: enzymatic parameters, cytofluorimetry (DNA/RNA content), cytokinetics
2. Cerebrospinal fluid cytology (cytocentrifugation or millipore filter technique)
3. X-Rays (chest, bone) and abdominal ultrasonography

Marker	T	B	Pre-B	Early Pre-B	Pre-T	Undifferentiated
E-rosettes	+	–	–	–	–	–
sIg	–	+	–	–	–	–
cIg	–	–	+	–	–	–
Ia (DR)	–	+	+	+	–	–
Monoclonal antibodies/T	+	–	–	–	+	±
Monoclonal antibodies/B	–	+	+	+	–	±
Common acute lymphoblastic leukaemia antigen (CALLA)	–	–	–	±	–	–
Frequency	15%	1%-3%	5%-10%	50%-60%		10%

35.3.2 Examinations Required for Treatment Monitoring

1. Diagnosis of infection; immunological status
2. Diagnosis of coagulation abnormalities
3. Evaluation of liver, kidney, and heart functions
4. Evaluation of nutritional and metabolic status
5. Electroencephalography, brain tomodensitometry (only if CNS disease)
6. HLA typing of patient and family (planning of a possible bone marrow transplantation)

35.4 Prognostic Factors

Make it possible to classify the patients in three groups: low-risk, high-risk and standard-risk. Major factors are underlined.

Prognostic factor	Favourable	Unfavourable
Age	3-7 years;	<2 years; >10 years
Race	White	Black
Sex	Female	Male
Leukaemic burden:		
Peripheral nodes	Absent	Enlarged
Hepatomegaly	Absent	Enlarged
Splenomegaly	Absent	Enlarged
Mediastinal mass[a]	Absent	Present

Prognostic factor	Favourable	Unfavourable
CNS disease	Absent	Present
Initial WBC/mm^3	$< 10^5$	$> 5 \times 10^5$
Hb level	< 7 g/dl	> 10 g/dl
FAB classification	L1	L2, L3
Surface markers[b]	Early pre-B CALLA+	T, B, pre-B
Immunoglobulins	Normal	Decreased
Cytogenetics	Hyperdiploidy	Pseudodiploidy Ph^1; t (8 ; 14) in ALL; and other chromosomal rearrangements
Response to induction therapy	M_1 marrow on day 14	M_3 marrow within 3-4 weeks

FAB, French-American-British

[a] An association of mediastinal mass and high WBC/mm^3 is correlated with poor prognosis.

[b] It has not been proved that T-markers, when not associated with other bad prognostic factors (e.g. mediastinal mass), are always correlated with poor prognosis.

35.5 Recommended Treatment Schedule for Acute Lymphoblastic Leukaemia (ALL) (See Also Sect. 13.11)

35.5.1 Remission Induction and Consolidation

1. Aim.

To achieve a prompt initial complete remission (within less than 3-4 weeks).

2. Methods.

Two major drugs are used:

a) Prednisone: 40-60 mg/m^2 daily p.o. for 3-4 weeks, then taper
b) Vincristine: 1.5-2 mg/m^2 i.v. weekly: three-five doses (maximum dose: 2 mg)

A third or a fourth drug may be added from onset to improve the percentage of cell kill, notably in unfavourable presentations: B-ALL, Ph^1-positive ALL, mediastinal mass combined with high leukocyte count and T-markers.

Commonly used drugs are: daunorubicin or doxorubicin, cytosine arabinoside, cyclophosphamide, teniposide (VM-26), high-dose or intermediate-dose i.v. methotrexate.

These three- or four-drug regimens are associated with higher toxicity and may require intensive supportive care. Consolidation treatment may influence duration of remission:

a) L-asparaginase, 500–1000 IU/kg i.v. × 10 days, is commonly prescribed, when M_1 marrow is obtained.
b) More aggressive schedules are under study, in high-risk patients, using intermediate- or high-dose i.v. methotrexate, high-dose cyclophosphamide, doxorubicin or daunorubicin.

3. Results. Remission is achieved in 95% of cases, no matter what the initial presentation.

35.5.2 CNS Prophylaxis

1. Aim.
a) To eradicate meningeal and cerebral microfoci of leukaemia cells and to decrease the risk of CNS relapse from 50% to 5%–10%.
b) To try to avoid neurological and endocrine disturbances

2. Conventional Method.
a) Whole-skull irradiation, 1800 rads in 9 fractions following induction and consolidation treatment
b) In association with four to six intrathecal (i.t.) injections of methotrexate 12 mg/m²/dose (maximum dose 12 mg) once a week, within the 5 weeks of induction and consolidation

3. Other Methods and Methods Under Study
a) Craniospinal irradiation without i.t. therapy
b) I.t. Methotrexate and/or cytosine alone
c) Intermediate- or high-dose i.v. methotrexate combined with i.t. methotrexate or cytosine without irradiation
d) Addition of nitrosoureas to consolidation treatment combined with i.t. therapy

35.5.3 Maintenance Treatment

1. Aim:
To prevent relapses, due to remaining leukaemic cells (G_0 or G_1 blocked cells), resistance to initial drugs, sanctuaries, and to avoid the development of drug-resistant cells.

2. Standard Method:
6-Mercaptopurine, 90 mg/m²/day p.o. each day combined with methotrexate 15–20 mg/m²/dose p.o. or i.m. once a week.

Reinduction with pulses of vincristine (two doses) and prednisone (1 week) is commonly added, every month during 1st year and every 3 months thereafter.

3. Other Approach:
Multiple drugs given intermittently in rotation.

4. Optimal Duration of Treatment:
3-5 years since first complete remission.

35.5.4 Under Study

The indications of intensive chemotherapy followed by bone marrow auto- or allograft in high-risk patients in first complete remission.

35.6 General Principles of Treatment of Relapses

35.6.1 Bone Marrow Relapse

Risk: 30% in standard-risk patients
80% in very high-risk patients

Use of conventional induction methods with three or four drugs, taking into account possible acquired cell resistance.

If failure, or in the event of subsequent relapses, some encouraging results have been obtained (but usually short-lasting) using:

a) High-dose i.v. methotrexate, high-dose cytosine arebinoside, etoposide (VP-16-213), m-AMSA (amsacrine)
b) Some combinations: VM-26-cytosine arabinoside; vincristine-L-asparaginase-methotrexate; L-asparaginase-cytosine arabinoside

Bone marrow relapse reintroduces the risk of CNS disease.

Due to the poor results obtained by conventional chemotheraphy to treat a medullary relapse, mainly in patients relapsing on therapy, a bone marrow allograft following high-dose chemotherapy and total-body irradiation must be planned, if possible, in early second remission; present results are very encouraging; bone marrow autograft with different modalities of purge is under study.

35.6.2 CNS Relapse

Risk $\leqslant 10\%$ in standard patients, after CNS prophylaxis. Weekly i.t. methotrexate (12 mg/m^2/dose) or cytosine arabinoside (30 mg/m^2) until CSF clearing, followed by periodic, monthly i.t. methotrexate, as maintenance.

Systemic chemotherapy must be maintained or reintroduced (in case of relapse off therapy).

Under Study:
Necessity of second cranial irradiation (high risk of leukoencephalopathy)
High-dose or intermediate-dose i.v. methotrexate
Injection of methotrexate into an Ommaya reservoir
Bone marrow transplantation

35.6.3 Testis Relapse

Risk: 10%–40% of cases, according to initial adverse prognostic factors. Radiotherapy (2400 rads) to both testes; reinforcement or reintroduction of systemic (and i.t.) chemotherapy. Bone marrow transplantation has to be planned in patients relapsing on therapy.

Under study: preventive irradiation of testes after remission induction in high-risk patients.

35.7 Follow-Up Procedures

35.7.1 During Maintenance Treatment

1. Complete clinical examination, height, weight, performance status
2. Blood-cell count: every 1–2 weeks
3. CSF examination: if clinical signs
4. Transaminase, alkaline phosphatase, creatinine levels, every 4–6 months
5. EEG and brain computerized axial tomographic (CAT) scan (useful only in cases of neurological or mental deterioration)

35.7.2 Before Stopping Treatment

1. Blood and bone marrow aspirate
2. CSF examination
3. Bilateral testis biopsy

35.7.3 After Stopping Treatment

1. Clinical evaluation every 2 months (2 years)
2. Blood cell count: every month (3-5 years)
3. Possible long-term sequelae: endocrine (growth, fertility), neurological [psychomotor function evaluation, EEG, computed tomography (CT) scan]

35.8 Prevention of Infections During Maintenance Therapy

1. Modification of drug dosages on the basis of granulocyte and lymphocyte count.
2. Stop maintenance treatment during viral disease due to: herpes zoster and varicella, herpes simplex, measles.
3. Prescribe zoster immunoglobulins or hyperimmune serum within 96 h of varicella or zoster contact.
4. The same approach should be used with standard immunoglobulins following measles contact.
5. Immunization with live vaccines is contraindicated; others are permissible.
6. Oral trimethoprim-sulfamethoxazole is effective in preventing pneumocystis carinii pneumonia in patients whose lymphocyte count is continuously under $1000/mm^3$.

35.9 Current Results

In 1968, less than 1% of patients were long-term survivors.

In 1985, 50% of patients are still in first remission 5 years after diagnosis.

A plateau is observed after 7 years of first remission.

Part IV

Management of Tumours of Special Significance in African and Asian Countries

36 "Mediterranean Abdominal Lymphoma" (Immunoproliferative Small-Intestine Disease)

Philip A. Salem

36.1 Definition

Immunoproliferative small-intestine disease (IPSID) is a distinct disease entity characterized by:

1. Clinical features:
   Chronic diarrhoea.
   Emaciation.
   Abdominal pain.
   Clubbing of fingers and toes.
   Occasionally - peripheral lymphadenopathy and palpable abdominal masses.
2. Radiological features:
   Malabsorption pattern on small-bowel radiological workup, mucosal fold thickening, segmentation and flocculation of barium mostly in jejunum, duodenum and less commonly the ileum.
3. Laboratory features:
   Evidence of malabsorption.
   Mild anaemia.
   Hypoalbuminaemia and hypocalcaemia.
4. Immunological abnormalities:
   Presence of an abnormal IgA globulin devoid of light chains and related to the Fc portion of the alpha heavy chain which is readily detectable in the serum, urine or intestinal fluid.
5. Pathological features:
   a) Gross:
      Diffuse disease of small bowel, most conspicuous in upper half. However, gross changes may not be apparent.
   b) Microscopic:
      In absence of malignant lymphoma. Diffuse lymphoplasmocytic cellular infiltrates in the intestinal mucosa or mesenteric nodes (sometimes benign in appearance).
      In presence of concomitant malignant lymphoma in the intestine

and/or mesenteric lymph nodes, two histopathological variants exist:

- Diffuse infiltration of the mucosa at sites away from tumoral masses by either pure plasmocytic or lymphoplasmocytic infiltration. This variety is associated with the immunoblastic sarcoma type of malignant lymphoma.
- Widespread follicular lymphoid hyperplasia in the small-intestine mucosa. The associated malignant lymphoma is usually diffuse and undifferentiated, often having a starry-sky appearance.

36.2 Diagnosis

1. Histopathological evidence.
2. Suggestive clinical findings.
3. Presence of alpha heavy chain protein. Absence of this protein does not exclude the diagnosis.

36.3 Relationship of IPSID to Alpha Heavy Chain Disease

Alpha heavy chain disease (HCD) is not a prerequisite for IPSID. In addition, IPSID may be associated with other paraproteins.

36.4 Epidemiology

1. Geographical distribution: Mediterranean and the non-Mediterranean Middle Eastern countries, South Africa. Occasionally in South America and Europe
2. Age: mean age - 25 years; age range - 15-40
3. Socio-economic profile: usually low socio-economic background, underprivileged rural communities
4. Diet: no nutritional factors yet recognized

36.5 Staging

36.5.1 Clinical

Bilateral pedal lymphangiography
Bone marrow biopsy

Complete radiological gastrointestinal workup
Liver scan

36.5.2 Pathological

Staging laparotomy when clinical stage is less than IV. Recommended procedures during laparotomy are the following:
- Gross examination of abdominal organs with special attention to small bowel, spleen, liver and lymph nodes
- Evaluation of intestinal involvement

1. In absence of gross tumour:
   a) Resection of a 10-cm-long segment of jejunum starting 20 cm from the ligament of Treitz (desirable but not compulsory). If not done, two wedge biopsies from the same area instead
   b) Three transmural wedge biopsies: one at 15 cm from the ileocaecal junction and the remaining two at approximately one-third and two-thirds of the way along the length of the small intestine
2. Gross tumour:
   a) Resection of involved segments
   b) As in 1 (b)
3. Wedge and multiple-needle liver biopsies
4. Excision of multiple lymph nodes from splenic pedicle, porta hepatis, mesentery and para-aortic region
5. Iliac-crest bone marrow biopsy
6. Bilateral oophoropexy in young female patients
7. Splenectomy only in the presence of gross nodular disease

36.5.3 Recommended Staging Classification

Stage 0[1]	Benign-appearing lymphoplasmocytic mucosal infiltrate. No evidence of malignancy
Stage I	Diffuse lymphoid infiltration of intestinal mucosa and malignant lymphoma in either intestine (Ii) or mesenteric lymph nodes (In), but not both
Stage II	Diffuse lymphoid infiltration of intestinal mucosa and malignant lymphoma in both intestine and mesenteric lymph nodes

[1] "Pre-malignant" phase of the disease. Should not be diagnosed short of adequate staging laparotomy. Stage 0 is potentially curable by prolonged antibiotic treatment.

Stage III	Diffuse lymphoid infiltration of intestinal mucosa, malignant lymphoma in abdomen and metastasis to retroperitoneal and/or extra-abdominal peripheral lymph nodes
Stage IV	Presence of metastasis in noncontiguous, nonlymphatic tissues in addition to abdominal lymphoma
Unknown	Exploratory laparotomy not done, no detectable extra-abdominal disease

36.6 Treatment and Results

Stage	Treatment	Results
0	No specific anticancer therapy indicated. Majority of patients cured by prolonged tetracycline treatment	Curable 80%-90%
I	Radiotherapy alone	Curable 40%-50%
II	Radiotherapy followed by six cycles of chemotherapy	Curable approximately 25%
III	Six cycles of chemotherapy followed by radiation therapy. In case of residual disease after radiation therapy, chemotherapy should be pursued	Cure rate is very low - medium survival is approximately 18 months
IV	Chemotherapy alone. Radiation therapy may be used to control local bulky disease	Medium survival is approximately 10 months

N.B. Radiotherapy should include whole abdomen with protection of kidneys and liver: 3000-3500 rads with localized boosting where necessary.

1. Evaluation of Treatment.
Small-bowel series
Absorption studies
Studies relating to alpha heavy chain protein in serum, intestinal juice, and at the cellular level with immunofluorescence
Multiple intestinal per-oral biopsies

36.7 Recommended Chemotherapy for IPSID

Adriamycin	40 mg/m^2 i.v.
Cyclophosphamide	600 mg/m^2 i.v.
Vincristine	1.4 mg/m^2 i.v.
Prednisone	40 mg/m^2/day × 5 p.o.

repeated every 3 weeks

37 Nasopharyngeal Carcinoma

John H. C. Ho

37.1 Epidemiology and Aetiology

1. Incidence highest in Southern Chinese, intermediate in Eskimos, Malays in Southeast Asia, Tunisians and Moroccans, and lowest in Caucasians
2. Male preponderance in incidence in all racial groups
3. Aetiology believed to be multifactorial:
   a) Genetically predetermined susceptibility
   b) Epstein-Barr virus infection
   c) Environmental factors in Southern China: salted fish and vitamin C deficiency in the diet in early life

37.2 Histology

Predominantly squamous cell carcinoma: undifferentiated or poorly differentiated type in 90% of cases in most races. In Caucasians, 30% are of the well-differentiated, keratinizing type, associated with poor prognosis.

37.3 Course of Disease and Prognostic Factors

37.3.1 Types of Spread

1. Locally invasive type (8%):
   Brain is vulnerable to direct spread from meningeal metastases or the primary tumour through base of skull (local pressure, brain softening and oedema) but not haematogenous spread
2. Metastatic type (33%):
   Early cervical lymph node metastases followed by distant nodal and haematogenous metastases, mainly bone (especially spine), lungs and liver

37.3.2 Prognosis

1. Best in metastatic type
2. Worst in combined type
3. Better for patients under 40 than 40 and over

37.3.3 Staging and Survival

Stage		5.-Year actuarial survival (%)	Disease-free survival (%)
I	Tumour confined to nasopharynx, i.e. T1, N0, M0	84	74
II	Tumour extended to nasal fossa, oropharynx or adjacent muscles or nerves below the base of skull, i.e. T2 and/or upper cervical nodal involvement, i.e. N1	66	52
III	Tumour extended beyond T2 limits or bone involvement, i.e. T3 and/or lower cervical nodal involvement, i.e. N2	39	31
IV	Supraclavicular nodal involvement irrespective of T	23	18
V	Distant spread present, i.e. M1	0	0

37.4 Treatment

37.4.1 Radiotherapy

Megavoltage radiation is the main form of therapy in stages I–IV.

1. Causes of treatment failure:
   a) Uncontrolled primary tumour or its intracranial extension
   b) Distant metastases
   and much less frequently
   c) Uncontrolled cervical nodal metastases with carcinoma "en cuirasse" supervening

37.4.2 Chemotherapy

1. Indications:
   As adjuvant to radiation therapy in stage IV disease or stage III with marked cervical nodal involvement with known risk of distant metastases

To shrink large cervical nodal metastases to facilitate subsequent radiation therapy
To treat visceral, not bone, metastases
To treat tumour recurrence in the neck when carcinoma "en cuirasse" has supervened
As radiosensitizers

2. Single agents effective:

Methotrexate Cyclophosphamide Bleomycin	Remission rate approximately 30% at 3-6 months

Other active agents: 5-Flouroracil (5-FU)
Cis-platinum

3. Multidrug chemotherapy:
Superiority to single agents has not yet been established

37.5 Recommended Chemotherapy

1. Cyclophosphamide - 1 g i.v. weekly
2. Methotrexate - 25 mg orally weekly
3. "COMF"

- Day 1:	Cyclophosphamide	500 mg i.v.	Inexpensive, well-tolerated and usable on out-patient basis
	Vincristine	1 mg i.v.	
	5-FU	750 mg i.v.	
- Day 8:	Cyclophosphamide	500 mg i.v.	
	Vincristine	1 mg i.v.	
	Methotrexate	50 mg i.v.	

repeated every 4 weeks

4. Methotrexate-bleomycin-Cis-platinum (II)

Day 1:	Bleomycin	10 mg/m^2 i.v.	repeated every 2 weeks for four cycles	Expensive, well-tolerated, but requires hospitalization
	Methotrexate	20 mg/m^2 i.v.		
Day 2:	Cis-platinum	80 mg/m^2 i.v.	repeated every 10 weeks	

38 Oesophageal Carcinoma

Zhao Ti Ping

38.1 Incidence

Frequent in certain regions of Asia, Africa, South Africa and Northern France

Annual age-adjusted death rate 100–150/10^5 in Linshein, Northern China, steadily increasing after 30 years, peaking at 60–69 years

38.2 Clinical Manifestations

1. Substernal distress
2. Choking
3. Dysphagia
4. Regurgitation
5. Bleeding
6. Rapid weight loss

38.2.1 Clinical Complication

1. Extension or perforation of oesophageal lesion to adjacent organs with possible recurrent nerve paralysis
2. Oesophagobronchial fistula and septic pneumonia
3. Distant metastatis to liver, lung and bone

38.3 Pathology

1. Anatomical distribution:
   Lower third: middle third: upper third = 2:2:1.
2. Histology:
   Mostly squamous cell carcinomas; except adenocarcinoma in the cardiac portion.

3. Spread:
   Infiltrative, polypoid or ulcerative. Circumferential and longitudinal spread may result in oesophageal stricture, torsion or abnormal motility.

38.4 Diagnosis

1. Radiological examination:
   Hypertrophy, interruption and distortion of mucosal pattern
   Small ulcer
   Circumscribed filling defect

N.B. By using double-contrast barium swallow, tumours of 0.5-1 cm are detectable

2. Fiberoptic oeosphagoscopy with biopsy
3. Exfoliative cytology by brushing.

38.5 Differential Diagnosis

1. Achalasia of oesophagus
2. Benign stricture
3. Oesophagitis

38.6 TNM Classification

1. Cervical and intrathoracic:
   T1 $\leqslant$ 5 cm/No obstruction
   T2 > 5 cm/obstruction/whole circumference
   T3 Extension outside oesophagus
2. Cervical:
   N1 Unilateral
   N2 Bilateral movable
   N3 Fixed
3. Intrathoracic:
   N1 Regional involvement on surgical exploration or mediastinoscopy
   NX Not explored

38.7 Treatment

38.7.1 Surgery and Radiotherapy

Upper third	Radiotherapy Resection and reconstruction in this region are difficult
Middle third	Radiotherapy followed by surgical resection with surgery alone, thorough clearance of paraoesophageal and hilar lymph nodes is difficult
Lower third	Surgical resection

N.B. In China, surgical resection has given 5-year survival rates of 25%-30%.

38.7.2 Chemotherapy

1. Single drugs active:

Methotrexate	0.5 mg/kg i.v. for 4 consecutive days
Bleomycin	10-15 mg/m^2 twice weekly up to maximum 300-400 mg
Cis-platinum	80 mg/m^2 once every 21 days
5-Fluorouracil (5-FU)	600 mg/m^2 weekly
Adriamycin	40 mg/m^2 i.v. for 2 consecutive days every 3 weeks. Total dose $\leqslant 550\ mg/m^2$

N.B. In patients with impaired condition, the following downward dose modifications can be applied:

Methotrexate	60 mg/m^2 i.v. once every 3 weeks, followed by citrovorum factor 10 mg/m^2 i.m. every 6 h for 3 days
Bleomycin	10 mg/m^2 i.m. once weekly up to a maximum 300-400 mg
Cis-platinum	60 mg/m^2 i.v. in perfusion, every 3 weeks
5-FU	600 mg/m^2 i.v. weekly
Adriamycin	40 mg/m^2 i.v. every 3 weeks - total dose $\leqslant 550\ mg/m^2$

2. Response rate:
   Less than 20%, with occasional improvement of obstruction of gullet but no long-term beneficial effect
3. Drug combinations:
   In recent years, combination chemotherapy such as vindesine + bleomycin + Cis-platinum; Cis-platinum + 5-FU have been reported in use together with radiotherapy or surgery, but results are not yet confirmed.

39 Hepatocellular Carcinoma in the Tropics

Charles L. M. Olweny

39.1 Incidence

Largely unknown – probably commonest malignant tumour affecting mankind:
High in sub-Saharan Africa, China, Philippines and Indonesia
Low in Europe and North America

39.2 Aetiology

1. Hepatotoxins:
   Especially aflatoxin produced by *Aspergillus flavus*. Evidence:
   a) Single dose induces liver cancer in rats.
   b) Heavy contamination with aflatoxin in areas where hepatocellular carcinoma (HC) is common.
   c) Significant association between ingested aflatoxin levels and HC demonstrated.
2. Hepatitis virus B:
   a) Significantly more HC patients are HBAg-positive than controls.
   b) Maternal transmission probably important.
3. Malnutrition:
   a) Baboons fed on pyridoxine-deficient diet develop liver nodules with features of malignancy.
   b) Animal experiments indicate that protein restriction potentiates effect of hepatotoxins.
   c) Protein malnutrition common in areas where HC prevalent.
4. Alcohol:
   a) HC commoner in alcoholics than non-alcoholics.
   b) Commoner in those who give up than those who continue drinking.
   c) In USA, alcoholic cirrhosis major factor in HC.
5. Alpha-1-Antitrypsin phenotypes:
   PIZ alleles carry increased risk of cirrhosis, fibrosis and ? HC.
6. Hormonal influence:
   a) Testosterone-treated mice more vulnerable to hepatic carcinogens; castration protective.

b) HC commoner in men than women.
c) Androgen therapy in aplastic anaemia associated with HC.
d) Oral contraceptives associated with hepatic adenomas.

39.3 Clinical Features

1. Symptoms commonly encountered:
   a) In Africa and Asia, history short (2–3 months)
   b) Right upper quadrant pain
   c) Right upper quadrant mass
   d) Weight loss
2. Commonest signs:
   a) Hepatomegaly
   b) Wasting
   c) Jaundice
   d) Signs of portal hypertension
   e) In Africa and Asia, patients 35–45 years vs 55–65 years in Europe or United States
3. Prognostic features:
   Wasting
   Venous collaterals
   Ascites
   Jaundice
4. Staging:

Stage	Characteristics	Survival at 3 months (%)
I	No wasting No jaundice No venous collaterals No ascites	80
II	No wasting No jaundice No collaterals Some ascites	20
III	Wasting Jaundice Venous collaterals Ascites	10

5. Metastasis:
   a) Lung
   b) Bone
   c) Lymph nodes

39.4 Diagnosis

1. Clinical suspicion - right upper quadrant mass and pain
2. Liver function tests - non-specific, but:

Alkaline phosphatase	elevated in 75%
Serum glutamicoxaloacetic transaminase (SGOT)	elevated in 50%
Bilirubin	elevated in 25%
Alpha-foetoprotein	positive in 60%

3. Enzyme gamma glutamyl transpeptidase markedly elevated in ascites
4. Isotopic and ultrasound scans helpful
5. Liver biopsy preferable during laparoscopy

39.5 Differential Diagnosis

1. Liver abscess - amoebic or pyogenic
2. Secondary deposits in liver rare in Africans as gastrointestinal tumours rare
3. Hydatid disease
4. Schistosomal fibrosis

39.6 Histology

1. Epithelial:
   a) Benign - Liver cell adenoma
      - Intrahepatic bile duct adenoma
      - Intrahepatic bile duct cystadenoma
   b) Malignant - Hepatocellular carcinoma
      - Cholangiocarcinoma
      - Bile duct cystadenocarcinoma
      - Combined hepatocellular/cholangiocellular
      - Hepatoblastoma

2. Non-epithelial:
   a) Haemangioma
   b) Haemangiosarcoma
   c) Embryonal sarcoma

39.7 Treatment

HC uniformly fatal - survival beyond 3 months in developing countries very rare

1. Surgery:
   a) Partial hepatectomy if localized, and liver non-cirrhotic
   b) Hepatic artery ligation - objective regression in 40%-45%. Contraindicated in portal vein thrombosis and advanced cirrhosis
   c) Hepatic artery ligation + chemotherapy
2. Chemotherapy:
   Drugs reported to produce objective responses:
   Adriamycin
   Neocarzinostatin
   Etoposide (VP-16-213)
   5-Fluorouracil + streptozotocin
   5-Fluorouracil + methyl-CCNU

39.8 Recommended Chemotherapy

Adriamycin is, so far, the only drug giving reproducible objective responses (40% on average):

Dose: 60- 75 mg/m^2 i.v. every 3 weeks
Maximum tolerable dose: 500-550 mg/m^2

Combination of Adriamycin with Other Drugs:
Combination with, e.g. dichloromethotrexate, razoxane (ICRF 159), cyclophosphamide and 5-azacytidine, has not increased response rate.

40 Bladder Cancer

Nazli Gad-El-Mawla

40.1 Epidemiology, Incidence and Aetiology

About 3% of all cancers
Incidence slowly increasing
Environmental factors: Cigarette smoking, aniline dyes, rubber additives, chronic bladder irritation due to schistosomiasis or chronic bacterial infection
N. B. Schistosomiasis explains high incidence of bladder cancer in Egypt (27.6% of all cancers), Iraq, Ghana and Nigeria.

40.2 Histology

97% of epithelial origin, often multifocal
Three histological types:
1. Transitional cell carcinoma (main type all over the world)
2. Squamous cell carcinoma (main type in area with schistosomiasis: in Egypt 75% of all cases)
3. Adenocarcinoma

40.3 Diagnosis

1. Symptomatology: dysuria, haematuria
2. Endoscopic examination
3. Rectal examination
4. Urine cytology
5. Lymphangiography
6. Intravenous pyelography
7. Computerized axial tomographic (CAT) scan, where available

40.4 Staging

Tis	In situ: "Flat tumour"
Ta	Papillary non-invasive
T1	Mobile mass, absent after transurethral resection (TUR)
T2	Indurated wall, absent after TUR
T3	Mass/induration, remains after TUR
T4	Fixed/extension to neighbouring organs
N1	Single homolateral regional
N2	Contra- or bilateral/multiple regional
N3	Fixed regional
N4	Juxta-regional
M1	Distant metastases

40.5 Prognosis According to Stage and Other Factors

Stage	5-year survival (%)
Tis-T1	70–80
T2	40–50
T3-T4	20–30

40.6 Therapy

Stage	Therapy
Tis	TUR, or local chemotherapy
Ta	TUR
T1	TUR
T2	Partial cystectomy
T3	Radical cystectomy
T4	Chemotherapy
N1	Pelvic adenectomy
N2	Pelvic adenectomy
N3	Chemotherapy
N4	Chemotherapy
M1	Chemotherapy

40.7 Chemotherapy

40.7.1 Single-Agent Chemotherapy

Agent	Remission rate (%)
5-Fluorouracil (5-FU)	Less than 35
Methotrexate	17-36
Adriamycin	16-37
Cis-platinum (DDP)	30-40
Other drugs not adequately studied:	
- Cyclophosphamide	
- Teniposide (VM-26)	
- Mitomycin C	

N. B. In bilharzial bladder cancer (squamous cell type), hexamethylmelamine, Cis-platinum, 5-FU and triaziquone (Trenimon), seem to be more effective than Adriamycin, methotrexate, bleomycin and VM-26.

40.7.2 Multidrug Chemotherapy

Drug combination	Remission rate (%)
Adriamycin/5-FU	35
Adriamycin/VM-26	19
Adriamycin/cyclophosphamide	33
Adriamycin/DDP/5-fluorouracil	65
DDP/Adriamycin/cyclophosphamide	43-50

40.7.3 Intravesical Chemotherapy

Indicated only for Stage 0 and A (multifocal, superficially spreading cancer):

Thiotepa	60 mg weekly for 4 weeks
Adriamycin	80 mg monthly
Epodyl	100 cm^3 of 1% solution, weekly for 12 weeks
DDP	60 mg monthly
Mitomycin C	40 mg weekly for 8 weeks

N. B. All drugs given in 100 cm^3 saline, retained in the bladder for 1 h. Response rate: 50%-70%

40.8 Recommended Chemotherapy and Comment

DDP 60–80 mg/m^2 i.v. every 3 weeks

N.B. To date, no drug combination has proved to be superior to DDP alone.

Appendices

Appendix A Common Abbreviations for the Most Widely Used Cytotoxic Agents

ACD	dactinomycin
Act-D	actinomycin D
AD-32	N-trifluoroacetyl adriamycin-14-valerate
ADM	Adriamycin (doxorubicin hydrochloride)
ADP	aminopterin
AGL	aminoglutethimide
ara-C	cytosine arabinoside
L-Asp	L-asparaginase
L-ASP	L-asparaginase
5-aza-C	5-azacytidine, NSC-102B16
BAF	triazinate
BCNU	carmustine, 1, 3-bis (2-chloroethyl)-l-nitrosourea
BLM, Bleo	bleomycin
BUdR	broxuridine
CA	cytarabine
CCNU	lomustine, 1- (2-chloroethyl)-3-cyclohexyl-l-nitrosourea
CDDP	Cis-platinum
CF	citrovorum factor
CLB	chlorambucil
CTX	cyclophosphamide, Cytoxan
DAG	dianhydrogalactitol
DBD	mitolactol, dibromodulcitol
DDP	Cis-platinum, diamminodichloroplatinum
DES	diethylstilboestrol
DEX	dexamethasone
DNM	daunomycin
DTIC	dacarbazine, imidazole carboxamide
EMP	extramustine phosphate
5-FU	5-fluorouracil
Hc	hydrocortisone
HDMTX	methotrexate, high-dose
HDMTX-CF	methotrexate, high-dose, + leucovorin rescue
HMM	hexamethylmelamine
HN2	mechlorethamine

HU	hydroxyurea
HXM	hexamethylmelamine
ICRF 159	razoxane
MAP	medroxyprogesterone
Me-CCNU	methyl-CCNU, 1- (2-chloroethyl)-3-(4-methyl-cyclohexyl)-l-nitrosourea
methyl-GAG	methylglyoxal bisguanylhydrazone
MGBG	methylglyoxal bisguanylhydrazone
MIT	mitomycin
MITOX	chlormethine
MNU	methylnitrosourea
6-MP	6-mercaptopurine
MTX	methotrexate
o,p'DDD	ortho-para'DDD, mitotane
L-PAM	melphalan
PRO, PCB, PCZ	procarbazine
PRD, PDN	prednisone
PTC	peptichemio
RCM	rufocromomycin
SZT	streptozotocin
TdR	thymidine
TEM	triethylene melamine
6-TG	6-thioguanine
β-TgdR	β-2'-deoxythioguanosine
ThioTEPA	triethylene thiophosphoramide, thiotepa
T-tepa	thiotepa
Umust	Uracil mustard
VCR	vincristine
VDS	vindesine
VBL	vinblastine
VM-26	teniposide
VP-16-213	etoposide

Acronyms of Most Commonly Used Drug Combinations

ABP	Adriamycin, bleomycin, prednisone
ABVD	Adriamycin, bleomycin, vinblastine, dacarbazine
ACM	Adriamycin, cyclophosphamide, methotrexate
ADIC	Adriamycin, dacarbazine
ADV	dactinomycin, dacarbazine, vincristine
ALOMAD	vincristine, methotrexate high dose + leucovorin rescue, Adriamycin, dacarbazine, chlorambucil, dactinomycin
A-OAP	Adriamycin, vincristine, cytosine arabinoside, prednisone
BACON	bleomycin, Adriamycin, cyclophosphamide, vincristine, nitrogen-musterol
BACOP	bleomycin, Adriamycin, cyclophosphamide, vincristine, prednisone
BACT	BCNU, cytarabine, cyclophosphamide, thioguanine
B-CAVe	bleomycin, CCNU, Adriamycin, vinblastine
BVCPP	BCNU, vinblastine, cyclophosphamide, procarbazine, prednisone
CAF_5	cyclophosphamide, Adriamycin, 5-fluorouracil
CHAD	cyclophosphamide, hexamethylmelamine, Adriamycin, Cis-platinum
CHAP	cyclophosphamide, hexamethylmelamine, Adriamycin, Cis-platinum
CHOP	cyclophosphamide, Adriamycin, vincristine, prednisone
CHOP(P)	cyclophosphamide, Adriamycin, vincristine, procarbazine, prednisone
CMF	cyclophosphamide, methotrexate, 5-fluorouracil
C-MOPP	cyclophosphamide, vincristine, procarbazine, prednisone
COAP	cyclophosphamide, vincristine, cytarabine, prednisone
COMA	cyclophosphamide, vincristine, methotrexate, cytarabine
COMB	cyclophosphamide, vincristine, Me-CCNU, bleomycin
COMF	cyclophosphamide, vincristine, methotrexate, 5-fluorouracil
COMP	CCNU, vincristine, methotrexate, procarbazine
COMPADRI I	cyclophosphamide, vincristine, Adriamycin, melphalan
COMPADRI II	cyclophosphamide, vincristine, Adriamycin, melphalan + methotrexate high dose
COMPADRI III	cyclophosphamide, vincristine, Adriamycin, melphalan + intensified Adriamycin
COP	cyclophosphamide, vincristine, prednisone
COPP	cyclophosphamide, vincristine, procarbazine, prednisone
CVP	cyclophosphamide, vincristine, prednisone
CVPP	CCNU, vinblastine, procarbazine, prednisone
CYVADACT	cyclophosphamide, vincristine, Adriamycin, dactinomycin
CYVADIC	cyclophosphamide, vincristine, Adriamycin, dacarbazine
FAM	5-fluorouracil, Adriamycin, mitomycin
FAMe	5-fluorouracil, Adriamycin, Me-CCNU

FMC	5-fluorouracil, mitomycin, cytarabine
FOAM	5-fluorouracil, vincristine, Adriamycin, mitomycin
Hexa CAF	hexamethylmelamine, cyclophosphamide, methotrexate, 5-fluorouracil
MAC	mitomycin, Adriamycin, cyclophosphamide
MOB	mitomycin, Adriamycin, bleomycin
MOF-strept	Me-CCNU, vincristine, 5-fluorouracil, streptozotocin
MOPP	nitrogen mustard, vincristine, procarbazine, prednisone
MVPP	nitrogen mustard, vinblastine, procarbazine, prednisone
OAP	vincristine, cytarabine, prednisone
POMP	methotrexate, vincristine, mercaptopurine, prednisone
PVB	Cis-platinum + vinblastine + bleomycin
SMF	streptozotocin, mitomycin, 5-fluorouracil
VAB I	vinblastine, dactinomycin, bleomycin
VAB II	vinblastine, dactinomycin, bleomycin, Cis-platinum
VAB III	vinblastine, dactinomycin, bleomycin, cyclophosphamide
VAC	vincristine, actinomycin-D, cyclophosphamide
VACAd	vincristine, dactinomycin, cyclophosphamide, Adriamycin
VADIC	vincristine, dactinomycin, dacarbazine
VAMP	vincristine, methotrexate, 6-mercaptopurine, prednisone
VAP	vincristine, actinomycin, prednisone

Appendix B Nomograms for Determination of Body Surface Area from Height and Weight

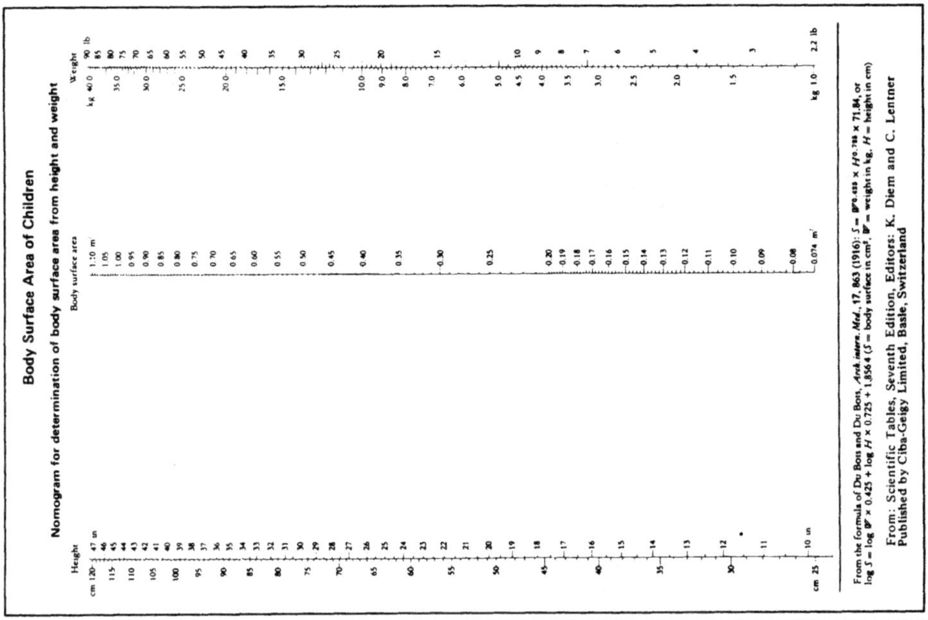

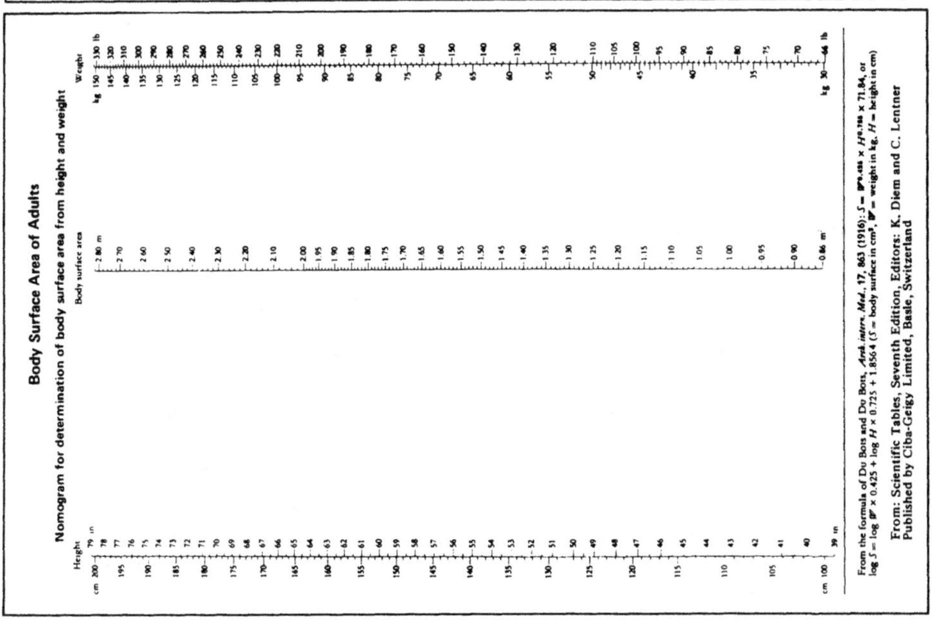

Appendix C List of Recommended Publications for Further Reading

Suggested Periodicals

Cancer – A Journal of the American Cancer Society
J. B. Lippincott Co., East Washington Square, Philadelphia, Pennsylvania 19105, USA
Cancer Treatment Reports
Public Health Service, National Institutes of Health, National Cancer Institute, Bethesda, Maryland 20014, USA
Cancer Treatment Reviews
Academic Press, Inc., 111 5th Avenue, New York, N. Y., 10003, USA
Medical and Pediatric Oncology
Liss, Inc., 150 5th Avenue, New York, N. Y. 10011, USA
Seminars in Oncology
Grune and Stratton, 6277 Sea Harbor Drive, Orlando, FL 32821
American Journal of Pediatric Hematology/Oncology
Masson Publishing, USA, East 60th Street, New York, N. Y. USA
British Journal of Cancer
MacMillan Press, Hound Mills, Basingstoke, UK
European Journal of Cancer and Clinical Oncology
Pergamon Press, Oxford, UK
Journal of Clinical Oncology
Grune and Stratton, 6277 Sea Harbor Drive, Orlando, FL 32821

Suggested Textbooks

Al Rashid RA (1979) Pediatric Cancer chemotherapy. Medical Examination Publishing, New York

Altman AS, Schwartz ID (eds) (1983) Malignant diseases of infancy, childhood and adolescence. W. B. Saunders Company

Becker FF (ed) (1977) Cancer – A comprehensive treatise. Vol 5: Chemotherapy, Plenum Press, New York

Bloom HJG, Lemerle J, Neidhardt MK, Voûte PA (eds) (1975) Cancer in children – Clinical Management. Springer-Verlag, Berlin

Brunner KW, Nagel GA (1976) Internistische Krebstherapie. Springer-Verlag, Berlin

Bucalossi P, Veronesi U (1973) Oncologia clinica, 3 volumes. Ambrosiana, Milan

Buyse ME, Staquet MJ, Sylvester RJ (1984) Cancer clinical trials – Methods and practice. Oxford University Press

Calman KC, Paul J (1978) An introduction to cancer medicine. MacMillan, London
Cancer Chemotherapy. Fundamental concepts and Recent advances. Yearbook Medical Publishers, Chicago, USA, 1976
Carter SK, Sakurai Y (1980) New anticancer drugs. Springer-Verlag, Berlin
Carter SK, Glatstein E, Livingston RB (1982) Principles of cancer treatment. McGraw-Hill, New York
Clarysse A, Kenis Y, Mathé G (1976) Cancer chemotherapy - Its role in the treatment strategy of hematologic malignancies and solid tumors. Springer-Verlag, Berlin
Devita VT, Hellman S, Rosenberg S (1985) Cancer-principles and practice of oncology. Lippincott, Philadelphia
Estevez RA, Alvarez CA, Chacon RD (eds) (1978) Oncologia clinica. Ediciones Universidad del Salvador, Buenos Aires
Estevez RA, Alvarez CA (eds) (1980) Drogas antineoplasicas. Catedra de oncologia, Facultad de Medicina, Universidad de Salvador, Buenos Aires
Haskell CM (ed) (1980) Cancer treatment. Saunders, Philadelphia
Horton J, Hill GJ (eds) (1977) Clinical oncology. Saunders, Philadelphia
Holland JF, Frei E (1982) Cancer medicine. Lea & Febiger, Philadelphia
Kücüksu MN, Ruacan SA (eds) (1978) Klinik onkoloji. Türk Kanser Arastirma ve Savas Kurumu Yayinlari, Ankara
Lawrence WJr, Terz JJ (1977) Cancer management. Grune Stratton, New York
Levine AS (ed) (1982) Cancer in the young. Masson Pub., USA
Manka I (ed) (1979) Klinicka onkologia. Osveta, Bratislava
Marsden HB, Steward JK (1976) Tumours in children. Recent results in cancer research. Springer-Verlag, Berlin
Mathe G, Oldham RK (1974) Complications of cancer chemotherapy. Springer-Verlag, Berlin
Mihich E, Eckhardt S (1980) Design of cancer chemotherapy. Experimental and clinical approaches. In series: Antibiotics and chemotherapy, 28. Karger, Basel
Miller DR, Baehner RL, McMillan CW (eds) (1984) Blood diseases of infancy and childhood. C. V. Moshy Company
Morra ME (ed) (1979) Cancer chemotherapy - treatment and care. Yale Comprehensive Cancer Center, New Haven
Molentius HW (1981) Manual of oncology. Urban & Schwarzenberg, Baltimore
Pinedo HM (1978) Clinical pharmacology of anti-neoplastic drugs. Elsevier, North Holland
Pinedo HM, Chabner BA (1985) Cancer chemotherapy 7. Elsevier, Amsterdam - New York - Oxford
Schimke RM (1978) Genetics and Cancer. Churchill Livingstone, London
Schweisguth O (1979) Tumeurs solides de l'enfant. Flammarion Médicine Sciences, Paris
Silver RT, Lauper RD, Jarowski CI (1977) A synopsis of cancer chemotherapy. Yorke Medical Books, New York
Simkovics JG (1979) Medical oncology. Marcel Decker, New York
Staquet MJ (1979) Cancer therapy. Prognostic factors and criteria of response. Raven Press, New York
Sutow WW, Vietti TJ, Fernbach DJ (1978) Clinical paediatric oncology. 2nd Edition
UICC Committee on Professional Education (1978) Clinical oncology - a manual for students and doctors. Springer Verlag, Berlin

GPSR Compliance

The European Union's (EU) General Product Safety Regulation (GPSR) is a set of rules that requires consumer products to be safe and our obligations to ensure this.

If you have any concerns about our products, you can contact us on ProductSafety@springernature.com

In case Publisher is established outside the EU, the EU authorized representative is:

Springer Nature Customer Service Center GmbH
Europaplatz 3
69115 Heidelberg, Germany

Batch number: 10704701

Printed by Printforce, the Netherlands